Molecular Applications in Cytology

Fernando C. Schmitt

Editor

Molecular Applications in Cytology

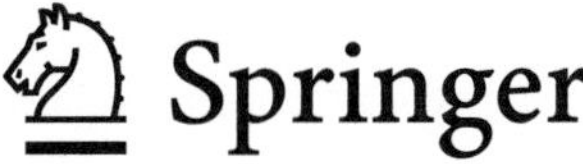 Springer

Editor
Fernando C. Schmitt
Medical Faculty of Porto University
Porto
Portugal

Instituto de Investigação e Inovação em Saúde
Universidade do Porto
Porto
Portugal

IPATIMUP, Institute of Molecular Pathology and Immunology of Porto University
Porto
Portugal

ISBN 978-3-030-09110-1   ISBN 978-3-319-74942-6   (eBook)
https://doi.org/10.1007/978-3-319-74942-6

This Springer imprint is published by the registered company Springer International Publishing AG part of Springer Nature.
The registered company address is: Gewerbestrasse 11, 6330 Cham, Switzerland

Preface

To do more with less… this is the great challenge for the pathology in the next decades. Recently many patients are managed based on diagnosis performed in small biopsies or cytology. Molecular techniques in the routine pathology are changing paradigms as did the introduction of immunohistochemistry some decades ago and are preferentially used on histological material. The goal of this book is to demonstrate that most of these techniques can be easily applied to the cytological material. In fact, cytological samples present numerous advantages over histological material. These include the ability to check the quality of the tissue immediately after harvesting, better preservation of RNA/DNA and the possibility of conducting extensively genomic studies on small amounts of cytological material obtained by fine-needle aspiration or from effusions, urine, among others. In turn, this minimizes the need for more invasive procedures and allows for more frequent re-sampling enabling monitoring of the disease along the time.

Molecular techniques in cytological samples have a wide array of applications. Depending on the method, they can be applied for diagnosis, subtype classification, and prognostic and predictive purposes. In this book we cover from the main aspects of pre-analytical phase, the applications in different organs and systems, through to the clinical integration of the results. Of course in this field of medicine knowledge advances so rapidly that a book cannot include all the more recent discoveries. However, the readers of this book can acquire very solid information in the different fields of molecular cytology that allow them to follow any new finding in the field. This book was written to the cytopathologists that even not practicing inside a molecular lab can acquire enough knowledge in the field that allow them to discuss the results and applications of different molecular techniques.

Now it is time to thank all those who have directly or indirectly collaborated for this book. For you the reader, it is time to relax, open the book and enjoy!

Porto, Portugal
Fernando C. Schmitt

Contents

Why Cytology for Molecular Testing? Pros and Cons

1

Lukas Bubendorf

1.1 Introduction

During the last decade, molecular pathology has grown to an important and indispensable subdiscipline of pathology, since diagnosis of an increasing number of tumor entities relies on molecular findings. At the same time, countless molecular targets and biomarkers related to new drugs in this era of personalized medicine have emerged requiring systematic testing in routine practice. This has been paralleled by rapidly evolving technical advances and testing platforms in molecular pathology making pathology a highly dynamic field. Today, different molecular methods such as polymerase chain reaction (PCR)-based techniques or next-generation sequencing (NGS) for mutation analysis and fluorescence in situ hybridization (FISH) for detection of DNA copy number alterations and gene rearrangements are in routine use in pathology laboratories. In addition, immunohistochemistry (IHC) has gained renewed clinical importance beyond its role to facilitate or narrow down a specific diagnosis. IHC can also identify the presence of therapeutic targets or surrogate markers for molecular alterations and/or be used to prescreen specimens for subsequent molecular testing. Most of the advances in predictive biomarker testing have initially been based on studies and clinical trials that relied on histological specimens. Accordingly, technical protocols and algorithms for evaluation or scoring had often been established for histological specimens, which raised the false impression that cytological specimens are not suitable for molecular testing by nature. This misconception among pathologists and clinicians was most prevalent in the early days of predictive marker testing and was further reinforced by the popular but imprecise term "tissue is the issue." Given the reality that a variably large fraction of cancers are diagnosed by cytology alone, this narrow, tissue-centered view has not survived for long. Reinforcing re-interventions in

L. Bubendorf
Institute of Pathology, University Hospital Basel, Basel, Switzerland
e-mail: Lukas.bubendorf@usb.ch

© Springer International Publishing AG, part of Springer Nature 2018
F. C. Schmitt (ed.), *Molecular Applications in Cytology*,
https://doi.org/10.1007/978-3-319-74942-6_1

patients despite informative cytological specimens only for the sake of possibly obtaining histological tumor specimens would not only be irrational but also unethical. Eventually, enough evidence has accumulated showing that in principle cytological preparations are equivalent to histological specimens for diagnostic and predictive molecular testing. One can even state that the reputation of cytology has taken a flying leap due to its now-recognized importance in predictive marker testing, not only among pathologist but also among clinicians. This is best exemplified in the field of biomarker analyses in lung cancer where current guidelines and recommendations emphasize the utility of cytological preparations for biomarker testing [1, 2]. Thus, there is no question whether or not molecular testing can be done on cytology. Cytology contains the same cells, the same RNA, DNA, and protein molecules as corresponding histology, yet cytological specimens have no tissue context, usually lack a stromal component, and are processed differently, which may require different approaches and modified protocols for molecular analysis. These and other differences provide challenges that are discussed in the following part of this chapter.

1.2   Little Material for Many Analyses

Most predictive molecular marker analyses need to be done from small biopsies or cytological specimens since curative tumor resection is not therapeutic in most patients with advanced tumors [3]. It is unrealistic to claim that a small biopsy is better than cytology just because it is histology. In diagnostic practice, one should not make a choice for or against cytology. Instead, it is critical to review all available material from one patient and to select the best suited ones for the different analyses. In fact, the triage and management of the available tumor material for the different analyses have become a new important task of pathologists and cytopathogists. This ideally implies that one person oversees all specimens of a patient at a given time or that cytopathologists and histopathologists at least work together very closely.

Cytopathologists often hesitate to use unique cytological slides for molecular testing because of legal obligations to retain diagnostic specimens. First and above all, however, specimens need to serve the patients and not the paragraphs. Notably, it is not necessary to destroy all evidence of a diagnostic specimen for molecular testing. First, one can capture still images or perform virtual slides prior to molecular testing. Second, there is no need to use all cells on a specimen, as part of the slide can easily be spared for documentation or future use. Third, in case of IHC, the cells on a slide remain intact and can be archived in a regular way. Even FISH does not destroy the cell nuclei, and the slides can be stored in the freezer for potential future DNA-based testing. Finally, an efficient use of the tumor cells and/or a stepwise molecular analysis helps to make most out of limited cytological material. Different areas on a highly cellular cytological smear may be used for different analyses. Thanks to the robustness of the DNA, even previously immune-stained slides are amenable to DNA testing including FISH and mutation analysis.

1.3 Analysis Based on Extracted DNA

Many molecular tests rely on the analysis of extracted DNA. The DNA quality in air-dried or ethanol-fixed cytological preparations is generally superior as compared to after formalin-fixed specimens, since formalin causes cross-linking and chemical modification and can therefore lead to false-negative and false-positive results [4, 5]. This is one of the reasons why mutation testing from ethanol-fixed cytological slides requires a lower minimum number of tumor cells both by traditional Sanger sequencing (50–100 cells) and NGS (200 cells) as compared to histological specimens, where at least 300–500 tumor cells are typically requested for mutation testing. In fact, it appears that DNA quality/integrity is perhaps more important than the DNA amount to obtain reliable results [4].

A minimum tumor cell proportion (TCP) is needed for mutation analysis, ranging from 10% to 20% for NGS and from 30% to 40% for Sanger sequencing. If these requirements are met, scratching off all cells from a cytological slide is equally straightforward as scratching off a formalin-fixed and paraffin-embedded (FFPE) tissue section for DNA extraction. In case of a lower TCP, there would be a high change to miss heterozygous mutations due to dilution with DNA from benign cells. Macro-dissection of areas with a high tumor cell proportion using a magnifying glass is an option in some cases but not feasible if there is tumor cells randomly admixed with predominating benign cells. Laser capture microdissection (LCMD) makes it possible to utilize such challenging specimens as it guarantees a TCP of least 80% after enrichment [6]. LCMD is particularly helpful in diagnostic cytological specimens, where small groups of tumor cells or individual tumor cells can be recorded for subsequent, supervised automated harvesting [7] (Fig. 1.1). In difficult cases with a high number of admixed benign cells on cytological slides, the tumors cells can first be flagged by IHC (e.g., TTF1 in case of pulmonary adenocarcinoma) to guarantee precise, interactive tumor cell collection. Taken together, cytological specimens allow to obtain high-quality DNA to test all predictive DNA mutations now and in the future.

1.4 FISH Analysis

Historically, FISH analysis in cancer cells was first applied to cell preparations including cell lines, and cell nuclei from human FFPE tissue blocks were dissociated prior to FISH analysis [8]. Therefore, it comes as little surprise that cytology is an ideal format for FISH analysis [9, 10]. The cells are intact and not truncated as in histology, so that the true number of FISH signals can be evaluated (Fig. 1.2). FISH on cytological slides often gives a clearer picture than FISH on histological sections. For example, a heterozygous deletion is clear since there is no unspecific background of pseudo-deletions as seen in histological sections due to lost signals by nuclear truncation. The lack of nuclear truncation in cytology results in higher gene or chromosome copy numbers by FISH in smears/cytospins/LBCs as compared to tissue or cell block sections. Therefore, mean gene or chromosome copy

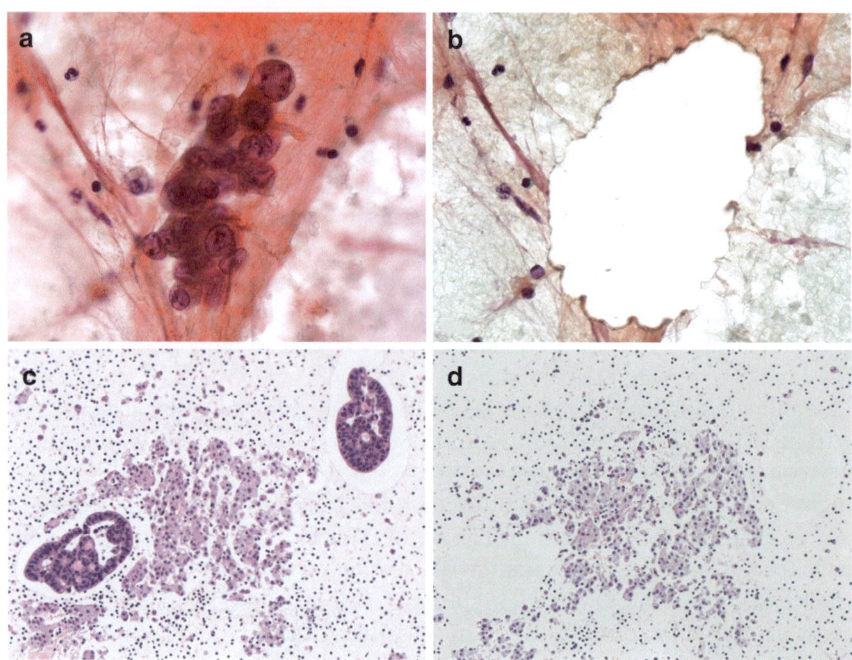

Fig. 1.1 Laser capture microdissection (LCMD) on cytological specimens (PALM Microlaser Technologies system). (**a**) Lung adenocarcinoma cells on a smear of from bronchial secretion cytology; ethanol fixed and Papanicolaou stained, ×400; (**b**) the same area after LCMD of the tumor cells. (**c**) Groups of lung adenocarcinoma cells and adjacent benign cells from the cellblock of a malignant pleural effusion; hematoxylin and eosin, ×200; and (**d**) empty areas after LCMD of the tumor cells on a subsequent section

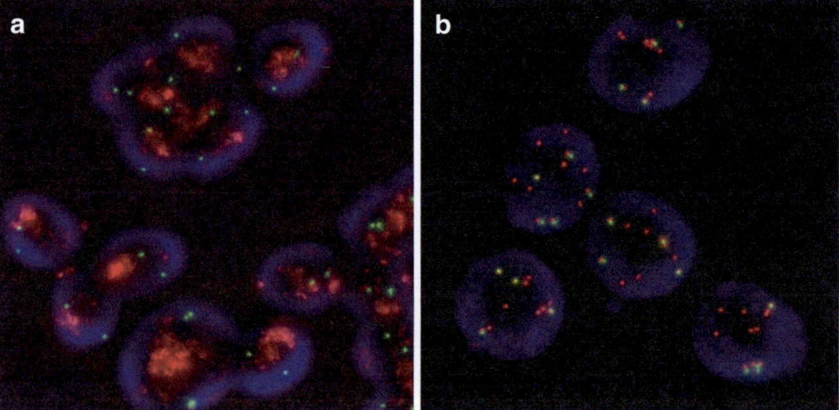

Fig. 1.2 Examples of FISH analysis on ethanol-fixed and previously Papanicolaou-stained cytological smears/cytospins, ×1000. Compressed z-stacked images showing the projection of all FISH signals in the intact cell nuclei. (**a**) Breast cancer cells with high-level *HER2* gene amplification: dense clusters of red *HER2* gene signals but only few green reference signals (centromer 17). (**b**) Cells of lung adenocarcinoma with *ALK* rearrangement: 6–8 rearranged *ALK* gene copies per cell showing a single red signal without a corresponding green signal and 3–4 non-rearranged gene copies with normal fusion signals; ALK break-apart FISH probe

numbers determined in smears/cytospins/LBCs need to be newly established for cytology or mathematically converted to use threshold that have been established for histological sections, as previously shown in case EGFR gene copy number [11]. As opposed to histology, FISH analysis of three-dimensional tumor cell aggregates can be challenging due to cell and signal overlap. However, this is not critical in case of deletions or high-level amplifications, where the relative proportion of the signals in an area of tumor cells is more important than the actual ratio on a cell-by-cell basis. Nevertheless, it is advised to analyze cells at the periphery of aggregates or search for adjacent single tumor cells. Provided that appropriate protocols are used, FISH on cytology provides brilliant results with less autofluorescent background than in histological specimens. Due to the robustness of DNA, FISH can be applied to diagnostic cytological specimens irrespective of fixation and type of stains. In our experience, previous May-Grünwald-Giemsa (MGG), hematoxylin and eosin (H&E), or Papanicolaou staining does not interfere with FISH analysis. Using pre-stained specimens allows selecting the optimal slides for FISH analysis based on cellular content and composition. Importantly, using automated relocation on an automated stage allow to relocate rare critical cell on a stained diagnostic slide to clarify the nature of atypical cells (Fig. 1.3). In our hands, evaluation of atypical cells by FISH is most helpful in the field of urinary, pancreatobiliary, and lung cytology [10, 12]. Such analyses in rare cells or cell groups are much more challenging in histological specimens due to change of the architecture on consecutive sections and artificial deletion of gene and chromosome copy numbers by nuclear truncation. It is also possible to use previously immunostained slides in case 3-amino-9-ethylcarbazole (AEC) has been used as a red chromogen. In contrast, the brown 3,3′-diaminobenzidine (DAB), instead, causes autofluorescence that interferes with FISH scoring. Using separate cellular areas on one slide allows two simultaneous FISH analysis on the same slide. Moreover, the same area can be re-hybridized with another FISH probe after the previous one has been washed off in case of limited material.

1.5 Immunohistochemistry

Immunohistochemistry (IHC), also referred to as immunocytochemistry when used in cytological specimens, is not a molecular method sensu stricto but still needs consideration because IHC findings can be directly related to diagnostic and predictive molecular and genetic alterations (Fig. 1.4) [13]. For example, ALK and ROS1 IHC has become standard practice to prescreen biopsy and cytology specimens for the respective gene rearrangements in non-small cell lung cancers (NSCLC). Similarly, there is specific antibody detecting V600E-mutated BRAF, and CMET IHC can be useful to prescreen for molecular MET testing regarding MET amplification or METex15 skipping mutation [14]. Notably, the European Medical Agency (EMA) typically prescribes a robust and well-validated methodology for predictive biomarker testing, respectively, but does not restrict it to a particular technique or histology. Although more data are needed, there is accumulating evidence that predictive IHC can be reliably applied to smears/cytospins/LBCs or cell blocks [15–20]. Similarly, PD-L1 staining and estimating the percentage of positive tumor cells

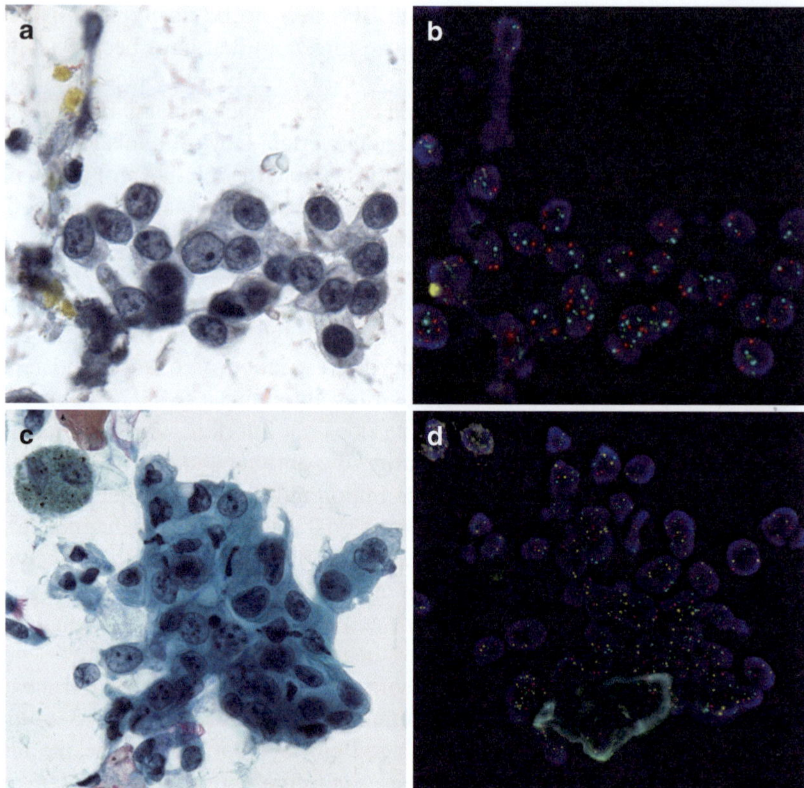

Fig. 1.3 Analysis of atypical cells by FISH after precise re-localization, Papanicolaou, ×630. Compressed z-stacked images showing the projection of all FISH signals in the intact cell nuclei. (**a**) FNA of the pancreato-biliary tract showing atypical cell suspicious of adenocarcinoma. (**b**) Multi-target FISH of the same cells showing normal copy numbers for chromosomes 3 (red), 17 (green), and 17 (aqua) (2 signals each) but complete loss of 9p21 (gold) proving clonality and epithelial neoplasia. (**c**) Atypical respiratory cells from bronchial brush cytology. Papanicolaou, ×600. (**d**) The same cells after multitarget FISH with probes for the EGFR gene (7p12, red), the MYC gene (8q24, gold), chromosome 5 (5p12, green), and chromosome 6 (centromere, aqua) showing normal copy numbers for all four probes (2 signals, each), being consistent benign reactive cells

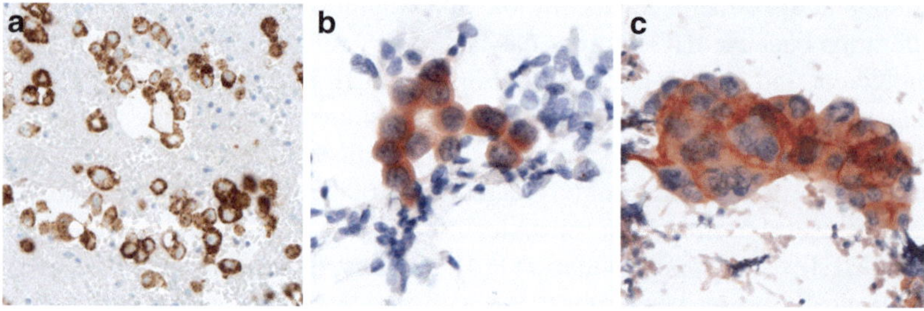

Fig. 1.4 Examples of predictive IHC on cytological specimens, ×400. (**a**) Melanoma cells expressing V6000E-mutated BRAF protein; cell block; VE1 antibody, Spring Bioscience. (**b**, **c**) IHC using Leica Bond-Max on conventional cytological specimens of lung adenocarcinomas showing (**b**) rare cells of a ROS1 tumor cells with cytoplasmic staining (D4D6 antibody, cell signaling) and (**c**) cytoplasmic and membranous PD-L1 staining (SP142 antibody, Ventana)

to select patients for PD1/PD-L1 inhibitors appear to be feasible in cytological preparations [3, 21, 22]. In smears/cytospins/LBC, membranous staining of tumor cells is less distinct than in FFPE tissue/cell block sections since the cells membranes are not cut but intact. Thus, staining of the horizontal cell membrane mostly appears as a diffuse surface staining. Quantitation of PD-L1-positive immune cells will be definitely more challenging if not impossible because of the lack of tissue context precluding proper assessment of interface activity of PD-L1-positive immune cells.

1.6 Diversity of Cytological Specimens

Pre-analytical variables including sample collection, triage, transportation, fixation, and handling are important factors that can directly impact the results of molecular testing and immunohistochemistry [23], as outlined in detail in Chap. 2. It has been shown that optimal molecular results can be obtained from a multitude of different cytological preparations [23, 24]. Therefore, both cell blocks and smears/cytospins/LBCs will be recommended as equally suitable as histology for lung cancer biomarker molecular testing in forthcoming 2016 update of the CAP/IASLC/AMP guideline. Pre-analytical factors are larger in number and less well defined in cytology than in histology, and there is a lack of standardization among laboratories for specimen collection, processing, and staining methodology [23]. Processing fresh cytological specimens to formalin-fixed and paraffin-embedded (FFPE) cell blocks helps to adjust cytology to tissue specimens and use the same analytical protocols, which is particularly practical for IHC. Therefore, using cell blocks is now common practice in cytology laboratories. Despite this advantage, it is not advised to replace ethanol-based preparations by cell blocks altogether, as one would give away the advantages that come with ethanol-fixed non-cell block preparations including superior morphological details, the high DNA quality, and the brilliance of FISH results. In addition, one should not rely on cell blocks alone for molecular analysis of cytological specimens, since cell blocks are not always available or may not contain enough tumor cells. It should also be kept in mind that there is currently more pre-analytical variability in cellblock than in FFPE tissue specimens due to different protocols being in use [25–30]. While fixation of tissue specimens in 10% formalin is a worldwide standard, there is no international consensus method for cell block preparation including different pre-fixation methods that could affect the results of molecular testing.

1.7 Professional Opportunity for Cytotechnicians

The quality of molecular analysis highly depends on specific skills of individuals involved in specimen selection and processing. This is also important in histology but particularly critical in cytology, which requires special skills in cytomorphology. This makes molecular analysis an exciting and rewarding new field of activity for cytotechnicians. They know how to identify tumor cells and have experience in laboratory work at the same time. Thus, cytotechnicians should embrace the opportunity to get involved in molecular cytology including the management of specimens for DNA extraction or FISH analysis. Especially the younger generation among them can easily handle interactive automated procedures such as LCMD, navigating a computer-guided automated stage for relocation of tumors cells on the slide or high-quality imaging of selected cells for analysis and documentation. In our experience, no one is better qualified for this work than well-trained cytotechnicians.

Conclusions

In case of advanced or recurrent cancer, incriminating surgical procedures should be avoided whenever possible. Fine-needle aspirates or body fluids can be obtained in a minimally invasive manner for cytological diagnosis and biomarker analysis. Given the published evidence and personal experience, the value and suitability of cytology specimens for comprehensive molecular marker testing are out of question. One can even anticipate that the role of cytology for the molecular search of targetable resistance mechanism in patients progressing under treatment with targeted drugs will increase in the future, together with liquid biopsies. This is not against or at the cost of histological specimens, since all available tumor material must be taken into account in order to cover all biomarker needs in the best possible way. Cytopathologists cannot hide in the back of surgical pathologists and molecular pathologists but must be familiar with the latest guidelines, the technical tools, and the minimum requirements for molecular testing of cytological specimens.

References

1. Kerr KM, Bubendorf L, Edelman MJ, Marchetti A, Mok T, Novello S, et al. Second ESMO consensus conference on lung cancer: pathology and molecular biomarkers for non-small-cell lung cancer. Ann Oncol. 2014;25(9):1681–90.
2. Roy-Chowdhuri S, Aisner DL, Allen TC, Beasley MB, Borczuk A, Cagle PT, et al. Biomarker testing in lung carcinoma cytology specimens: a perspective from members of the pulmonary pathology society. Arch Pathol Lab Med. 2016. Apr 15 (Epub ahead of print).
3. Bubendorf L, Lantuejoul S, de Langen AJ, Thunnissen E. Nonsmall cell lung carcinoma: diagnostic difficulties in small biopsies and cytological specimens: number 2 in the series "Pathology for the clinician" edited by Peter Dorfmuller and Alberto Cavazza. Eur Respir Rev. 2017;26(144). https://doi.org/10.1183/16000617.0007-2017.
4. da Cunha Santos G. Standardizing preanalytical variables for molecular cytopathology. Cancer Cytopathol. 2013;121(7):341–3.
5. Moelans CB, Oostenrijk D, Moons MJ, van Diest PJ. Formaldehyde substitute fixatives: effects on nucleic acid preservation. J Clin Pathol. 2011;64(11):960–7.
6. Cheng L, Zhang S, MacLennan GT, Williamson SR, Davidson DD, Wang M, et al. Laser-assisted microdissection in translational research: theory, technical considerations, and future applications. Appl Immunohistochem Mol Morphol. 2013;21(1):31–47.
7. Bubendorf L, Savic S, Ruiz C. Molecular techniques. In: Bibbo M, Wilbur DC, editors. Comprehensive cytopathology. 4th ed. Philadelphia: Elsevier Saunders; 2015. p. 912–25.
8. Sauter G, Moch H, Moore D, Carroll P, Kerschmann R, Chew K, et al. Heterogeneity of erbB-2 gene amplification in bladder cancer. Cancer Res. 1993;53(10 Suppl):2199–203.

9. Sauter G, Feichter G, Torhorst J, Moch H, Novotna H, Wagner U, et al. Fluorescence in situ hybridization for detecting erbB-2 amplification in breast tumor fine needle aspiration biopsies. Acta Cytol. 1996;40(2):164–73.
10. Savic S, Bubendorf L. Common fluorescence in situ hybridization applications in cytology. Arch Pathol Lab Med. 2016;140(12):1323–30.
11. Zlobec I, Raineri I, Schneider S, Schoenegg R, Grilli B, Herzog M, et al. Assessment of mean EGFR gene copy number is a highly reproducible method for evaluating FISH in histological and cytological cancer specimens. Lung Cancer. 2010;68(2):192–7.
12. Vlajnic T, Somaini G, Savic S, Barascud A, Grilli B, Herzog M, et al. Targeted multiprobe fluorescence in situ hybridization analysis for elucidation of inconclusive pancreatobiliary cytology. Cancer Cytopathol. 2014;122(8):627–34.
13. Zhou F, Moreira AL. Lung carcinoma predictive biomarker testing by immunoperoxidase stains in cytology and small biopsy specimens: advantages and limitations. Arch Pathol Lab Med. 2016;140(12):1331–7.
14. Lee GD, Lee SE, Oh DY, Yu DB, Jeong HM, Kim J, et al. MET Exon 14 skipping mutations in lung adenocarcinoma: clinicopathologic implications and prognostic values. J Thorac Oncol. 2017;12(8):1233–46.
15. Bubendorf L, Buttner R, Al-Dayel F, Dietel M, Elmberger G, Kerr K, et al. Testing for ROS1 in non-small cell lung cancer: a review with recommendations. Virchows Arch. 2016;469(5):489–503.
16. Bubendorf L, Lantuejoul S, Yatabe Y. Analysis in cytology. In: Tsao MS, Hirsch FR, Yatabe Y, editors. IASLC Atlas of ALK and ROS1 testing in lung cancer. 2nd ed. North Fort Myers: International Association for the Study of Lung Cancer, Editorial Rx Press; 2016.
17. Pisapia P, Lozano MD, Vigliar E, Bellevicine C, Pepe F, Malapelle U, et al. ALK and ROS1 testing on lung cancer cytologic samples: perspectives. Cancer. 2017;125(11):817–30.
18. Savic S, Bode B, Diebold J, Tosoni I, Barascud A, Baschiera B, et al. Detection of ALK-positive non-small-cell lung cancers on cytological specimens: high accuracy of immunocytochemistry with the 5A4 clone. J Thorac Oncol. 2013;8(8):1004–11.
19. van der Wekken AJ, Pelgrim R, t Hart N, Werner N, Mastik MF, Hendriks L, et al. Dichotomous ALK-IHC is a better predictor for ALK inhibition outcome than traditional ALK-FISH in advanced non-small cell lung cancer. Clin Cancer Res. 2017;23(15):4251–8.
20. Wang W, Tang Y, Li J, Jiang L, Jiang Y, Su X. Detection of ALK rearrangements in malignant pleural effusion cell blocks from patients with advanced non-small cell lung cancer: a comparison of Ventana immunohistochemistry and fluorescence in situ hybridization. Cancer Cytopathol. 2015;123(2):117–22.
21. Skov BG, Skov T. Paired comparison of PD-L1 expression on cytologic and histologic specimens from malignancies in the lung assessed with PD-L1 IHC 28-8pharmDx and PD-L1 IHC 22C3pharmDx. Appl Immunohistochem Mol Morphol. 2017;25(7):453–9.
22. Thunnissen E, Yatabe Y, Lantuejoul S, Bubendorf L. Immunohistochemistry for PD-L1. In: Tsao MS, Kerr KM, Dacic S, Yatabe Y, Hirsch FR, editors. IASLC Atlas for PD-L1 immunohistochemistry testing in lung cancer. North Fort Myers: International Association for the Study of Lung Cancer, Editorial Rx Press; 2017.
23. da Cunha Santos G, Saieg MA. Preanalytic specimen triage: smears, cell blocks, cytospin preparations, transport media, and cytobanking. Cancer. 2017;125(S6):455–64.
24. Knoepp SM, Roh MH. Ancillary techniques on direct-smear aspirate slides: a significant evolution for cytopathology techniques. Cancer Cytopathol. 2013;121(3):120–8.
25. Balassanian R, Wool GD, Ono JC, Olejnik-Nave J, Mah MM, Sweeney BJ, et al. A superior method for cell block preparation for fine-needle aspiration biopsies. Cancer Cytopathol. 2016;124(7):508–18.
26. Crapanzano JP, Heymann JJ, Monaco S, Nassar A, Saqi A. The state of cell block variation and satisfaction in the era of molecular diagnostics and personalized medicine. CytoJournal. 2014;11:7.
27. Jain D, Mathur SR, Iyer VK. Cell blocks in cytopathology: a review of preparative methods, utility in diagnosis and role in ancillary studies. Cytopathology. 2014;25(6):356–71.

28. Lindsey KG, Houser PM, Shotsberger-Gray W, Chajewski OS, Yang J. Young investigator challenge: a novel, simple method for cell block preparation, implementation, and use over 2 years. Cancer. 2016;124(12):885–92.
29. Tian SK, Killian JK, Rekhtman N, Benayed R, Middha S, Ladanyi M, et al. Optimizing workflows and processing of cytologic samples for comprehensive analysis by next-generation sequencing: memorial Sloan Kettering cancer center experience. Arch Pathol Lab Med. 2016.
30. van Hemel BM, Suurmeijer AJ. Effective application of the methanol-based PreservCyt fixative and the cellient automated cell block processor to diagnostic cytopathology, immunocytochemistry, and molecular biology. Diagn Cytopathol. 2013;41(8):734–41.

How to Prepare Cytological Samples for Molecular Testing

2

Claudio Bellevicine, Umberto Malapelle, Elena Vigliar,
Pasquale Pisapia, Carlo Ruosi, and Giancarlo Troncone

2.1 Introduction

Molecular cytopathology, a rapidly evolving field of modern cytopathology, features an increasing number, variety, breadth and depth of tests, which underlines the effective interplay between genomics and cytology [1]. Challenging cases classified as atypical or as of undetermined significance may be further stratified into high- and low-risk groups by the demonstration of specific oncogenic mutations [2]. Moreover, by the development of personalized/precision medicine, cancer gene testing on cytological samples from patients with surgically unresectable, high-stage locally advanced, recurrent or metastatic malignancies is crucial [3]. Although fine-needle aspiration (FNA) biopsy, a rapid, efficient and minimally invasive technique, and core needle biopsy (CNB) represent complementary methods to sample superficial and deep-seated lesions, the use of FNA for gene testing is advantageous over CNB in several respects. Despite a wide range of cytopreparations, fixation and staining techniques, FNA have higher tumour fraction, ensure a wider sampling of the targeted lesion and offer a better quality DNA and an effective triage for ancillary studies when coupled with rapid on-site evaluation [2]. More recently, cytological specimens have also been validated for next-generation sequencing (NGS) to simultaneously screen different types of mutations in multiple genes and in multiple patient samples using small amounts of input material [4].

C. Bellevicine · U. Malapelle · E. Vigliar · P. Pisapia · C. Ruosi · G. Troncone (✉)
Department of Public Health, University of Napoli Federico II, School of Medicine,
Naples, Italy
e-mail: giancarlo.troncone@unina.it

© Springer International Publishing AG, part of Springer Nature 2018

F. C. Schmitt (ed.), *Molecular Applications in Cytology*,
https://doi.org/10.1007/978-3-319-74942-6_2

2.2   The Cytopathologist's Role

The cytopathologist is responsible of those multiple actions cumulatively referred to as pre-analytical processing (Fig. 2.1). He has to review cytopathology reports and archived materials to select best quality smears or representative cell-block sections to determine the cellularity and purity of the tumour sample being submitted for biomarker testing, having the responsibility to cancel the request for molecular assay whenever the cellularity is below the analytical sensitivity of the molecular assay. Similar to surgical pathologists, there is a wide interobserver variation also among cytopathologists in estimating tumour fraction, and even in the same

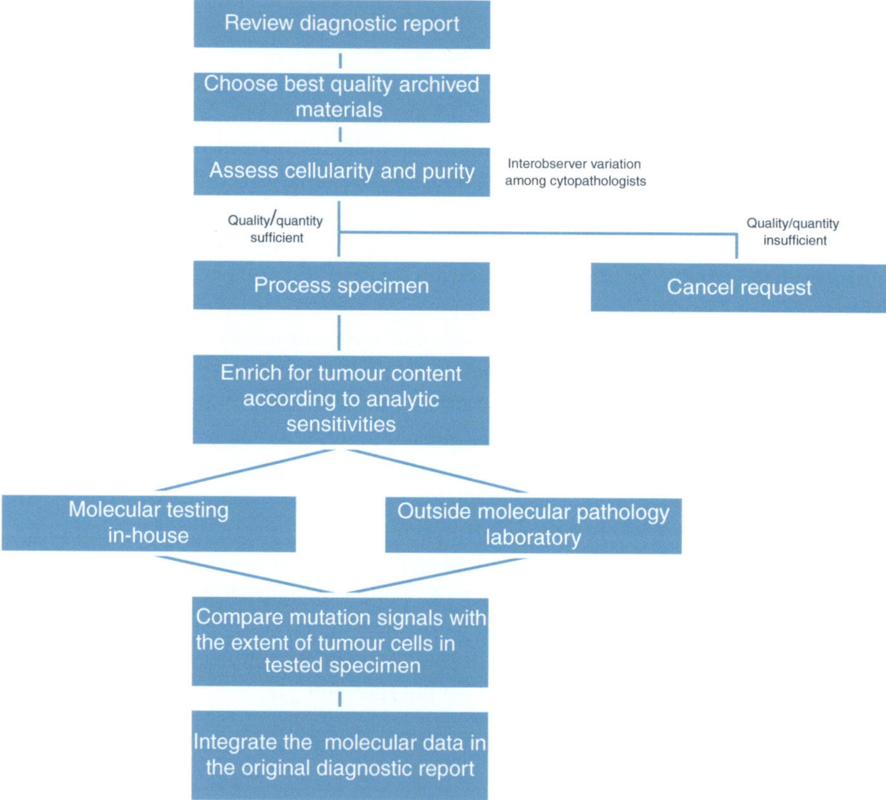

Fig. 2.1 Cytopathologist role in molecular testing. The cytopathologist has to review cytopathology reports and archived materials to select the best quality sample among several preparation types with varying suitability, having the responsibility to cancel the request for molecular assay whenever the cellularity, even after tumour cell enrichment, is below the analytical sensitivity of the molecular assay. Regardless of the test being performed in-house or in referral laboratories, the cytopathologist needs to evaluate critically the results before integration in the original cytological diagnostic report

institution, cancellation rates vary widely among cytopathologists [5]. Care should be taken to identify viable tumour areas in which the tumour ratio is optimal and the percentage inflammatory cells and of potentially amplification inhibitors (such as mucin, melanin and tumour cell necrosis) is minimal [2]. Since various mutational assays have different analytic sensitivities, the cytopathologist (or the technician) should enrich for tumour content to a level that is acceptable for the assay being used. Once the results of the genotyping analysis are received, the cytopathologist needs knowledge of the molecular diagnosis and of available treatment strategies; on occasion, the cytopathologist may also compare the mutation signals with the extent of tumour cells in the tested specimen, carefully evaluating the quality processes employed to ensure confidence in the results, taking care to integrate the molecular data in its original diagnostic report.

2.3 Test Request

As a general rule, the test request should be made appropriately to ensure that every patient who needs a test is offered one in a timely manner while avoiding unnecessary procedures. The test is usually requested by the oncologists and less frequently by other specialists, including surgeons and interventional radiologists. Ideally, rather than by a single specialist, test request should be made multidisciplinary (tumour board) [6]. Also in light of the increased awareness among patients and their families of the novel technological and therapeutic opportunities, the tumour board should ensure that the needs of a precise cytological diagnosis and of multiple predictive assays would simultaneously be met [6]. Thus, the effective communication between the laboratory, the oncologists and the cytopathologist is crucial to plan effective sampling strategies to ensure that adequate tissue amount is obtained [7]. As a matter of the fact, the cytopathologist may not know whether the patient is a candidate for surgery or for targeted therapy. Thus, the cytological sample is not the optimal testing approach when a larger resection specimen is subsequently available for analysis [7]. Similarly, for diagnoses made on a metastatic or recurrent lesion, the cytopathologist should be informed whether any prior specimen of the same patient has already been tested. Previous chemotherapy regimens can change gene expression and mutation status and should be documented on the request form. In some cases, patients with poor performance status may still be considered candidates for testing, as clinical response without significant side effects may follow the detection of a targetable genomic alteration [7].

Rather than on oncologist's demand, the automatic (reflex) testing by cytopathologists, based on diagnosis and tissue availability, can be more efficient. Reflex testing avoids the costs in time and money of specimen retrieval from pathology archives and the treatment delay for patients who are found to harbour a targetable molecular alteration [8]. However, molecular testing is expensive, and as molecular biomarkers are evolving rapidly over time, new targets may be identified in the interval between diagnosis and recurrence.

2.4 The Integrated and Standardized Cytopathology-Molecular Report

One of the main goals for a successful multidisciplinary approach to the oncologic patient is a clear communication between the different members of the care team. Considering the importance of the cytological approach for the diagnosis and treatment of different types of cancers, particular attention should be paid to the redaction of the cytopathology report, the most important way of communication for the cytopathologist. Besides the microscopic, morphologically based diagnosis, the cytology specimens are increasingly tested by genetic analysis, but the incorporation of the molecular results into the original cytopathology report is not standardized and depends on the local practice habit. In particular, when the molecular test are performed "in-house", the results are usually incorporated as *addendum* to the original microscopic diagnosis and signed out either by the original cytopathologist who diagnosed the case or, in academic settings, together with the molecular pathologist or the biologist who actually performed the molecular test. Conversely, when the molecular tests are externalized, a separate report is sent back to the oncologist or pathologist and may not be recorded or added to the cytology report. In this latter case, the lack of integration between the microscopic and molecular cytological diagnosis in a single, comprehensive report leaves to the requesting physician the responsibility of the correct interpretation of these two pieces of the diagnosis. However, the integration of cancer phenotype and genotype is not a simple exercise of data sum-up because it provides accurate information on the biology of the tumour, with important repercussion on the diagnostic accuracy, prognosis and treatment. Thus, these integration efforts should be made by the cytopathologist who is aware of the microscopy as well as of the molecular results. Moreover, the demand for a timely and complete diagnosis is becoming increasingly common since many tumours are now tested for a wide range of actionable mutational targets. Thus, the availability of genetic information at the same time of the microscopic diagnosis in a single, integrated and standardized cytopathology report allows a clearer and more rapid communication between the cytopathologist and the oncologist [9].

2.5 Reference Laboratories

The cytopathologist may perform the molecular testing in-house, which is a frequent procedure in the United States, supervising the activity of his/her Clinical Laboratory Improvement Amendment (CLIA)-accredited intramural molecular pathology laboratory [7]. Conversely, in Europe not all pathology departments are equipped to run molecular testing, and a greater number of cytopathologists refer to outside molecular pathology laboratories [10].

Processes should be established to ensure that specimens with a final cytopathology diagnosis are sent to external molecular pathology laboratories within three working days of receiving requests. However, in our practice, the mean time between the oncologist's request and specimen dispatching is nearly double the recommended time (5.8 working days) [10]. Noteworthy, delivery times are longer for larger-volume pathology departments than for smaller laboratories. Budget, the availability of technical personal and reimbursement issues may be factors influencing these differences. However, once the cytopathologists are made aware of the delays in the processing of the request and the shipping of the tumour samples, corrective actions can be obtained [11]. The breakage of slides during transport is also a potential issue; nonetheless, careful packing of slides can prevent this to be a serious drawback to the use of smears.

When determining the centre to select for outside molecular testing, the cytopathologist should ensure that the laboratory is accredited either at the national or at the international level [7]. The laboratory should join external quality assurance assessment once or twice a year; however, as only histological samples are usually included in the proficiency testing schemes, the assessment of the quality of testing on cytology remains problematic. It is also relevant that the laboratory staff would include anatomic pathology-certified pathologists who verify specimen quantity and quality and supervise specimen selection, interface with clinicians and troubleshoot problems [7].

The cytopathologist should be aware of the minimum tumour percentage required by the reference laboratory to accept a specimen. While the analytic sensitivity dictates the burden of tumour that must be present in the tested sample, it is also necessary that the method used has sufficient reference range for a wide spectrum of mutations. The cytopathologist should control whether the reference laboratory routinely microdissects samples and the method of microdissection used. Another key issue to consider are the cytopreparation types validated and accepted for testing [7]. Most laboratories will accept cytology cell blocks, while an additional option that has already reached widespread adoption is the use of direct smears.

2.6 Cell Block

Formalin-fixed, paraffin-embedded (FFPE) cell blocks (CBs) were first introduced in the early 1970s, as an aid to microscopic diagnosis, by highlighting tumour architectural organization not readily appreciated on other cytological preparations [12]. Later, CBs have traditionally been employed by cytopathological laboratories to perform ancillary immunocytochemical stainings. CBs, similar to the traditional histological blocks, do not require additional molecular assay validation [13]; given the regulatory requirement for archival slides retention and the concern to use direct smears, they represent a useful banked tissue archive [2]. As most molecular testing clinical practice guideline panels include expert molecular histopathologists, the use of cell-block sections is usually recommended over smears. Neutral buffered formalin, the fixative most commonly used for tissue preservation, induces the methylene bridging of bases and the formation of cross-links between nucleic acids and available proteins and random polymerase errors in nucleotide incorporation, usually being C-T or G-A transitions [14]; these sequencing artefacts mainly occur when the amounts of template DNA are low, as in the case of DNA obtained from microdissected sections, and DNA treatment with *Escherichia coli* uracil *N*-glycosylase before amplification and genotyping on shorter amplicons may be a way to avoid artefactual mutations [14]. As far as RNA extraction is concerned, relatively harsh conditions with the inclusion of proteinase K digestion followed by heating steps are employed in an effort to break the methylene bridges. Even with optimized digestion and heating steps, however, it is not possible to completely remove all chemical modifications such as residual methyl groups from FFPE-extracted RNA [15].

Cellularity is evaluated by examining a haematoxylin-eosin (H&E)-stained section prepared from the cell block; thus, the percentage of tumour cells in deeper sections of the cell block used for molecular testing is assessed in an extrapolative fashion inferred but not actually known. When the tumour cellularity is high and more than sufficient for testing, paraffin scrolls can simply be placed directly into a tube for extraction without microdissection, and cellularity assessment of an H&E section taken after the scrolls (postcurl section) may be unnecessary [16]. More often, however, cell blocks feature a low tumour content [17], and in a recent electronic survey among the members of the American Society of Cytopathology and other pathologists, many laboratories shared dissatisfaction with their cell-block preparation methods [18]. In addition, across institutions there is extreme variability in cell-block preparation techniques and lack of uniformity with some practices including additional dedicated passes for cellular enrichment [18]. Thus, with cell blocks with low tumour content, unstained sections should be lined up with a corresponding tumour-mapped haematoxylin-eosin-stained slide, with circled tumour-rich areas as a guide for macrodissection or microdissection. Noteworthy, the standard 4–5 µ cell-block sections do not represent the entire nuclei from the cell and are likely to have lower nucleic acid yields for molecular testing per cell than the whole cells obtained from other non-formalin-fixed cytologic substrates [16]. Cutting extra, unstained cell-block sections upfront to avoid refacing block would be ideal to save as much tumour tissue as possible for molecular testing, avoiding that ancillary studies are requested in a piecemeal fashion [19].

A main disadvantage of using cell blocks is the inability to assess cellularity and adequacy at the time of procedure, because processing is not usually complete until the following day (Table 2.1). Thus, the adequacy assessment of cell-block preparations is largely based on the rapid on-site evaluation (ROSE) performed on the corresponding direct smears, which may or may not be entirely representative of the cell-block cellularity [17, 18]. Usually the cell block represents a pooled specimen from multiple passes, and therefore the tumour cell population from high-yield needle passes are diluted by background benign elements in off-target needle passes. This is problematic because the analytic sensitivity of molecular diagnostic assays depends on a percentage tumour cellularity threshold, below which false-negative results will occur (i.e. contaminating benign tissue will be negative for the molecular abnormality being tested).

Table 2.1 Advantages and disadvantages of different cytological preparations for mutation testing

	Direct smears	Cell blocks	Liquid-based cytology
Advantages	High-quality DNA Visualization of malignant cells ROSE feasible The areas of optimal tumour/benign ratio are easier to find and delineate	Diagnostic smears preserved Standardized for immunostainings Guidelines recommended Useful for image-guided procedure	Eliminates the need for slide preparation by clinicians Material maximized Optimal yield and quality of CytoLyt-derived DNA
Disadvantages	Additional rigorous validation Loss of diagnostic material Delay due to coverslip removal LCM may be needed	Poor DNA quality ROSE unfeasible Pooled sample Unsatisfactory cell-block preparation method	ROSE unfeasible Pooled sample Suboptimal yield and quality of Cytorich Red-derived DNA

2.7 Direct Smears

Unlike cell blocks, the additional rigorous validation for each individual molecular assay performed on smear preparations for clinical reporting poses the biggest challenge in using these specimen preparations for ancillary studies [17]. However, when a cell block is not available, the smears used for diagnosis are the only source of tumour cells testable for molecular studies. As far as manual microdissection is concerned, the direct smears are typically superior to the cell blocks, because the smeared sample is more dispersed with a greater variation in the proportion of tumour/benign in different areas of the slide (Table 2.1). Therefore, it is easier to find and delineate areas of tumour enrichment on smears, even in cases with overall low tumour fraction [17].

Two are the usual methods of tissue selection either via the scraping of the smear or by cell lifting [20]. The first procedure is carried out by a flat, single-edge scalpel blade to collect all material into a small clump, which is pushed to a corner of the slide. The corner of the slide is placed over the open end of an Eppendorf collecting tube, and the scraped tissue is gently pushed into the tube with the tip of the scalpel blade or a pipette tip. The tissue selection by cell lifting exploits the Pinpoint solution of the Pinpoint Slide DNA Isolation System (Zymo Research) that is applied over the selected area [21]. The quantity of Pinpoint solution required is based on the dimension of the tissue area and is calculated according to the manufacturer's instructions. The solution is spread evenly over the area of interest with the side of a pipette tip and was allowed to air-dry for approximately 30–45 min. After the solution is completely dry and had formed a thin blue film, the embedded tissue together with the dried film is loosened, with a razor blade used to cut around the edge of the film. The film is then peeled from the slide, transferred to an Eppendorf tube and centrifuged briefly so that the tissue could be collected at the bottom of the tube [20].

More recently, molecular testing has been validated on DNA extracted from cancer cells isolated from routine smears by cell-transfer technique [22, 23]. This method had already been employed to enable immunohistochemical stainings, and it is based on the use of a special media (Mount Quick) commercially available (Daido Sangyo, Tokyo, Japan). This latter is spread uniformly over the top of the cellular material on de-coverslipped smears. After slide heating the media is hardened, cut and placed in an Eppendorf tube for DNA extraction and molecular testing [22]. This method has several advantages, being inexpensive, easily performed by a cytotechnologist and enabling multiple analyses in selected slide areas, which can be useful when dealing with different cancer cell population components [23].

Both alcohol-fixed and air-dried smears are suitable for the readily isolation of reasonably stable high-quality DNA and a sound choice for long-term DNA storage, although heat and humidity are potential problematic issues [24]. Non-cross-linking alcoholic reagents yield superior results as RNA fixatives in comparison with aldehydes because they cause little chemical change and typically provide higher-quality nucleic acids for molecular testing than do FFPE sections [15]. Most studies using previously stained cytology smears have shown that molecular testing can be performed successfully using both Diff-Quik- as well as Papanicolaou-stained slides. However, a recent study by Killian et al. [25] suggests that Diff-Quik-stained smears should be preferred to Papanicolaou-stained slides. While these latter featured DNA degradation as a function of age, the Diff-Quik-stained smears provided high-quality DNA even if archived for a prolonged period, allowing for the performance of sophisticated molecular diagnostic studies such as high-resolution comparative genomic hybridization assays [25]. Conversely, even more recently in a cell line-based study, Papanicolaou-stained smears yielded optimal DNA yield and fragment length [26]. Interestingly, several studies showed that Diff-Quik smears are as good as cell blocks and Papanicolaou for NGS testing without significant differences in the total number of reads, the percentage of reads mapping to the target region or the coverage of target regions in the gene set.

Although the process of removing the coverslip of archival smears does not compromise the quality of the DNA isolated for molecular studies, it is time-consuming [26]. To avoid any delay, ROSE, at the time of the FNA procedure, enables the best triage of the sample for diagnosis and ancillary studies and the selection of a representative slide that it is maintained uncoverslipped for immediate DNA extraction [21]. Alternatively, da Cunha Santos et al. proposed the "freezer method" [27]. Once that the slide is frozen, a blade is used to lift off the coverslip, and after xylene soaking, the slide can be then sent for manual microdissection. This method is very fast and could be an important tool for molecular analysis performed on cytology smears [28].

When most of the diagnostic cells are on a single slide, the molecular testing will destroy the evidence of tumour cells, which might have medicolegal consequences. To mitigate the medicolegal constraints, smears can be digitally scanned, to record the cytomorphology of representative diagnostic microscopic fields for the archives. In our practice we experienced that to record the three-dimensional groups and tissue material of variable thickness is required, the use of a z-axis scanner that unlike whole slide imaging of histology slides is time-consuming and results in relatively large digital image files [5].

2.8 Liquid-Based Cytology

ROSE for tumour cell adequacy is crucial to ensure that the obtained material is sufficient and properly preserved not only for the identification of malignancy but also for biomarker testing [2]. This can be successfully performed either by a cyto-pathologist or by a properly trained cytotechnologist or even by a pulmonologist [29]. Unfortunately, due to budget and staff limitation, ROSE is not always feasible [30]. In this setting, liquid-based cytology (LBC) represents a valid alternative to traditional cytology, avoiding the possibility that untrained clinicians may improperly smear and triage the aspirated material, thus limiting artefacts [31].

The specimen is simply expelled in its entirety into an alcohol-based fixative, such as CytoLyt (Hologic, Bedford, Massachusetts) or CytoRich Red (Fisher Scientific UK Ltd., Loughborough, Leicestershire, England) solutions, and by proprietary instruments, a cell monolayer slide is prepared [31]. In our experience, although direct smears show a higher DNA yield and are more cell-rich than LBC slides, the differences in adequacy and in mutant rate between the two samples are minimal [31]. This may probably reflect the similar effect of methanol-based CytoLyt and ethanol-based smear fixation on DNA preservation (Table 2.1). Conversely, LBC samples fixed with CytoRich Red have shown poorer DNA preservation due to the presence of a small amount (<1%) of formaldehyde that may cause DNA degradation and modification by the cross-linking of cytosine residues on either strands [17]. In addition, residual material from CytoLyt samples has been shown to feature optimal RNA integrity being suitable for nucleic acid isolation and subsequent analysis by RT-PCR. However, RNA degradation was reported in specimens stored for 12 months at room temperature, and long-term storage requires −80 °C [15].

Several studies have described using LBC specimens for molecular analysis, either by scraping off cells from the LBC slides or extracting DNA directly from the rinse solution [32, 33]. In a recent survey, we reported that the referring cytopathologists more frequently outsource LBC slides rather than vials to referral laboratories; in fact, LBC vial dispatching is unpractical as the vials are stored only for a limited period of time with limited long-term DNA stability and often the residual solution is not sufficient for testing [31]. In addition, the possibility of directly visualizing neoplastic cells is preferable, also when comparing the mutation signals with the extent of tumour cells in the tested slide [33]. When the low-sensitive direct sequencing method is employed, neoplastic cell enrichment is mandatory [13]; however, manual microdissection on LBC slides is difficult, as neoplastic and non-neoplastic components from different in- and off-target fine-needle aspiration passes are pooled together and homogeneously distributed during processing. Laser capture microdissection is expensive and time-consuming and hardly feasible in routine clinical setting [32]. Alternatively, highly sensitive molecular techniques, such as real-time PCR methods, can be used directly on the DNA extracted from the preservant solution of the vial, without slide preparation [31].

2.9   Fresh Cells

Fresh, unfixed cells may be processed for immediate nucleic acid extraction with excellent results [2]. The advantage of a short acquisition time for molecular processing is mostly required to ensure high-integrity RNA for some molecular applications such as complementary DNA (cDNA) labelling for microarray analysis and transcriptome analysis [15]. In contrast, RT-PCR or qRT-PCR analysis for fusion gene detection is more tolerant of partially degraded RNA because the design can be based on an analysis of smaller regions of RNA [15]. For long-term storage, aliquots can be frozen at 80 °C RNA later or similar RNA-stabilizing solutions and stored in freezers [34]; fresh cells can also be stored at room temperature for months in Whatman filter paper cards (GE Healthcare Life Sciences, Buckinghamshire, England) [35]. This latter method is an easy, fast, inexpensive and operative-friendly procedure and ensures high quality of nucleic acid for molecular testing, but the amount of genetic material that can be extracted from the FTA cards is limited [36]. Moreover, the disadvantage of using fresh/frozen/FTA-collected cells is the lack of direct microscopic examination of the tissue specimen from which the DNA/RNA is isolated, and false negatives can commonly occur if the sample tested does not have an adequate tumour fraction [24].

2.10   Nucleic Acid Sample Quantity and Quality Assessment

The accurate analysis of input nucleic acid sample quantity, purity and integrity is crucial, especially on scant routine cytological samples. Several techniques should be used in a complementary manner, as none of them, alone, can provide all the information required to fully characterize the DNA/RNA sourced from a cytological sample [34, 37],

Spectrophotometer analysis based on ultraviolet (UV) light absorption of a diluted nucleic acid samples read at 260 nm and 280 nm is largely used to quantified DNA or RNA. Between nucleic acid correlation and absorbance (A), there is a linear correlation able to predict the DNA or RNA quantity in the solution. Pure RNA has an A260/A280 of 2.1, whereas pure DNA will have an A260/A280 of 1.8. Currently, miniaturized automatic platforms, such as NanoDrop Spectrophotometer, allow accurate analyses also of small sample sizes (0.5–2 μL) [37].

Fluorimetric assays represent an alternative to spectrophotometric methods [37]. The binding of fluorescent dyes to nucleic acids measures the subsequent changes in fluorescence levels. With respect to spectrophotometry, fluorescence-based quantification is more sensitive and precise and may be specific for the nucleic acid of interest. Since fluorometers measure fluorescence in relative rather than absolute units, the measurement is first calibrated with a known concentration of a standard nucleic acid solution with characteristics similar to the sample to be measured. Following calibration, a single measurement can establish the concentration of nucleic acid in the solution, but typically a standard curve will be required to ascertain the linearity of the assay in the range measured. Automated systems such as the Qubit 2.0 fluorometer (Life Technologies) can be used with a range of different fluorescence-based quantification assays for the measurement of nucleic acid concentration in solution. The assays demonstrate a wide dynamic range for detection and are capable of accurately analysing small samples. It is critical to observe that the OD reading is a measure of absorption and provides a measure of quantity and not quality or sample integrity.

Nucleic acid samples can be analysed and compared using instrumentation such as the Agilent 2100 BioAnalyzer, Bio-Rad Experion or the last developed Agilent TapeStation 4200 [38]. These instruments use a lab-on-a-chip approach, combining capillary electrophoresis with fluorescent detection. The electrophoretic process carried out on the chip is based on traditional gel electrophoresis principles that have been miniaturized, which reduces sample consumption and separation time. The chip (or the cartridges for TapeStation 4200 only) accommodates wells for samples, gel and an external standard (fragment size ladder) [38]. During manufacturing, microchannels are fabricated in glass to create interconnected networks among the wells. These micro-channels are then filled with a sieving polymer and fluorescence dye. Electrodes are inserted in the wells and the chip becomes an integrated electrical circuit. Charged biomolecules such as DNA or RNA are driven through the matrix in response to a voltage gradient. Due to a constant mass-to-charge ratio and the presence of a sieving polymer matrix, the molecules are separated by size such that smaller fragments migrate faster than larger ones. Dye molecules intercalate into nucleic acid strands, and these complexes are detected by laser-induced fluorescence. Data is then translated into electronic gel-like images and electropherograms. The informatics suites that support these instruments are used to determine a relative integrity number (RIN) for the DNA (only TapeStation 4200) and RNA samples. Intact nucleic acid has a RIN of 10, whereas completely degraded nucleic acid has a RIN of 1. In this way, interpretation of an electropherogram is facilitated and comparison of samples is possible.

2.11 DNA Input

Reliable, consistent, robust and accurate results from molecular tests using cytological samples will depend on standardized protocols for maximizing DNA yield and quality, and pre-analytical variables will have a direct impact on the analysis [17].

Although very small quantities of input material can be successfully amplified for molecular evaluation thanks to the exponential increase of target DNA via polymerase chain reaction, the yield of DNA is a critical pre-analytic factor that determines the success of molecular analysis. Thus, assay validation with low-input

DNA levels is crucial to reliably process cytological samples [2, 7]. In fact, a test that confidently detects a mutation with a specified quantity of input DNA relies on the fact that the tested DNA contains a minimum burden of the mutation. As the input quantity is decreased, the total mutation burden may drop below the lower threshold of detection for the assay. Whenever the tested specimens, which do not meet the validated input requirement, have a negative result, a disclaimer in the molecular pathology report is needed to indicate that the analytic sensitivity of the assay may be compromised by reduced nucleic acid input [7].

A number of variables associated with cytologic samples, including the type of fixative, slide, mounting medium and the tissue-extraction methodology, can affect the yield and quality of DNA. A detailed study carried out on cell lines by Dejmek et al. [26] reported that spray or ethanol-fixed slides provide better results in terms of DNA yield and fragment length over air-dried slides. While in these latter amplicon sizes of 388 bp could be consistently amplified and while amplification of a 578-bp amplicon proved to be difficult, in the spray-fixed samples, bands from the longest 760-bp amplicon could be observed in most samples [26]. Slide type can also have an effect on the DNA yield [20]. Clinical laboratories may use a variety of glass slides for the routine processing of smears from aspirates. Fully frosted (FF) slides are useful in low-cellularity aspiration samples, since their high cellular adhesion capability prevents cell loss during fixation in alcohol-based fixative solutions. Conversely nonfrosted (NF) slides have no specialized surface or coating to enhance cellular adhesion, being used when adequate cellularity is not an issue. The positively charged (PC) slides have a specialized surface that electrostatically enhances the adhesion of cellular material. A recent study reported a lower DNA yield for FF slides in comparison with NF and PC, which likely reflects the difficulty in dislodging cells from the crevices of FF slides [20]. Thus, although FF slides show better cell retention than other slides, they are more difficult to use for tissue extraction and are not optimal for the DNA yield.

Similarly, when cells are directly scraped off from previously stained archival direct smears and cytospin preparations by dissection, the DNA yield is higher than that obtained by cell lifting employing the Pinpoint solution [20]. Noteworthy, a significantly higher DNA yield was obtained with slides mounted with the low-hazard, organic, polymer-based mounting medium EcoMount (BioCare Medical LLC, Concord, Calif) when compared with the xylene-based mounting medium Pertex (CellPath Ltd., Newtown, Powys, UK) [26].

2.12 Cytopathology Informatics and Bioinformatics

The management of the increasing number of data derived by the molecular tests performed on cytopathology specimens has required the implementation of laboratory information systems (LIS). LIS are informatic databases used to facilitate the workflow through the different phases of the molecular tests (pre-analytical, analytical and post-analytical), delivering accurate and timely electronic results to the physician who is treating the patient. The LIS can also be useful to track the specimens in the different parts of the laboratory. In fact, with the increased complexity of information derived from a single cytology specimen, the samples could be split to perform ancillary testing to refine the microscopic diagnosis (e.g. immunocytochemistry) and to define by molecular test a treatment tailored to the patient, avoiding time delay. The LIS can assist the pathologist to place all of the test orders and to add supplemental results on the same cytological report. In fact, considering the different types of available tests, multiple results are usually reported as addenda to an original cytology diagnosis. This workflow might make it difficult for clinicians to manage their patients since they usually prefer to timely receive unified reports. To this end, the LIS can be helpful to produce an integrated cytological and molecular diagnostic report, quickly delivering it as electronic file on remote dispositive such as notepads or smartphones.

An increasing number of pathology laboratories are offering NGS testing on cytology samples. In diagnostic settings, NGS is usually employed as targeted multigene sequencing to detect pharmacologically actionable mutations. However, the "dry bench" analysis of the huge amount of sequencing data generated for each NGS run requires different steps to reliably identify a mutation. In particular, after the alignment of sequencing reads against the human reference genome sequence, each base is checked to find a significant sequence alteration called *variant*. The variant calls are usually performed by a bioinformatic software that allows the automatic recognition of these genomic alterations. Unfortunately, when the DNA extracted has low quality or its quantity is below the input requested by the NGS platform employed, suboptimal NGS postsequencing metrics may be generated. In this setting, the NGS may produce sequences that could not be adequately analysed automatically by the software. Thus, a skilled and dedicated bioinformatician should help the biologist to examine the sequence directly by using a genome viewer software that allows the visual inspection of the generated reads and recognition of clinical significant variants [39, 40].

2.13 Future Directions

As technology is advancing at rapid pace, a range of novel techniques is emerging. In particular NGS and fully automated platforms may necessitate specific sample requirements and dedication from cytopathologist to develop special cytopreparation protocols.

In particular, establishing the minimum number of cells needed to allow a next-generation sequencing approach from cytology sample is a crucial point. The studies that applied NGS to cytological material had usually a retrospective design, and only samples that featured at least 20% of neoplastic cells were selected, which may not fully reflects current practice. In any case, sample requirement depends on target capture, gene panel and platform types. Illumina NGS required 15,000 cells when following hybridization capture or 5000 cells when preceded by PCR-based capture, while Ion Torrent NGS needed between 100 and 1000 cells. As far as DNA input is concerned, Illumina NGS required from 50 to 170 ng, following

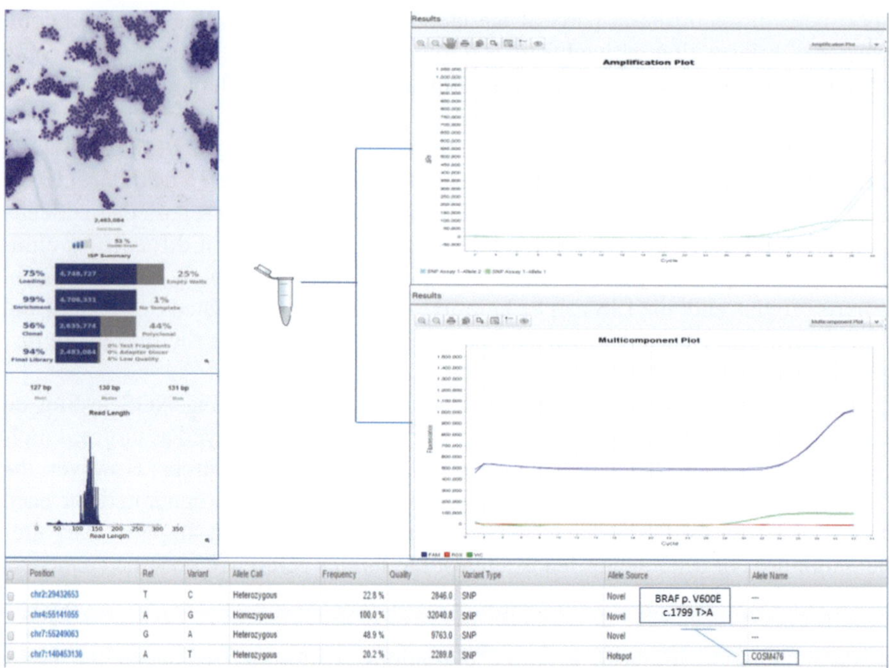

Fig. 2.2 NGS on a direct smear. (**a**) Thyroid FNA diagnosed as malignant, papillary thyroid cancer. Note the high cellularity (direct smears, Diff-Quik staining, 20× magnification); (**b**) Main metrics generated during the NGS processing. (**c**) Here is reported the histogram of the distribution of generated reads. Note that the majority of reads is distributed in the expected amplicon size range (75–150 bp), indicating a smear featuring good-quality DNA. (**d**) Genomic variant (BRAFV600E) identified by the variant caller software. (**e**) The BRAFV600E mutation was orthogonally confirmed by real-time PCR

hybridization capture or 30 ng downstream of multiplex PCR. Conversely, Ion Torrent sequencing of PCR products only needs 10 ng of DNA and precisely 12 μl of diluted DNA at a concentration of 0.8 ng/μL. An example of direct smear from a thyroid FNA, successfully processed by NGS, is reported in Fig. 2.2. Even more recently, it was shown that lowering the input DNA concentration below the manufacturer's recommended threshold of 10 ng (>0.8 ng/μL) is feasible leading to a marked increase in the NGS success rate from 58.6% to 89.8% [5, 41].

More relevant than DNA input is the percentage of neoplastic cells; in a low cancer cell background, the preferential amplification of a small number of DNA molecules may be representative only of the benign component, leading to a false-negative result. As a matter of the fact, most NGS assays have a lower limit of mutation detection of 10%, which requires at least 20% of neoplastic cells [42]. However, a more recent NGS approach, based on the use of narrower gene panel focused on a limited number of targets, enables the detection of low abundant mutations with a specificity of 100% [43].

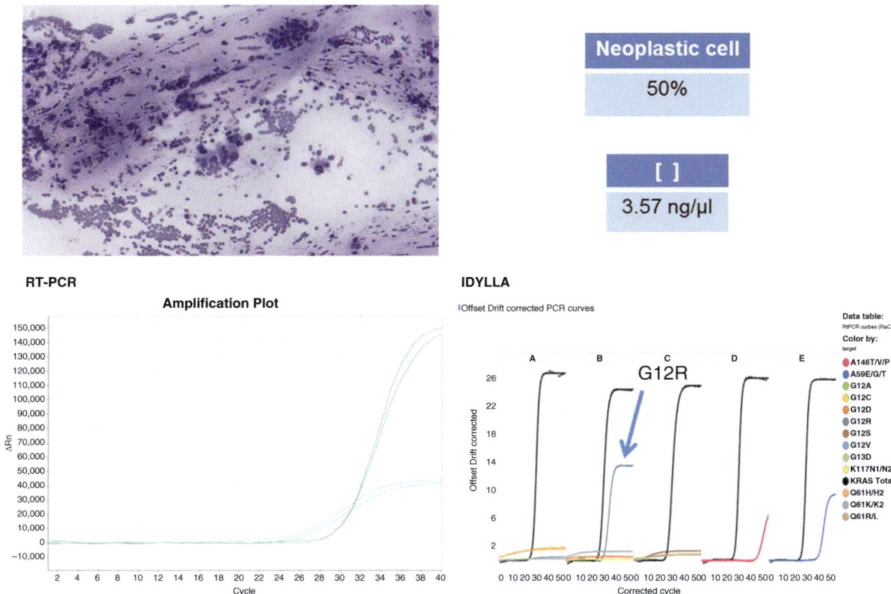

Fig. 2.3 Archivial DNA was extracted from a Diff-Quik-stained smear of pancreatic cancer featuring 50% of neoplastic cells and a concentration of 3.57 ng per microlitre. Representative graphs of standard RT-PCR and of Idylla are reported both showing G12R KRAS mutation

Besides NGS technological improvements, automated allele-specific real-time PCR technology is also advancing at rapid pace. In particular, the fully automated molecular diagnostics system Idylla (Biocartis, Mechelen, Belgium) is a fascinating technology [44, 45]. Sample preparation is combined with PCR thermocycling and fluorescence detection of target sequences. Without needing highly skilled staff, within approximately 90 min, the European Community (CE) in vitro diagnostic use (IVD) marked Idylla mutational tests can genotype relevant biomarkers. Although, the Idylla tests were designed for use with FFPE sections, the Idylla system can also process DNA preparations from cytological samples [46, 47]. To this end, only 10 ng of archival DNA, directly pipetted into the cartridge, is sufficient to obtain results in most samples (Fig. 2.3). Conversely, further technological refinements are needed to process scraped cells and to better adapt the automated extraction modalities to stained cytological material.

In conclusion, the cytopathologist not only provides the specimen for molecular diagnostics, among several preparation types with varying suitability, but also establish when, where and how biomarker testing should be performed [10]. To this end, modern cytotechnologists and cytopathologists should be dedicated to optimizing and standardizing cytological sample preparation methods not only for cytomorphology but also to preserve biomolecular integrity [3].

References

1. Idowu MO. Epidermal growth factor receptor in lung cancer: the amazing interplay of molecular testing and cytopathology. Cancer Cytopathol. 2013;121(10):540–3.
2. Bellevicine C, Vita GD, Malapelle U, Troncone G. Applications and limitations of oncogene mutation testing in clinical cytopathology. Semin Diagn Pathol. 2013;30(4):284–97.
3. Clark DP. Seize the opportunity: underutilization of fine-needle aspiration biopsy to inform targeted cancer therapy decisions. Cancer Cytopathol. 2009;117(5):289–97.
4. Vigliar E, Malapelle U, de Luca C, Bellevicine C, Troncone G. Challenges and opportunities of next-generation sequencing: a cytopathologist's perspective. Cytopathology. 2015;26(5):271–83.
5. Roy-Chowdhuri S, Stewart J. Preanalytic variables in cytology: lessons learned from next-generation sequencing-the MD Anderson experience. Arch Pathol Lab Med. 2016;140:1191–9.
6. Lopez-Rios F, Angulo B, Gomez B, Mair D, Martinez R, Conde E, Shieh F, Tsai J, Vaks J, Current R, Lawrence HJ, Gonzalez de Castro D. Comparison of molecular testing methods for the detection of EGFR mutations in formalin-fixed paraffin-embedded tissue specimens of non-small cell lung cancer. J Clin Pathol. 2013;66(5):381–5.
7. Aisner DL, Sams SB. The role of cytology specimens in molecular testing of solid tumors: techniques, limitations, and opportunities. Diagn Cytopathol. 2012;40(6):511–24.
8. Lindeman NI, Cagle PT, Beasley MB, Chitale DA, Dacic S, Giaccone G, Jenkins RB, Kwiatkowski DJ, Saldivar JS, Squire J, Thunnissen E, Ladanyi M. Molecular testing guideline for selection of lung cancer patients for EGFR and ALK tyrosine kinase inhibitors: guideline from the College of American Pathologists, international association for the study of lung cancer, and association for molecular pathology. J Thorac Oncol. 2013;8(7):823–59.
9. Pitman MB, Black-Schaffer WS. Post-fine-needle aspiration biopsy communication and the integrated and standardized cytopathology report. Cancer. 2017;125(S6):486–93.
10. Vigliar E, Malapelle U, Bellevicine C, de Luca C, Troncone G. Outsourcing cytological samples to a referral laboratory for EGFR testing in non-small cell lung cancer: does theory meet practice? Cytopathology. 2014;26(5):312–7.
11. Janssens A, De Droogh E, Lefebure A, Kockx M, Pauwels P, Germonpre P, van Meerbeeck JP. Routine implementation of EGFR mutation testing in clinical practice in Flanders: 'HERMES' project. Acta Clin Belg. 2014;69(2):92–7.
12. Loukeris K, Vazquez MF, Sica G, Wagner P, Yankelevitz DF, Henschke CI, Cham MD, Saqi A. Cytological cell blocks: predictors of squamous cell carcinoma and adenocarcinoma subtypes. Diagn Cytopathol. 2012;40(5):380–7.
13. Malapelle U, Bellevicine C, Zeppa P, Palombini L, Troncone G. Cytology-based gene mutation tests to predict response to anti-epidermal growth factor receptor therapy: a review. Diagn Cytopathol. 2011;39(9):703–10.
14. Marchetti A, Felicioni L, Buttitta F. Assessing EGFR mutations. N Engl J Med. 2006;354(5):526–8.
15. Bridge JA. Reverse transcription-polymerase chain reaction molecular testing of cytology specimens: pre-analytic and analytic factors. Cancer Cytopathol. 2016;125(1):11–9.
16. da Cunha SG, Wyeth T, Reid A, Saieg MA, Pitcher B, Pintilie M, Kamel-Reid S, Tsao MS. A proposal for cellularity assessment for EGFR mutational analysis with a correlation with DNA yield and evaluation of the number of sections obtained from cell blocks for immunohistochemistry in non-small cell lung carcinoma. J Clin Pathol. 2016;69(7):607–11.
17. Roy-Chowdhuri S, Aisner DL, Allen TC, Beasley MB, Borczuk A, Cagle PT, Capelozzi V, Dacic S, da Cunha Santos G, Hariri LP, Kerr KM, Lantuejoul S, Mino-Kenudson M, Moreira A, Raparia K, Rekhtman N, Sholl L, Thunnissen E, Tsao MS, Vivero M, Yatabe Y. Biomarker testing in lung carcinoma cytology specimens: a perspective from members of the pulmonary pathology society. Arch Pathol Lab Med. 2016;140:1267–72.
18. Crapanzano JP, Heymann JJ, Monaco S, Nassar A, Saqi A. The state of cell block variation and satisfaction in the era of molecular diagnostics and personalized medicine. CytoJournal. 2014;11:7.

19. Bellevicine C, Malapelle U, de Luca C, Iaccarino A, Troncone G, Pantanowitz L. EGFR analysis: current evidence and future directions. Diagn Cytopathol. 2014;42(11):984–92.
20. Roy-Chowdhuri S, Chow CW, Kane MK, Yao H, Wistuba II, Krishnamurthy S, Stewart J, Staerkel G. Optimizing the DNA yield for molecular analysis from cytologic preparations. Cancer Cytopathol. 2016;124(4):254–60.
21. Hookim K, Roh MH, Willman J, Placido J, Weigelin HC, Fields KL, Pang J, Betz BL, Knoepp SM. Application of immunocytochemistry and BRAF mutational analysis to direct smears of metastatic melanoma. Cancer Cytopathol. 2012;120(1):52–61.
22. Wu HH, Eaton JP, Jones KJ, Cramer HM, Randolph ML, Post KM, Malek A, Bilbo S, Sen JD, Chen S, Cheng L. Utilization of cell-transferred cytologic smears in detection of EGFR and KRAS mutation on adenocarcinoma of lung. Mod Pathol. 2014;27(7):930–5.
23. Shi Q, Ibrahim A, Herbert K, Carvin M, Randolph M, Post KM, Curless K, Chen S, Cramer HM, Cheng L, Wu HH. Detection of BRAF mutations on direct smears of thyroid fine-needle aspirates through cell transfer technique. Am J Clin Pathol. 2015;143(4):500–4.
24. Knoepp SM, Roh MH. Ancillary techniques on direct-smear aspirate slides: a significant evolution for cytopathology techniques. Cancer Cytopathol. 2013;121(3):120–8.
25. Killian JK, Walker RL, Suuriniemi M, Jones L, Scurci S, Singh P, Cornelison R, Harmon S, Boisvert N, Zhu J, Wang Y, Bilke S, Davis S, Giaccone G, Smith WI Jr, Meltzer PS. Archival fine-needle aspiration cytopathology (FNAC) samples: untapped resource for clinical molecular profiling. J Mol Diagn. 2010;12(6):739–45.
26. Dejmek A, Zendehrokh N, Tomaszewska M, Edsjo A. Preparation of DNA from cytological material: effects of fixation, staining, and mounting medium on DNA yield and quality. Cancer Cytopathol. 2013;121(7):344–53.
27. da Cunha Santos G, Schroder M, Zhu JB, Saieg MA, Geddie WR, Boerner SL, McDonald S. Minimizing delays in DNA retrieval: the "freezer method" for glass coverslip removal. Letter to the editor regarding comparative study of epidermal growth factor receptor mutation analysis on cytology smears and surgical pathology specimens from primary and metastatic lung carcinomas. Cancer Cytopathol. 2013;121(9):533.
28. Rao A, Khode R, Sayage-Rabie L. Reply to comparative study of epidermal growth factor receptor mutation analysis on cytology smears and surgical pathology specimens from primary and metastatic lung carcinomas. Cancer Cytopathol. 2013;121(9):534.
29. Gasparini S. It is time for this 'ROSE' to flower. Respiration. 2005;72(2):129–31.
30. Natu S, Hoffman J, Siddiqui M, Hobday C, Shrimankar J, Harrison R. The role of endobronchial ultrasound guided transbronchial needle aspiration cytology in the investigation of mediastinal lymphadenopathy and masses, the North Tees experience. J Clin Pathol. 2010;63(5):445–51.
31. Bellevicine C, Malapelle U, Vigliar E, de Luca C, Troncone G. Epidermal growth factor receptor test performed on liquid-based cytology lung samples: experience of an academic referral center. Acta Cytol. 2014;58:589–94.
32. Malapelle U, de Rosa N, Bellevicine C, Rocco D, Vitiello F, Piantedosi FV, Illiano A, Nappi O, Troncone G. EGFR mutations detection on liquid-based cytology: is microscopy still necessary? J Clin Pathol. 2012;65(6):561–4.
33. Malapelle U, de Rosa N, Rocco D, Bellevicine C, Crispino C, Illiano A, Piantedosi FV, Nappi O, Troncone G. EGFR and KRAS mutations detection on lung cancer liquid-based cytology: a pilot study. J Clin Pathol. 2012;65(1):87–91.
34. Ladd AC, O'Sullivan-Mejia E, Lea T, Perry J, Dumur CI, Dragoescu E, Garrett CT, Powers CN. Preservation of fine-needle aspiration specimens for future use in RNA-based molecular testing. Cancer Cytopathol. 2011;119(2):102–10.
35. da Cunha Santos G, Liu N, Tsao MS, Kamel-Reid S, Chin K, Geddie WR. Detection of EGFR and KRAS mutations in fine-needle aspirates stored on Whatman FTA cards: is this the tool for biobanking cytological samples in the molecular era? Cancer Cytopathol. 2010;118(6):450–6.
36. Peluso AL, Cascone AM, Lucchese L, Cozzolino I, Ieni A, Mignogna C, Pepe S, Zeppa P. Use of FTA cards for the storage of breast carcinoma nucleic acid on fine-needle aspiration samples. Cancer Cytopathol. 2015;123(10):582–92.

37. Simbolo M, Gottardi M, Corbo V, Fassan M, Mafficini A, Malpeli G, Lawlor RT, Scarpa A. DNA qualification workflow for next generation sequencing of histopathological samples. PLoS One. 2013;8(6):e62692.
38. Pop LA, Puscas E, Pileczki V, Cojocneanu-Petric R, Braicu C, Achimas-Cadariu P, Berindan-Neagoe I. Quality control of ion torrent sequencing library. Cancer Biomark. 2014;14(2–3):93–101.
39. Hanna MG, Pantanowitz L. The role of informatics in patient-centered care and personalized medicine. Cancer. 2017;125(S6):494–501.
40. Bellevicine C, Sgariglia R, Malapelle U, Vigliar E, Nacchio M, Ciancia G, Eszlinger M, Paschke R, Troncone G. Young investigator challenge: can the Ion AmpliSeq Cancer Hotspot panel v2 be used for next-generation sequencing of thyroid FNA samples? Cancer Cytopathol. 2016;124(11):776–84.
41. Roy-Chowdhuri S, Goswami RS, Chen H, Patel KP, Routbort MJ, Singh RR, Broaddus RR, Barkoh BA, Manekia J, Yao H, Medeiros LJ, Staerkel G, Luthra R, Stewart J. Factors affecting the success of next-generation sequencing in cytology specimens. Cancer Cytopathol. 2015;123(11):659–68.
42. Kanagal-Shamanna R, Portier BP, Singh RR, Routbort MJ, Aldape KD, Handal BA, Rahimi H, Reddy NLG, Barkoh BA, Mishra BM, Paladugu AV, Manekia JH, Kalhor N, Chowdhuri SR, Staerkel GA, Medeiros LJ, Luthra R, Patel KP. Next-generation sequencing-based multi-gene mutation profiling of solid tumors using fine needle aspiration samples: promises and challenges for routine clinical diagnostics. Mod Pathol. 2014;27(2):314–27.
43. Paweletz CP, Sacher AG, Raymond CK, Alden RS, O'Connell A, Mach SL, Kuang Y, Gandhi L, Kirschmeier P, English JM, Lim LP, Janne PA, Oxnard GR. Bias-corrected targeted next-generation sequencing for rapid, multiplexed detection of actionable alterations in cell-free DNA from advanced lung cancer patients. Clin Cancer Res. 2016;22(4):915–22.
44. Colling R, Wang LM, Soilleux E, Melchior L, Grauslund M, Bellosillo B, Montagut C, Torres E, Moragon E, Micalessi I, Frans J, Noten V, Bourgain C, Vriesema R, van der Geize R, Cokelaere K, Vercooren N, Crul K, Rudiger T, Buchmuller D, Reijans M, Jans C, Janku F, Claes B, Huang HJ, Falchook GS, Devogelaere B, Kockx M, Bempt IV, Reijans M, Naing A, Fu S, Piha-Paul SA, Hong DS, Holley VR, Tsimberidou AM, Stepanek VM, Patel SP, Kopetz ES, Subbiah V, Wheler JJ, Zinner RG, Karp DD, Luthra R, Roy-Chowdhuri S, Sablon E, Meric-Bernstam F, Maertens G, Kurzrock R. Automated PCR detection of BRAF mutations in colorectal adenocarcinoma: a diagnostic test accuracy study. J Clin Pathol. 2015;69:398–402.
45. Melchior L, Grauslund M, Bellosillo B, Montagut C, Torres E, Moragon E, Micalessi I, Frans J, Noten V, Bourgain C, Vriesema R, van der Geize R, Cokelaere K, Vercooren N, Crul K, Rudiger T, Buchmuller D, Reijans M, Jans C. Multi-center evaluation of the novel fully-automated PCR-based Idylla BRAF mutation test on formalin-fixed paraffin-embedded tissue of malignant melanoma. Exp Mol Pathol. 2015;99(3):485–91.
46. de Biase D, de Luca C, Gragnano G, Visani M, Bellevicine C, Malapelle U, Tallini G, Troncone G. Fully automated PCR detection of KRAS mutations on pancreatic endoscopic ultrasound fine-needle aspirates. J Clin Pathol. https://doi.org/10.1136/jclinpath-2016-203696.
47. De Luca C, Gragnano G, Pisapia P, Vigliar E, Malapelle U, Bellevicine C, Troncone G. EGFR mutation detection on lung cancer cytological specimens by the novel fully automated PCR-based Idylla EGFR mutation assay. J Clin Pathol. 2016;70(4):295–300.

Molecular Tests Use in Cytological Material (Analytical Phase)

3

Zsofia Balogh and Philippe Vielh

3.1 Introduction

Molecular techniques are increasingly important as diagnostic, prognostic, and predictive tools in daily cytology practice. However, these techniques are only effective when preceded by a careful morphological examination. In majority of the cases, the neoplastic cells are readily recognized by an experienced (cyto)pathologist. Only selected cases classified as atypical or as of undetermined significance may be further stratified into high- and low-risk groups by the demonstration of specific oncogenic characteristics, in order to confirm, supplement, and refine morphological information [1]. Moreover, they may be useful in decision-making to identify the right drug for the right patient (personalized or precision medicine) and to integrate diagnosis with and provide feedback from treatment efficiency (theranostic applications).

3.2 qPCR and RT-PCR

The abbreviation of qPCR should be used for quantitative real-time PCR, and the RT-qPCR should be used for reverse transcription-qPCR according to the Minimum Information for Publication of Quantitative Real-Time PCR Experiments (MIQE) guidelines [2]. The acronym "RT-PCR" commonly denotes reverse transcription polymerase chain reaction and not real-time PCR.

Z. Balogh (✉)
Gustave Roussy, Villejuif, France
e-mail: zsofia.balogh@gustaveroussy.fr

P. Vielh
Laboratoire National de Santé, Dudelange, Luxembourg
e-mail: philippe.vielh@lns.etat.lu

© Springer International Publishing AG, part of Springer Nature 2018
F. C. Schmitt (ed.), *Molecular Applications in Cytology*,
https://doi.org/10.1007/978-3-319-74942-6_3

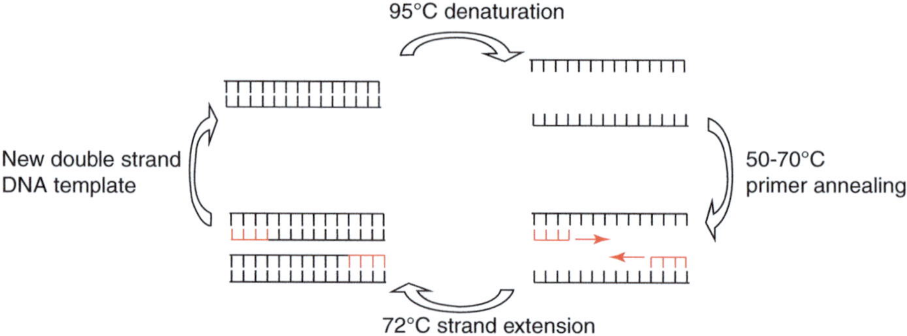

Fig. 3.1 Polymerase chain reaction (PCR) is a technique based on amplification for DNA detection. The standard protocol involves heat denaturation at 95 °C to separate the DNA strands, lowering the temperature to 50–70 °C to allow the oligonucleotide primers to hybridize (annealing) and then increasing the temperature to 72 °C, the optimum of the DNA polymerase, for primer extension. This process is repeated cyclically, creating high number of copies of the target sequence

The real-time polymerase chain reaction (qPCR) is a molecular technique based on polymerase chain reaction (PCR) (Fig. 3.1). It monitors the amplification of a targeted DNA molecule during along the reaction in "real time," thus immediately and simultaneously, and not only at its end point, in contrary to the conventional PCR. Real-time PCR may be used quantitatively, semiquantitatively, or qualitatively.

Reverse transcription polymerase chain reaction (RT-PCR) may be used for measuring gene expression (Fig. 3.2). The characterization of gene expression in cells with the measurement of mRNA levels has long been of interest, both in terms of which genes are expressed in which tissues and at what levels, even though it has been shown that due to posttranscriptional gene regulation events, such as RNA interference, there is not necessarily always a strong correlation between the abundance of mRNA molecules and the corresponding protein levels [3]. The measurement of mRNA expression is still a useful tool in determining the activity of the transcriptional machinery of the cells in the presence of external signals, such as drug treatment, to compare a healthy state to a diseased state or to refine diagnosis [4–7].

Thus, on one hand, qPCR combined with RT-PCR (RT-qPCR) offers robust approach to measure gene expression levels in biological samples. On the other hand, the combination of PCR-based mutation detection methods with qPCR offers sensitive techniques to detect point mutations. This information may be useful in understanding the exact mechanism of drug resistance and cancer evolution. Furthermore, in particular cases, when cytomorphological study alone does not provide enough certainty for a definitive diagnosis, such as for small round cell tumors, the diagnosis can be confirmed by ancillary techniques like detection of fusion transcripts, which can also be performed on cytological material [8]. The combination of RT-PCR and fine-needle aspiration (FNA) cytology, the FNA-PCR might result in superior sensitivity as compared to FNA cytology or ultrasound B-scan. As an example, tyrosinase FNA-PCR has been shown to be particularly useful in the

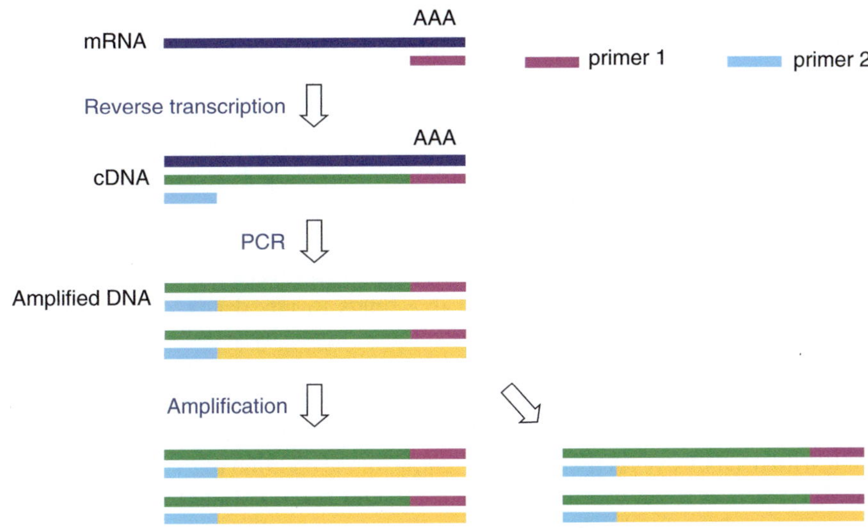

Fig. 3.2 Reverse transcription polymerase chain reaction (RT-PCR), a variant of polymerase chain reaction (PCR), is a technique used to qualitatively detect gene expression. In RT-PCR, the RNA template is first converted into a complementary DNA (cDNA) using a reverse transcriptase enzyme. The cDNA is then used as a template for exponential amplification using PCR. Abbreviations: mRNA, messenger RNA; AAA, poly-A tail

management of melanoma lesions with diameters below 10 mm [9]. Furthermore, the quantification of PDX-1 mRNA in FNA samples may be helpful to improve the diagnosis of pancreatic cancer [10].

3.2.1 Background

qPCR uses fluorochromes to detect the level of gene expression.

In order to amplify small amounts of DNA, the same methodology is used as in conventional PCR using a DNA template, at least one pair of specific primers, deoxyribonucleotides, a suitable buffer solution, and thermostable DNA polymerase. A substance labeled with a fluorochrome is added to the PCR mix in a thermal cycler that contains a detector for measuring the emission of fluorescence after the fluorochrome has been excited by a laser beam with appropriate wavelength. The three successive steps of the PCR cycle are (1) heat denaturation of the double-stranded DNA, (2) annealing of primers allowing them to hybridize to their complementary sequences, and (3) strand extension catalyzed by the DNA polymerase. These three successive steps are repeated 35–40 times to generate 2^{35}–2^{40} copies of the target sequence [11] (Fig. 3.1). To robustly detect and quantify gene expression from small amounts of RNA, gene transcript amplification is necessary. For messenger RNA (mRNA)-based PCR, the RNA sample is first reverse transcribed to complementary DNA (cDNA) with an RNA-dependent DNA polymerase, also known as the reverse transcriptase enzyme. The cDNA is then amplified by PCR using non-specific (random hexamers or oligo-dT primers) or preferably with specific primers of the target of interest.

There are two different approaches for PCR product detection in real-time PCR: (1) real-time PCR with double-stranded (ds) DNA-binding dyes as reporters and (2) fluorescent reporter probe method.

3.2.1.1 qPCR with dsDNA-Binding Dyes as Reporters

A non-specific intercalating fluorescent dye binds to any dsDNA product during PCR which leads to an increase in the fluorescence intensity at each cycle. However, dsDNA dyes such as SYBR™ Green or ethidium bromide (EtBr) will bind to all dsDNA PCR products, including primer dimers, which are non-specific by-products in PCR. This can hinder the accurate monitoring of the intended target sequence. The qPCR with dsDNA dyes is prepared as usual, with the addition of fluorescent dsDNA dye. The reaction is run in a qPCR instrument, and the fluorescent intensity is measured after each cycle; the dye only emits fluorescence when bound to the dsDNA (the PCR product). The advantage of this method is that it only needs a pair of primers to carry out the amplification, which keeps the costs down. However, only one target sequence can be monitored in an assay; the reaction cannot be multiplexed.

3.2.1.2 Fluorescent Reporter Probe Method

Sequence-specific oligonucleotide DNA probes are labeled with a fluorescent reporter molecule permitting the detection of the probe only after being hybridized to its complementary sequence. The fluorescent reporter probe method relies on an oligonucleotide probe attached at one end to a fluorescent reporter and at the other end to a fluorescent quencher. The technique is based on the fluorescence resonance energy transfer (FRET). Briefly, a reporter fluorochrome is excited and emits a specific wavelength in the absorption range of the quencher fluorochrome. The close physical distance between the reporter and the quencher molecules prevents detection of any fluorescence. After the hybridization of the reporter probes to the complementary DNA strand, the probe is broken down by the $5'–3'$ exonuclease activity of the Taq polymerase. This allows the release and physical separation of the reporter from the proximity of the quencher and thus enables the unquenched emission of fluorescence. After excitation at the required wavelength with an appropriate laser beam, this fluorescence can be detected. At each cycle of the PCR, the increase of the PCR product targeted by the probe therefore causes a proportional increase of the fluorescence intensity (Fig. 3.3).

Fluorescent reporter probes detect only the DNA containing the sequence complementary to the probe; therefore the detection is much more specific than with the dsDNA-binding dyes, and this probe gives the possibility to perform the technique even in the presence of other dsDNA. With the use of differently colored fluorochromes, reporter probes can be applied in multiplex assays for monitoring several target sequences in the same reaction. The high specificity of the probes has also the advantage to prevent the interference of the measurements caused by primer dimers.

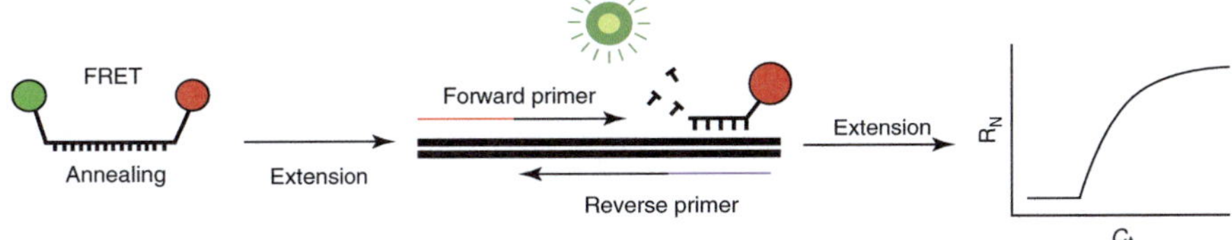

Fig. 3.3 Reaction mechanism of real-time polymerase chain reaction (qPCR) based on fluorescent reporter probe technology. The probe is an oligonucleotide probe that has a fluorescent reporter at the 5′ end and a quencher attached to the 3′ end. Once hybridized to the target sequence during annealing, the probe is cleaved by DNA polymerase, which separates the fluorescent reporter from the quencher. Once they are separated, the signal is emitted and detected in the real-time machine. The intensity of fluorescence is proportional to the amount of PCR product produced. FRET: Fluorescence resonance energy transfer. Rapid and quantitative detection of hepatitis B virus, Yue-Ping Liu, Chun-Yan Yao, Department of Laboratory Medicine, Southwest Hospital, the Third Military Medical University, Chongqing 400038, China. Copyright ©The Author(s) 2015. Published by Baishideng Publishing Group Inc. All rights reserved. World J Gastroenterol. Nov 14, 2015; 21(42): 11954–11,963. Published online Nov 14, 2015. doi: https://doi.org/10.3748/WJG.v21.i42.11954

3.2.2 Data Analysis

qPCR has the advantage that it does not need subsequent gel electrophoresis. Furthermore, in contrast to classical end-point PCR, qPCR allows monitoring of the target quantity at any point in the amplification process by measuring fluorescence. A commonly performed method of DNA/RNA quantification relies on plotting fluorescence intensity against the number of cycles on a logarithmic scale. A threshold for the signal detection is usually set three- to fivefold of the standard deviation of the noise above background. The number of cycles at which the fluorescence exceeds the threshold is the threshold cycle (C_t) [12]. During the exponential amplification phase, the target DNA quantity doubles each cycle. Over 20–40 cycles, the amount of PCR product reaches a plateau not directly correlated with the amount of DNA in the initial PCR mix. However, the amplification efficiency is often variable among primers and templates. Therefore, a titration experiment with serial dilutions of DNA template to create a standard curve is advised. The slope of the linear regression curve is used to determine the efficiency of the amplification.

In order to quantify the level of gene expression, the C_t of a target gene is subtracted from the C_t of the housekeeping reference gene in the same sample with the purpose of normalizing the variation in the amount and quality of RNA between different samples. This normalization approach is commonly known as the ΔC_t method [13] and has the advantage to allow the comparison of the expression of a gene of interest among different samples. However, for such comparison, the expression level of the reference gene must be constant across the different samples, like a function related to basic cellular survival [12, 14]. Another reason for the application of reference gene is to correct non-specific variation like the differences in the quality and quantity of RNA used and the efficiency of reverse transcription.

Thus, choosing a reference gene fulfilling this criterion is of major importance and often challenging to find a gene showing equal levels of expression across a range of different conditions or tissues [15]. The most commonly used reference genes are those that code for the following enzymes: tubulin, glyceraldehyde-3-phosphate dehydrogenase, albumin, cyclophilin, and ribosomal RNAs [16].

3.3 FISH

3.3.1 Background

Fluorescent *in situ* hybridization (FISH) uses (DNA, RNA, or peptide nucleic acid—PNA) fluorescently labeled probes to target homologous nucleic acid sequences (DNA, less frequently RNA such as mRNA, lncRNA, and miRNA) with high degree of sequence complementarity [17]. The technique was developed in the early 1980s [18] and is used to detect and localize the presence or absence of specific DNA sequences on chromosomes. It can assay both interphase and metaphase nuclei. The fluorescent probes require a microscope equipped with fluorescent filter sets and a UV source for interpretation. Another option is if the probes are labeled with a chromogene allowing the use of a light microscope (chromogenic or silver *in situ* hybridization, CISH or SISH, respectively). It is traditionally used in onco-hematological diagnostics complementing or not karyotyping, but its application became much broader from solid tumor analysis through prenatal diagnostics to constitutional genetics. The main advantage of (F)ISH compared to classical karyotyping is that it can be performed on fixed or archived samples, such as fine-needle aspiration (FNA) cytological samples [19–21] (Fig. 3.4), formalin-fixed paraffin-embedded (FFPE) tissues, circulating tumor cells (CTCs) [22], frozen tissue sections, or touch preparations. Furthermore, it does not require dividing cells; therefore it provides both prospective and retrospective information [23].

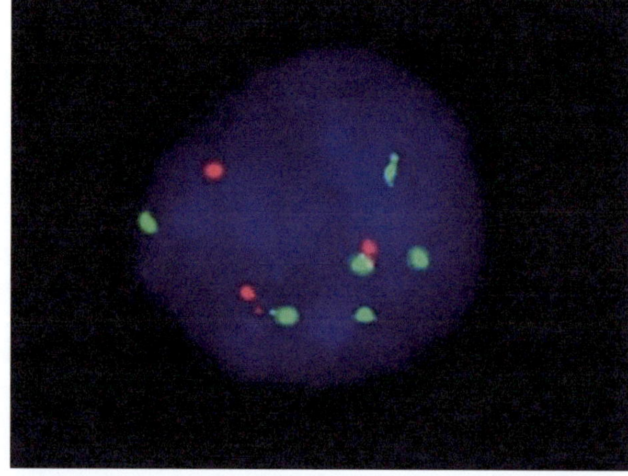

Fig. 3.4 Fluorescent *in situ* hybridization (FISH) on a fine-needle aspiration (FNA) cytology sample from a thyroid lesion of a patient with follicular carcinoma using ZytoLight 1p36 (red)/1q25 (green) and ZytoVision probe mix showing loss of 1p36 compared to the control region 1q25

3.3.2   Process of Preparation and Hybridization

The basic principles of the FISH experiment to localize a gene in the nucleus are simple: the use of a specific probe that is detectable and the hybridization of that probe to its target (Fig. 3.5). The detection of nucleic acids relies on complementary base pairing between the probe and the target sequences. The final step is the visualization of the nucleic acid of interest by microscopy.

First, a probe is constructed or commercially prepared which may be from different origin, such as oligonucleotide sequences, bacterial artificial chromosomes (BAC), plasmid artificial chromosome (PAC), yeast artificial chromosomes (YAC),

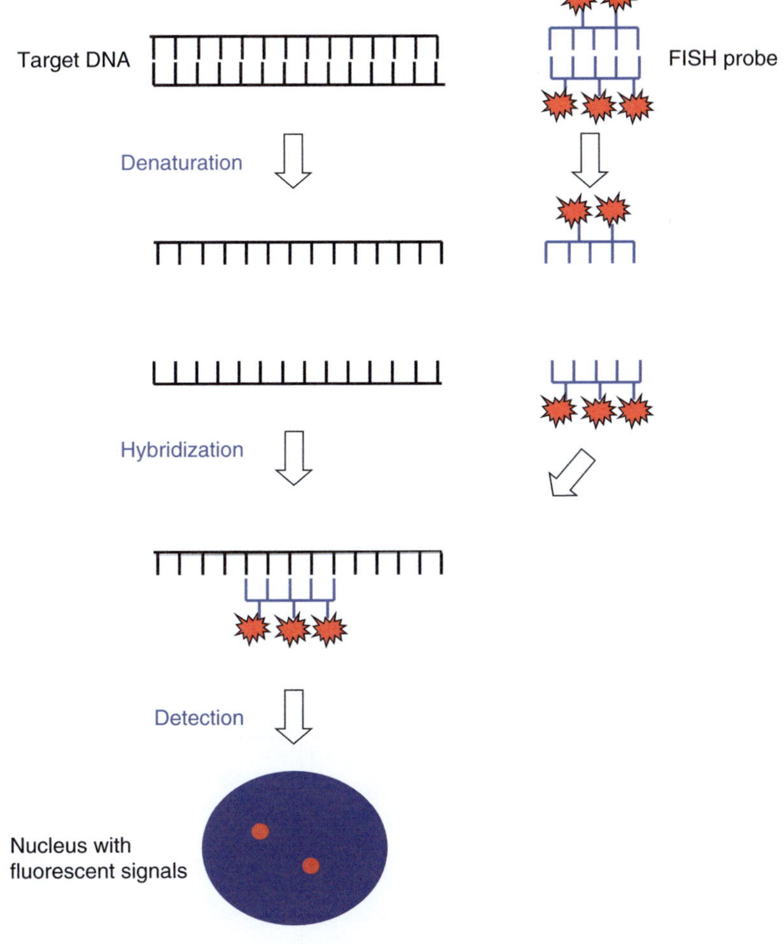

Fig. 3.5   The basic principles of the fluorescent *in situ* hybridization (FISH) technique to localize a gene in the nucleus are the following: the use of a fluorescently labeled, specific probe and the hybridization of that probe to its target sequence

or cosmids. The probe must be large enough to hybridize specifically with its target but not so large as to hinder the hybridization process. The probe is labeled directly with fluorochromes or indirectly with targets for antibodies or with biotin. Labeling can be performed in various ways, such as nick translation, random-primed PCR, or degenerate oligonucleotide-primed PCR (DOP-PCR) using conjugated nucleotides. To prevent cross hybridization based on the presence of repetitive elements, the addition of COT-1 DNA or the removal of repetitive sequences of the probe is advised.

Then, an interphase or metaphase chromosome preparation is produced. The chromosomes are firmly attached to a substrate, usually glass. Repetitive DNA sequences must be blocked by adding short fragments of DNA to the sample. The probe is then applied to the chromosome DNA and incubated between 4 and 16 h while hybridizing. Several wash steps remove all non-hybridized, partially hybridized, or non-specifically hybridized probes to reduce the background noise. The results are then visualized and quantified using a microscope that is capable of exciting the dye and recording images.

3.3.3 Data Analysis

Different sort of probes may be applied according to the type of chromosomal alterations (Fig. 3.6): (1) numerical aberrations can be detected by (a) centromeric

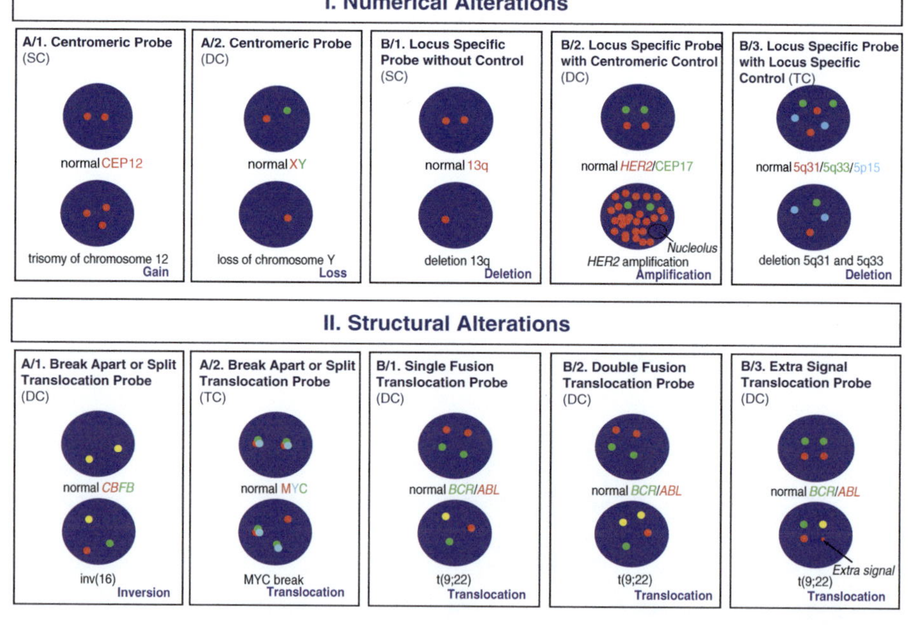

Fig. 3.6 Different FISH probe designs and their interpretation. *SC* single color, *DC* double color, and *TC* triple color

(α-satellite) probes specific to highly repetitive juxtacentromeric heterochromatin to preferentially observe gains and losses of entire chromosomes (aneusomies) and (b) locus-specific probes targeting a region of interest used to test gene duplications, amplifications, or deletions (probe mixes may be single, dual, or triple color depending on the presence or absence of centromeric or other controls); (2) structural aberrations such as chromosomal translocations or inversions (a) break apart, or split (translocation) probes are used for identifying chromosomal translocations of genes which have unknown or a large number of possible translocation partners (e.g., *KMT2A* gene with more than 80 already identified translocation partners) and (b) "fusion" translocation probes (single fusion, double fusion, and extra signal probes) are used for detecting chromosomal translocations in case both translocation partners are known and characteristic for a tumor entity.

Finally, it is also possible to combine immunohistochemistry (IHC) with FISH to increase sensitivity and specificity of the reaction or to apply alternative methods combining fluorescent immunophenotyping and ISH.

3.4 Sequencing

3.4.1 DNA Sequencing

Sequencing is a technique to determine the primary structure of an unbranched biopolymer, resulting in a symbolic linear depiction called the sequence. DNA sequencing is the process of determining the order of nucleotides in a given DNA fragment.

Most classical DNA sequencing has been performed using the Frederick Sanger's method, known as the chain termination method. This technique applies sequence-specific termination of DNA synthesis by modified nucleotide molecules (Fig. 3.7).

Chain termination sequencing is initiated by using a short oligonucleotide primer complementary to the template at a specific site on the template DNA. The oligonucleotide primer is extended by an enzyme that replicates DNA, the

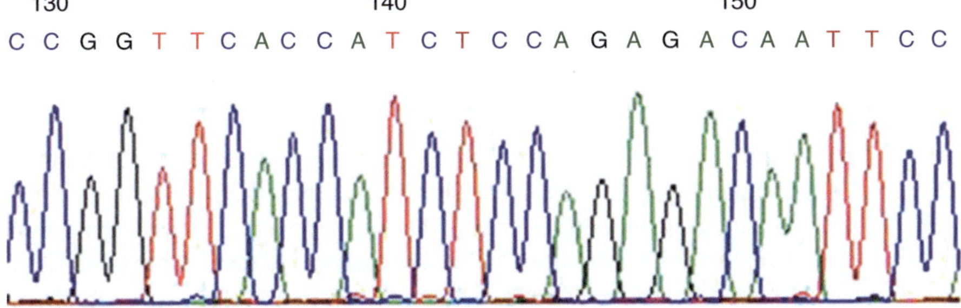

Fig. 3.7 Sanger sequencing. Part of the immunoglobulin gene (Ig) heavy-chain variable domain (IgV$_H$) sequence of a patient with chronic lymphocytic leukemia with increased prolymphocytes (CLL/PL)

DNA-dependent DNA polymerase. In the presence of the primer, the DNA polymerase, the reaction contains also the four deoxynucleotide bases, along with a low concentration of a chain-terminating nucleotide (commonly dideoxynucleotide). Limited incorporation of the chain-terminating nucleotides results in a series of related DNA fragments that are terminated only at positions where that particular nucleotide is used. The fragments are then size-separated by electrophoresis in a gel or more commonly in a capillary filled with a polymer.

An alternative method, called the dye-terminator sequencing, has the major advantage that the complete sequencing set can be performed in a single reaction, rather than the four needed with the previous approach. Thus, each of the dideoxynucleotide chain terminators is labeled with a separate fluorescent dye emitting fluorescence at a different wavelength. A problem related to this technique may be that it can produce uneven data peaks with different heights due to template-dependent difference in the incorporation of the large dye chain terminators. However, this problem has been minimized with the introduction of new enzymes and dyes that minimize incorporation variability [24]. The use of this technique for the vast majority of sequencing reactions is changing rapidly due to the increasing cost-effectiveness of second- and third-generation systems (Illumina, Roche, Thermo Fisher Scientific, and others).

3.4.2 RNA Sequencing

RNA is less stable in the cell than DNA and also more prone to breakdown by nucleases. As the RNA molecules are generated by transcription from DNA, this information is already available in the cell's DNA code. However, by sequencing RNA molecules, it is possible to reach additional of information. While DNA sequencing gives the genetic profile of the cells, RNA sequencing reflects only the sequences that are actively expressed at a given moment. In order to sequence RNA, the usual method is first to reverse transcribe the RNA extracted from the sample to produce cDNA fragments. These cDNA fragments can be sequenced as described previously (Fig. 3.8). Most of the RNAs expressed in cells are ribosomal RNAs or small RNAs which are most often not in the focus of the study. This RNA fraction can be removed from the RNA extract *in vitro* to enrich for messenger RNA which is usually in the scope of interest. Derived from exons, these mRNA molecules are later translated to proteins that support cellular functions. Thus, the expression profile of the cells indicates cellular activity, particularly desired in the studies of diseases, cellular behavior, and response to treatments or stimuli. RNA sequencing is used to analyze the continuously changing cellular transcriptome; specifically, this method facilitates the ability to look at alternative gene spliced transcripts, posttranscriptional modifications, gene fusions, mutations, SNPs, and changes in gene expression [25]. In addition to mRNA transcripts, RNA sequencing may provide information about different RNA populations, such as total RNA and small RNAs, like miRNA, tRNA, and ribosomal RNA [26]. The technique can also be used to determine exon/intron borders and verify previously annotated borders. As reverse transcription of RNA

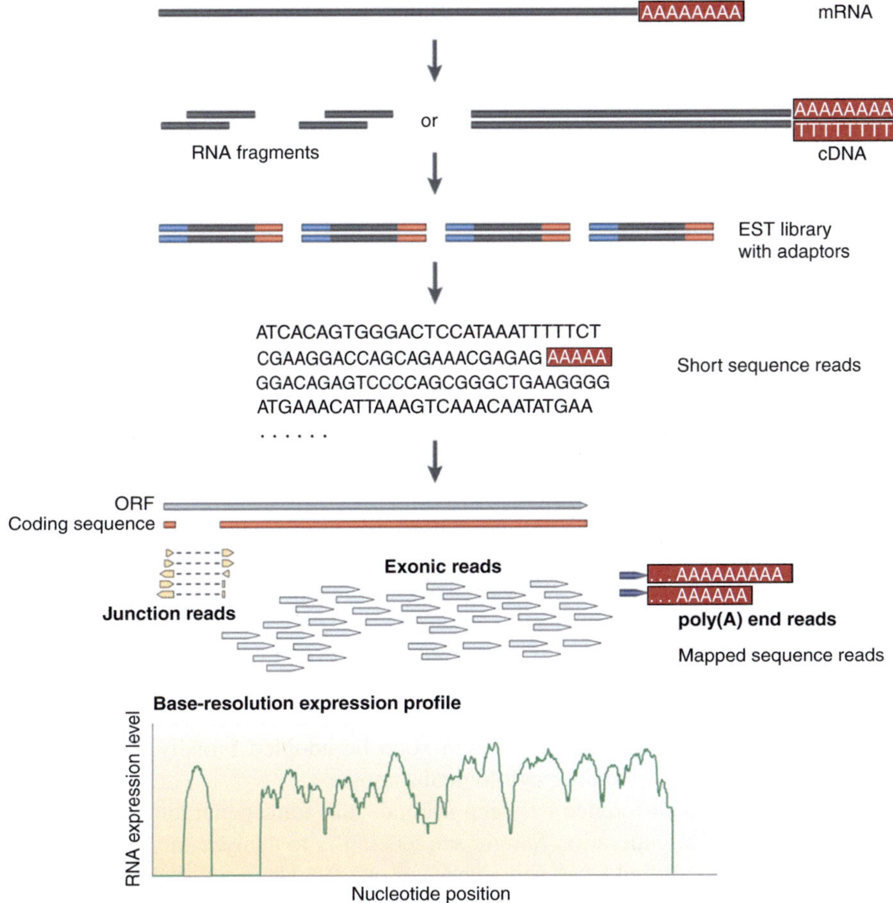

Fig. 3.8 A typical RNA-Seq experiment. Briefly, long RNAs are first converted into a library of cDNA fragments through either RNA fragmentation or DNA fragmentation. Sequencing adaptors (blue) are subsequently added to each cDNA fragment, and a short sequence is obtained from each cDNA using high-throughput sequencing technology. The resulting sequence reads are aligned with the reference genome or transcriptome and classified as three types: exonic reads, junction reads, and poly(A) end-reads. These three types are used to generate a base-resolution expression profile for each gene, as illustrated at the bottom; a yeast ORF with one intron is shown (Reprinted with permission from Nature Publishing Group. Zhong Wang, Mark Gerstein, and Michael Snyder. RNA-Seq: a revolutionary tool for transcriptomics Nat Rev. Genet. 2009 Jan; 10(1): 57–63. doi: https://doi.org/10.1038/nrg2484. License N°: 3956491042838)

into cDNA has been shown to introduce biases and artifacts that may interfere with proper characterization and quantification of RNA transcripts, single-molecule direct RNA sequencing technique is developed; thus RNA molecules are sequenced directly in a massively parallel manner without RNA to cDNA conversion [27].

Fusion genes caused by different structural modifications of the genome have gained attention because of their relationship with cancer [28]. As RNA sequencing has the advantage to analyze a sample's whole transcriptome in an unbiased manner, it makes this technique an attractive tool to find fusion genes related to different kinds of cancer [25].

3.4.3   Large-Scale Sequencing

Whereas the above-described sequencing techniques are used to analyze limited sized fragments, separate related terms are used when a large portion of the genome is sequenced. There are platforms developed to perform exome sequencing, thus to analyze a subset of all DNA across all chromosomes that encode genes, or whole genome sequencing, which is the sequencing of all nuclear DNA of a human.

3.5   Next-Generation Sequencing (NGS)

At the moment of the appearance of next-generation sequencing (NGS) techniques, platforms were capable to serve only for large-scale applications, focused on whole-genome sequencing, with protocols, consumable costs, and a turnaround time unsuitable for the needs of diagnostic laboratories. With the development of miniaturized technology by benchtop NGS sequencers, test costs decreased, moving NGS from a few large sequencing core centers to a method widely available in individual diagnostic laboratories. Currently, most pathology departments are equipped with a NGS benchtop sequencer; thus NGS will soon be adopted broadly as a tool for molecular diagnostics, including cytological samples.

The fundamental difference between second- and third-generation sequencing platforms to the first-generation Sanger sequencing is to analyze hundreds of millions of clonally amplified DNA sequences simultaneously in a parallel manner, as compared to a one amplified DNA segment per capillary, per reaction approach (Fig. 3.9). The term next-generation sequencing applies to genome sequencing, transcriptome profiling (RNA sequencing), DNA-protein interaction analysis (ChIP sequencing), and epigenome characterization [29].

In the past couple of years, numerous NGS-based methods for genome analysis have emerged leading to the discovery of a large number of new mutations and fusion transcripts in cancer. RNA sequencing data could help researchers interpreting "personalized transcriptome" so that it will help in understanding the transcriptomic changes, ideally identifying driver mutations causing a disease. However, the feasibility of this technique is dictated by the costs in terms of time and money.

MicroRNA sequencing, a type of RNA sequencing, is the use of next-generation sequencing or massively parallel high-throughput sequencing to sequence microRNAs, also called miRNAs. MicroRNA sequencing differs from other forms of RNA sequencing in that input material is often enriched for small RNAs. This technique enables to examine tissue-specific expression patterns, disease associations, and different isoforms of miRNAs and to discover previously uncharacterized miRNAs. The fact that dysregulated miRNAs play a role in disease development and

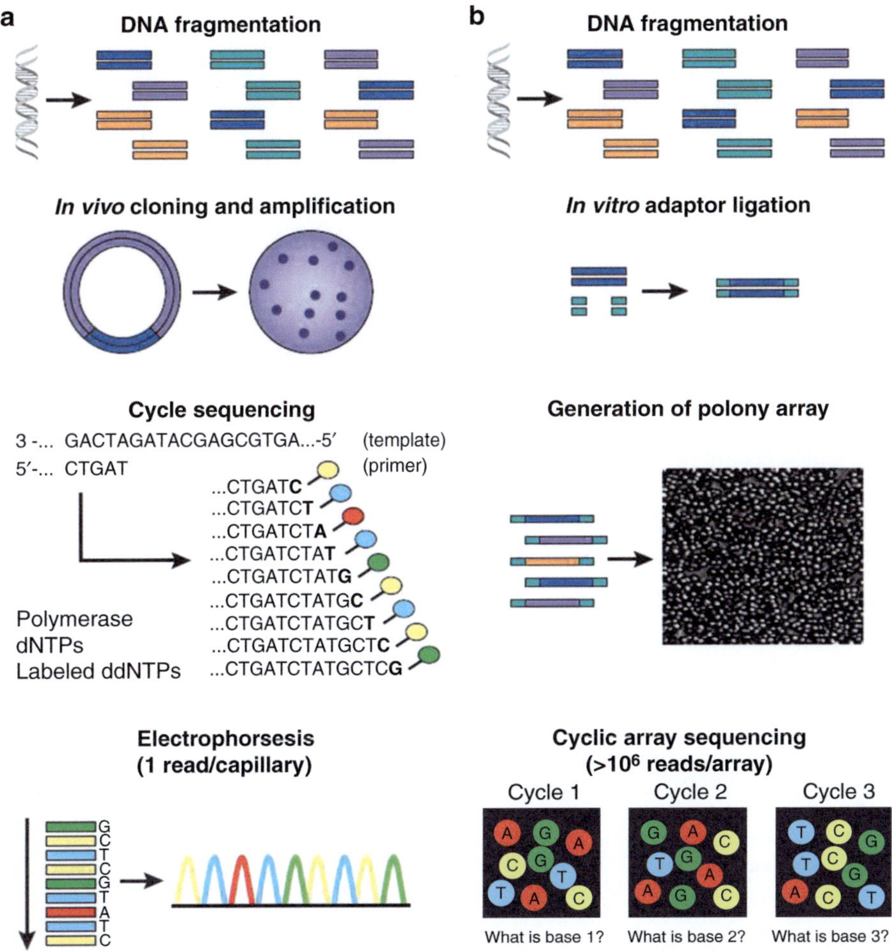

Fig. 3.9 Workflow of conventional versus second-generation sequencing. (**a**) With high-throughput shotgun Sanger sequencing, genomic DNA is fragmented and then cloned to a plasmid vector and used to transform *E. coli*. For each sequencing reaction, a single bacterial colony is picked and plasmid DNA isolated. Each cycle sequencing reaction takes place within a microliter-scale volume, generating a ladder of ddNTP-terminated, dye-labeled products, which are subjected to high-resolution electrophoretic separation within 1 of 96 or 384 capillaries in one run of a sequencing instrument. As fluorescently labeled fragments of discrete sizes pass a detector, the four-channel emission spectrum is used to generate a sequencing trace. (**b**) In shotgun sequencing with cyclic-array methods, common adaptors are ligated to fragmented genomic DNA, which is then subjected to one of several protocols that results in an array of millions of spatially immobilized PCR colonies or "polonies." Each polony consists of many copies of a single shotgun library fragment. As all polonies are tethered to a planar array, a single microliter-scale reagent volume (e.g., for primer hybridization and then for enzymatic extension reactions) can be applied to manipulate all array features in parallel. Similarly, imaging-based detection of fluorescent labels incorporated with each extension can be used to acquire sequencing data on all features in parallel. Successive iterations of enzymatic interrogation and imaging are used to build up a contiguous sequencing read for each array feature (Reprinted with permission from Nature Publishing Group. Shendure J, Ji H. Next-generation DNA sequencing. Nat Biotechnol. 2008 Oct;26(10):1135–45. doi: https://doi.org/10.1038/nbt1486. License N°: 3956460603963)

progression, such as cancer, has positioned miRNA sequencing to potentially become an important tool for helping diagnostics and prognostics [30–32].

Regardless of the specific features of any single platform type, the NGS workflow is composed of four consecutive steps: (1) the generation of a short fragment DNA library, (2) single fragment clonal amplification (emulsion PCR; see below), (3) massive parallel sequencing, and (4) sequencing data analysis [33].

3.5.1 Emulsion or Droplet Digital PCR: A Tool for Single Fragment Clonal Amplification

Emulsion PCR, also known as droplet digital PCR (ddPCR), is a method for performing digital PCR that is based on water-oil emulsion droplet technology. A sample is fractionated into 20,000 droplets, and PCR amplification of the template molecules occurs in each individual droplet. ddPCR technology uses reagents and workflows similar to those used for most standard assays. The key difference between ddPCR and traditional PCR lies in the method of measuring nucleic acid amounts. ddPCR, similarly to traditional PCR, carries out a single reaction within a

Fig. 3.10 Next-generation sequencing technologies that use emulsion PCR. (**a**) A four-color sequencing by ligation method using Life/APG's support oligonucleotide ligation detection (SOLiD) platform is shown. Upon the annealing of a universal primer, a library of 1,2-probes is added. Unlike polymerization, the ligation of a probe to the primer can be performed bidirectionally from either its 5′-PO4 or 3′-OH end. Appropriate conditions enable the selective hybridization and ligation of probes to complementary positions. Following four-color imaging, the ligated 1,2-probes are chemically cleaved with silver ions to generate a 5′-PO4 group. The SOLiD cycle is repeated nine more times. The extended primer is then stripped, and four more ligation rounds are performed, each with ten ligation cycles. The 1,2-probes are designed to interrogate the first (x) and second (y) positions adjacent to the hybridized primer, such that the 16 dinucleotides are encoded by four dyes (colored stars). The probes also contain inosine bases (z) to reduce the complexity of the 1,2-probe library and a phosphorothioate linkage between the fifth and six nucleotides of the probe sequence, which is cleaved with silver ions. Other cleavable probe designs include RNA nucleotides and internucleosidic phosphoramidates, which are cleaved by ribonucleases and acid, respectively. (**b**) A two-base encoding scheme in which four dinucleotide sequences are associated with one color (e.g., AA, CC, GG, and TT are coded with a blue dye). Each template base is interrogated twice and compiled into a string of color-space data bits. The color-space reads are aligned to a color-space reference sequence to decode the DNA sequence. (**c**) Pyrosequencing using Roche/454's Titanium platform. Following loading of the DNA-amplified beads into individual PicoTiterPlate (PTP) wells, additional beads, coupled with sulfurylase and luciferase, are added. In this example, a single type of 2′-deoxyribonucleoside triphosphate (dNTP)—cytosine—is shown flowing across the PTP wells. The fiber-optic slide is mounted in a flow chamber, enabling the delivery of sequencing reagents to the bead-packed wells. The underneath of the fiber-optic slide is directly attached to a high-resolution charge-coupled device (CCD) camera, which allows detection of the light generated from each PTP well undergoing the pyrosequencing reaction. (**d**) The light generated by the enzymatic cascade is recorded as a series of peaks called a flowgram. PPi, inorganic pyrophosphate (Reprinted with permission from Nature Publishing Group. Michael L. Metzker. Sequencing technologies—the next generation. Nature Reviews Genetics 11, 31–46 (January 2010)|doi:https://doi.org/10.1038/nrg2626. License N°: 3956470943742)

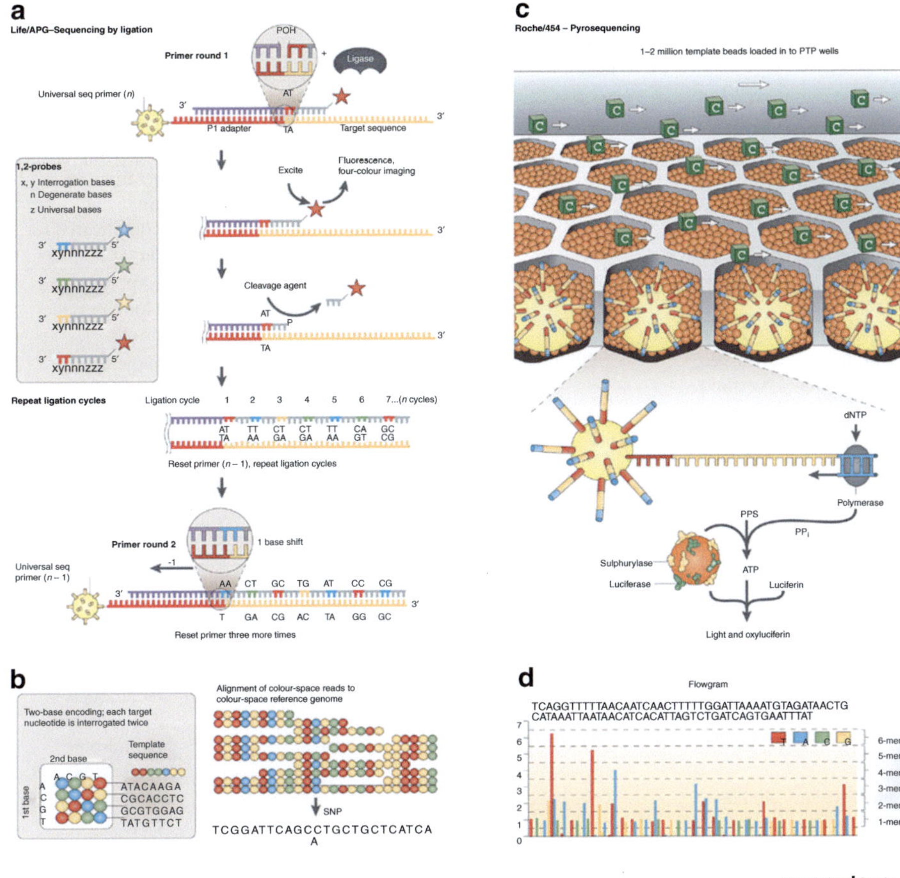

sample; however, the sample is separated into a large number of partitions, and the reaction is performed in each partition individually. This separation allows a more reliable collection and sensitive measurement of nucleic acid amounts. The method is routinely used for clonal amplification of samples for NGS [34] (Fig. 3.10).

The different sequencing techniques are summarized and compared in Table 3.1.

3.5.2 454 Pyrosequencing

The technique amplifies DNA inside water droplets in an oil solution (emulsion PCR), with each droplet containing a single DNA template attached to a single primer-coated bead that then forms a clonal colony. The technique relies on the detection of pyrophosphate release during nucleotide incorporation. Pyrosequencing uses luciferase enzyme to generate light for detection of the individual nucleotides added to the growing DNA strand, and the combined data are used to generate sequence readouts [35] (Figs. 3.10 and 3.11).

Table 3.1 Comparison of different sequencing techniques

Method	Read length	Single read accuracy (%)	Reads per run	Advantages	Disadvantages
Sanger sequencing	400–900 bp	99.9	N/A	Long individual reads	More expensive, requires more time, and complicated for larger projects
Pyro sequencing	700 bp	99.9	1 million	Fast. Long read size	Expensive runs. Homopolymer errors
Illumina sequencing	MiniSeq, NextSeq, 75–300 bp; MiSeq, 50–600 bp; HiSeq 2500, 50–500 bp; HiSeq 3/4000, 50–300 bp; HiSeq X, 300 bp	99.9	MiniSeq/MiSeq, 1–25 million; NextSeq, 130–260 million; HiSeq2500,300million–2 billion; HiSeq 3/4000 2.5 billion; HiSeq X, 3 billion	High sequence yield potential	Expensive equipment. Requires high concentrations of DNA
SOLiD sequencing	50 + 35 or 50 + 50 bp	99.9	1.2–1.4 billion	Low cost per base	Slower than other techniques. Troubles with palindrome sequences
Ion Torrent sequencing	400 bp	98	80 million	Fast. Less expensive equipment	Homopolymer errors
Single-molecule real-time sequencing	10,000 bp to 15,000 bp avg.; maximum read length >40,000 bases	87	500–1000 megabases	Longest read length. Fast. Detects 4mC, 5mC, 6mA	Expensive equipment. Moderate throughput

3.5.3 Illumina (Solexa) Sequencing

The method is based on reversible dye-terminator technology and engineered polymerases [36]. Thus, DNA molecules and primers are first attached on a slide or flow cell and amplified with polymerase so that local clonal DNA colonies, so-called DNA cluster, are formed. To determine the sequence, four types of reversible terminator bases are added, and non-incorporated nucleotides are washed away. A camera takes images of the fluorescently labeled nucleotides. After, the dye, together with the terminal 3′ blocker, is removed from the DNA chain, allowing for the next cycle to begin. Unlike pyrosequencing, the DNA chains are extended one nucleotide

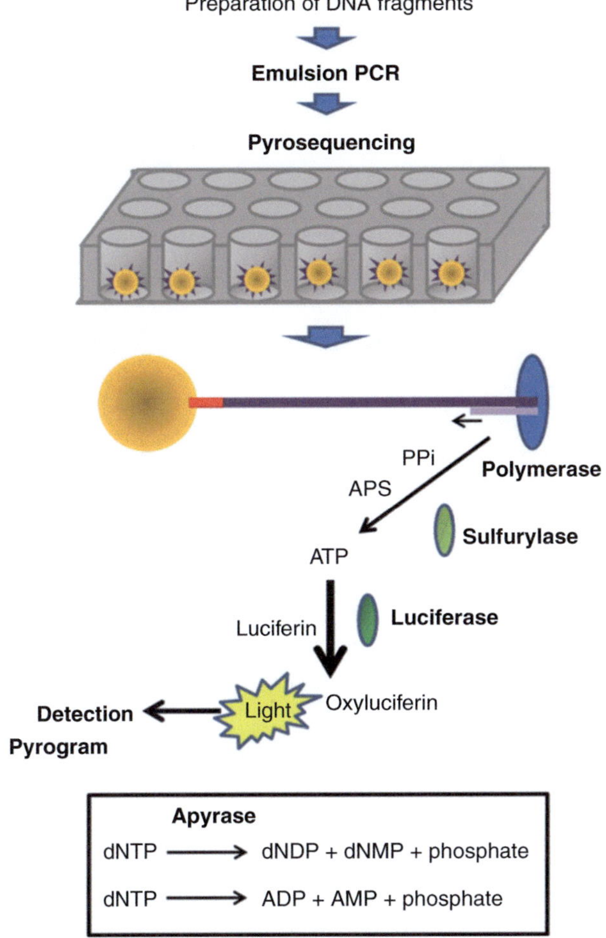

Fig. 3.11 The 454 pyrosequencing approach. Pyrosequencing as a tool for better understanding for human microbiomes, José F. Siqueira, Jr., Ashraf F. Fouad, and Isabela N. Rôças: Department of Endodontics and Molecular Microbiology Laboratory, Dental School, Estácio de Sá University, Rio de Janeiro, RJ, Brazil; Department of Endodontics, Prosthodontics and Operative Dentistry, Dental School, University of Maryland, Baltimore, MD, USA Copyright © 2012 José F. Siqueira et al. J Oral Microbiol. 2012; 4: https://doi.org/10.3402/jom.v4i0.10743. Published online 2012 Jan 23. doi: https://doi.org/10.3402/jom.v4i0.10743

at a time, and image acquisition can be performed at a delayed moment, allowing for very large arrays of DNA colonies to be captured by sequential images taken from a single camera. Decoupling the enzymatic reaction and the image capture allows an optimal throughput and a theoretically unlimited sequencing capacity (Fig. 3.12).

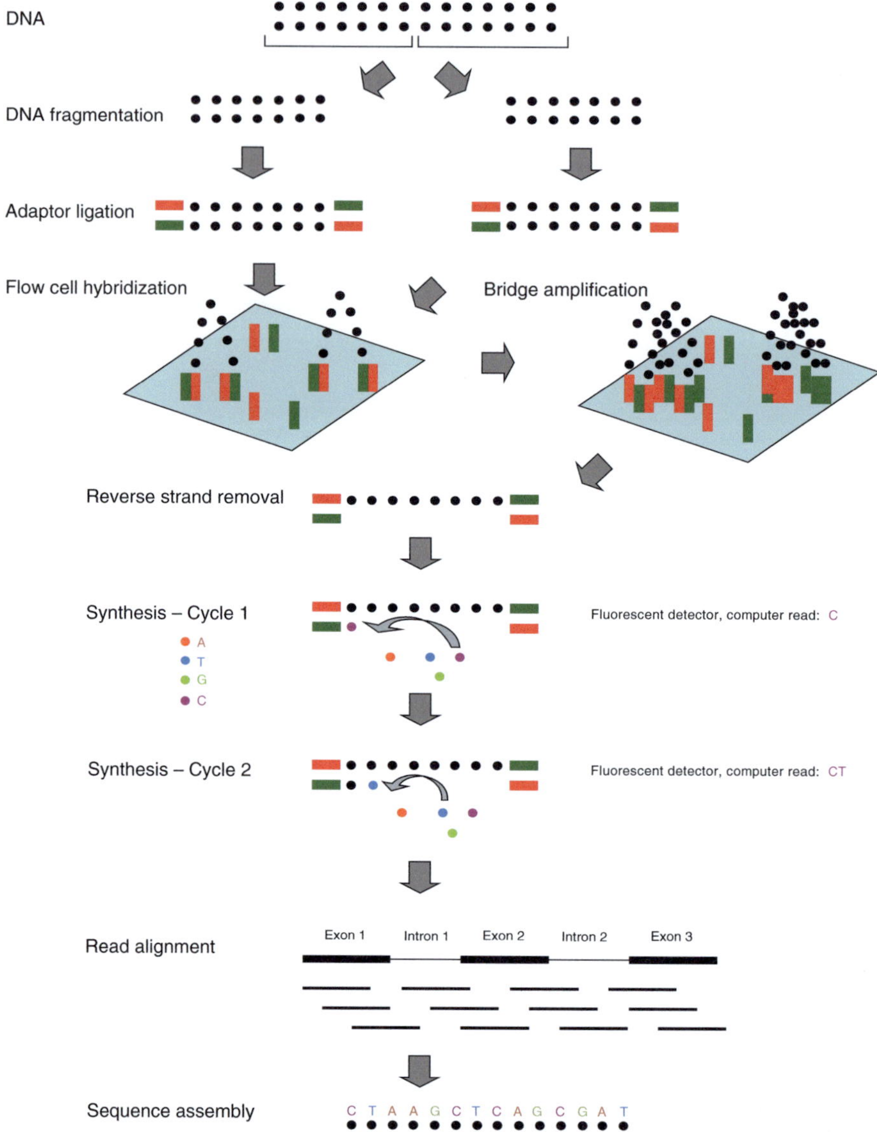

Fig. 3.12 Overview of DNA next-generation sequencing using the Illumina platform. First, DNA is fragmented into smaller input-sized fragments by enzymes or by sonication. The ends of these fragments are repaired, and specific adapters are ligated to the ends of the fragments, allowing hybridization to a flow cell. An amplification step (bridge amplification) is performed to create a "cluster" of fragments with the same sequence. One strand of DNA is removed, and fluorescently labeled nucleotides are passed by each cluster. An image of the flow cells is recorded for each cycle and a computer processes which nucleotide was incorporated at each cluster's coordinates. The fluorescent label is cleaved, and the next round of fluorescently labeled nucleotides is passed by each cluster. Again, the nucleotide is recorded, and each cycle leads to the sequence of each fragment (a "read"). These reads are then aligned to a reference genome sequence. By merging short reads together, it is therefore possible to reconstruct the unfragmented original sequence [37]

3.5.4   SOLiD Sequencing

The method is based on sequencing by oligonucleotide ligation. Thus, a pool of all possible oligonucleotides of a fixed length is labeled according to the sequenced position. Oligonucleotides are annealed and ligated by DNA ligase for matching sequences result in a signal informative of the nucleotide at that position. Before sequencing, the DNA is amplified by emulsion PCR. The resulting beads, each containing a single copy of the same DNA molecule, are deposited on a glass slide (Fig. 3.10). This method has been reported to face difficulties when sequencing palindromic sequences [38].

3.5.5   Ion Torrent Semiconductor Sequencing

The system is based on using standard sequencing chemistry but with a novel, semiconductor-based detection system. In contrast to the traditional optical detection, this method measures the hydrogen ions that are released during DNA polymerization. A microwell containing a template DNA strand to be sequenced is flooded with a single type of nucleotide. If the nucleotide is complementary to the template, it is incorporated into the growing strand. The reaction causes the release of a hydrogen ion that triggers the sensor. In case a homopolymer repeat is present in the template sequence, multiple nucleotides will be incorporated in a single cycle. This will lead to the release of an equal number of hydrogen ions and a proportionally higher electronic signal [39] (Fig. 3.13).

3.5.6   Single-Molecule Real-Time Sequencing (Pacific Biosciences)

This is the first commercially available sequencer which is able to sequence single molecules in real time. It is also capable to exceed read length greater than 1 kb (Fig. 3.14).

3.5.7   Cytological Implementation of NGS

A recent study shows that endoscopic ultrasound FNA cytology genotyping represents a suitable surrogate and may complement the conventional stratification criteria in decision-making for therapies, and targeted NGS may guide future biomarker-driven therapeutic development in pancreatic adenocarcinoma [40]. Another study on thyroid lesion shows that molecular testing provides great promise in reducing the diagnostic uncertainty of cytologically indeterminate thyroid nodules, as it is one of many factors that contribute to the overall probability of malignancy for a patient. Accordingly, the decision to use ancillary molecular testing, the selection of the appropriate molecular test, and the interpretation of its

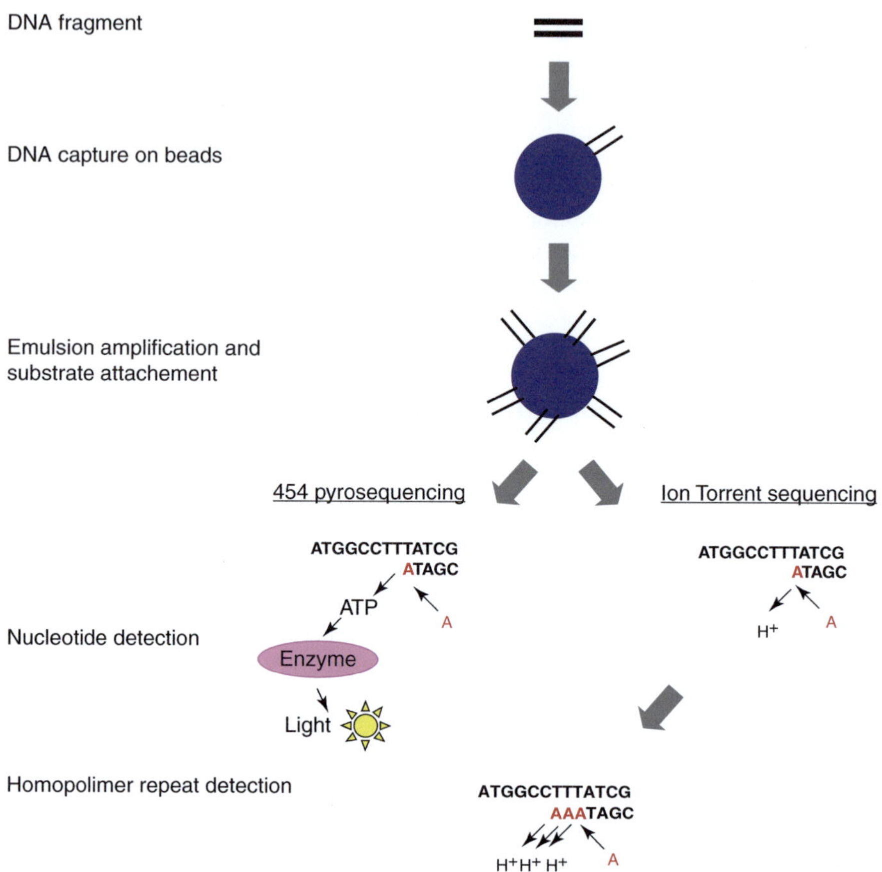

Fig. 3.13 Comparison of 454 pyrosequencing and Ion Torrent semiconductor sequencing. Both 454 pyrosequencing and Ion Torrent sequencing immobilize DNA fragments onto beads. In both platforms, template molecules are first immobilized on a bead which is emulsified so that subsequent amplification can occur clonally within the droplet. After clonal amplification, enrichment for DNA-positive beads is performed. Enriched beads are deposited at the bottom of a well, and sequencing is performed by flowing one base at a time over the templates. 454 pyrosequencing uses a cascade of reactions resulting from pyrophosphate being released from each incorporation reaction, which leads to a photon being emitted by the enzyme luciferase. Whereas in Ion Torrent, an incorporation event is measured by a pH change from the release of protons resulting from the incorporation. In Ion Torrent sequencing, if homopolymer repeats of the same nucleotide are present (AAA), multiple hydrogen ions will be released, generating a higher electrical signal. This is subsequently interpreted as multiple identical nucleotides being present in the sequence [37]

results should always be performed within the context of cytological, clinical, and ultrasonographic findings [41].

Data generated by NGS technologies have a pivotal role in precision medicine. These high-throughput techniques are preferentially performed on fresh tissue, but there is an increasing need for protocols adapted to materials derived

Pacific Biosciences – Real-time sequencing

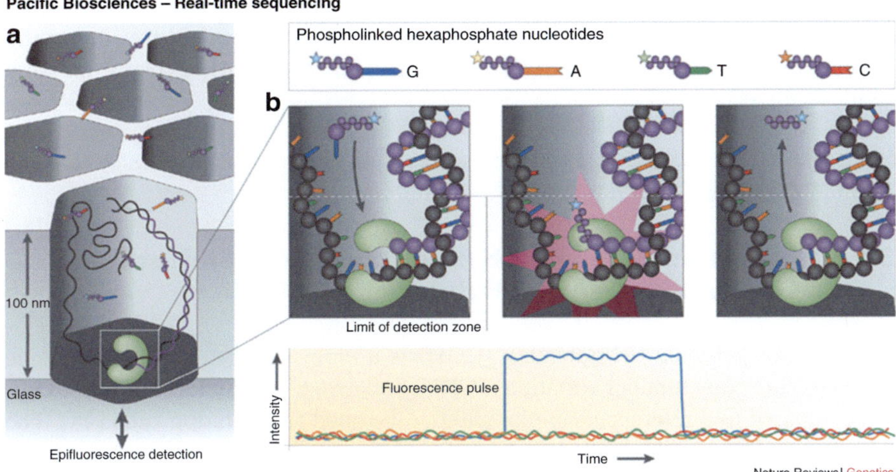

Fig. 3.14 Real-time sequencing. Pacific Biosciences' four-color real-time sequencing method is shown. (**a**) The zero-mode waveguide (ZMW) design reduces the observation volume, therefore reducing the number of stray fluorescently labeled molecules that enter the detection layer for a given period. These ZMW detectors address the dilemma that DNA polymerases perform optimally when fluorescently labeled nucleotides are present in the micromolar concentration range, whereas most single-molecule detection methods perform optimally when fluorescent species are in the pico- to nanomolar concentration range. (**b**) The residence time of phospholinked nucleotides in the active site is governed by the rate of catalysis and is usually on the millisecond scale. This corresponds to a recorded fluorescence pulse, because only the bound, dye-labeled nucleotide occupies the ZMW detection zone on this timescale. The released, dye-labeled pentaphosphate by-product quickly diffuses away, dropping the fluorescence signal to background levels. Translocation of the template marks the interphase period before binding and incorporation of the next incoming phospholinked nucleotide (Reprinted with permission from Nature Publishing Group. Michael L. Metzker. Sequencing technologies–the next generation. Nature Reviews Genetics 11, 31–46 (January 2010)|doi:https://doi.org/10.1038/nrg2626. License N°: 3956500798445)

from formalin-fixed paraffin-embedded tissues and stained cytology specimens [42]. The work performed by Piqueret-Stephan *et al.* shows that the quality of DNA extracted from routinely processed cytological smears is compatible with a multi-target sequencing of a large series of genes of interest with methods such as array-based genomic analysis and whole-exome sequencing [43]. With the application of NGS, a deeper understanding of disease, genome instability, and intra-tumor heterogeneity, will allow us to reach greater therapeutic precision [44–46].

The majority of mutation detection assays used for solid tumor profiling use DNA sequencing to interrogate somatic point mutations because they are relatively easy to identify and interpret. Many cancers, however, including high-grade serous ovarian, esophageal, and small-cell lung cancer, are driven by somatic structural variants that are not measured by these assays. Therefore, there is currently an unmet need for clinical assays that can cheaply and rapidly profile structural variants in solid tumors. Low-cost, shallow, whole-genome sequencing is emerging as a promising clinical sequencing strategy for structural variant-driven tumors. Furthermore, algorithmic advances are improving sequencing efficiency by extracting additional information from existing sequencing assays [47].

3.6 Others

3.6.1 Comparative Genomic Hybridization (CGH) and Array Comparative Genomic Hybridization (aCGH)

Comparative genomic hybridization (CGH) is a molecular cytogenetic technique for analyzing copy number variations (CNVs) relative to ploidy level of a test sample compared to a reference sample, without the need for culturing cells [48]. The advantage of this method is to quickly and efficiently compare two genomic DNA samples arising from two sources, which are most often closely related, because it is suspected that they contain differences in terms of either gain or losses of either whole chromosomes or sub-chromosomal regions (Fig. 3.15). CGH is only able to detect unbalanced chromosomal abnormalities. This is because balanced chromosomal abnormalities, such as reciprocal translocations, inversions, or ring chromosomes, do not affect copy number, thus what is detected by CGH technique. CGH does, however, allow for the exploration of all human chromosomes in a single experiment and the discovery of deletions and duplications, which may lead to the

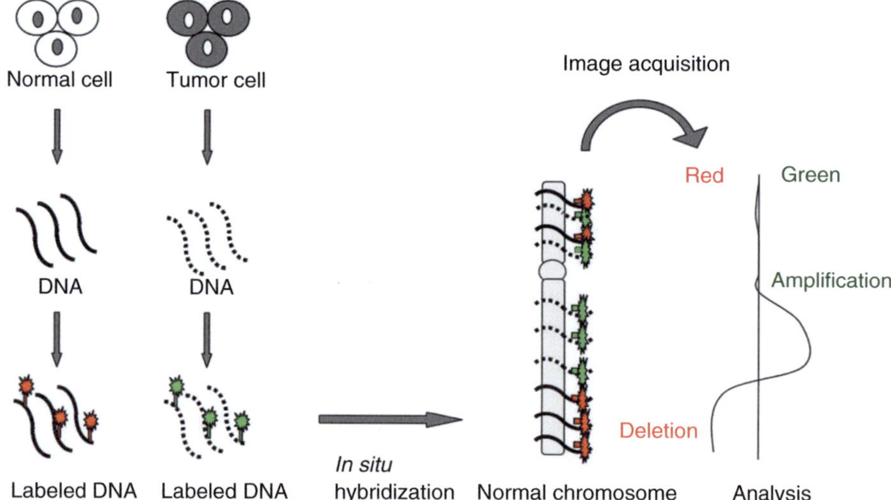

Fig. 3.15 Comparative genomic hybridization (CGH). DNA samples isolated from normal and tumor tissue are fluorescently labeled and hybridized to normal male chromosomes. With the measurement of the green to red fluorescent intensity ratios along the axis of each chromosome, the regions of amplifications and deletions of the tumor sample can be identified

identification of candidate genes to be further explored by other molecular cytological methods [49]. Through the use of DNA (oligonucleotide) microarrays together with CGH method, the more specific form of array CGH (aCGH) has been developed, allowing for the locus-by-locus analysis of CNVs with an increased resolution of 100 kb [50].

3.6.2 SNP Array

The basic principles of single-nucleotide polymorphism (SNP) array are the same as the DNA microarray. These are the convergence of DNA hybridization, fluorescence microscopy, and solid surface DNA capture. The three mandatory components of the SNP array are (1) an array containing immobilized allele-specific oligonucleotide probes, (2) fragmented nucleic acid sequences of target which is labeled with fluorescent dyes, and (3) a detection system that records and interprets the hybridization signal. The SNP chips are generally described by the number of SNP positions they assay. Two probes must be used for each position to detect both alleles; if only one probe was used, experimental failure would be indistinguishable from homozygosity of the non-probed allele.

SNP array is a useful tool for detecting slight variations between whole genomes. The most important applications of SNP arrays are the determination of disease susceptibility and the measurement of the efficacy of drug therapies. SNP array can also be used to generate a virtual karyotype to determine the copy number of each SNP on the array and then align the SNPs in chromosomal order. Furthermore, SNP is a valuable tool to study genetic abnormalities in cancer, such as to search for loss of heterozygosity (LOH). LOH occurs when one allele of a gene is mutated in a damaging way and the normally functioning allele is lost. LOH develops commonly during oncogenesis, frequently with the involvement of tumor suppressor genes. Other array-based techniques, such as comparative genomic hybridization, can detect genomic gains and losses leading to LOH. SNP arrays, however, have the additional advantage of allowing the detection of copy-neutral LOH, such as uniparental disomy and gene conversion. Copy-neutral LOH is a form of allelic imbalance. In copy-neutral LOH, one allele or a whole chromosome from a parent is missing, resulting in the duplication of the other parental allele, which might be pathological and often involved in imprinting disorders.

3.6.3 Combined SNP and CGH Array

While only SNP arrays enable the detection of copy number-neutral regions of LOH, they have limited ability to detect single-exon CNVs due to the distribution of SNPs across the genome. Thus, combining SNP probes and exon-targeted array CGH into one platform provides clinically useful genetic screening in an efficient manner [51]. The technique is also commercially available.

3.6.4 NanoString Method

NanoString's nCounter technology is a variation of DNA microarray. It uses molecular "barcodes" and microscopic imaging to detect and count up to several hundred unique transcripts in one hybridization reaction. Each color-coded barcode is attached to a single target-specific probe corresponding to a gene of interest. Advantages of the tool are the reproducibility, sensitivity, and low background signal and also that NanoString does not require amplification of target molecules. Disadvantages are the up-front cost of the necessary instruments and that at least three probes should be used per potential target, which would greatly increase cost and reduce the maximum multiplexing of the technology. NanoString represents a middle ground between quantitative PCR and other hybridization microarray technologies [52].

3.7 Perspectives

Molecular techniques complementing cytomorphology are increasingly used for diagnostic, prognostic, predictive, and theranostic purposes. The cytopathologist's involvement and coordination in this rapidly evolving field are crucial for the effective implementation of molecular tools in our present and future cytological practices [53–56]. Similarly to the initial application of immunocytochemical, flow, and static cytometric techniques, pathologists should know the basic principles, main applications, and pitfalls of molecular methods in order to use them timely.

References

1. Schmitt FC, Vielh P. Molecular biology and cytopathology. Principles and applications. Ann Pathol. 2012;32(6):e57–63.
2. Bustin SA, Benes V, Garson JA, Hellemans J, Huggett J, Kubista M, Mueller R, Nolan T, Pfaffl MW, Shipley GL, Vandesompele J, Wittwer CT. The MIQE guidelines: minimum information for publication of quantitative real-time PCR experiments. Clin Chem. 2009;55(4):611–22.
3. Greenbaum D, Colangelo C, Williams K, Gerstein M. Comparing protein abundance and mRNA expression levels on a genomic scale. Genome Biol. 2003;4(9):117.
4. Chevillard S, Ugolin N, Vielh P, Ory K, Levalois C, Elliott D, Clayman GL, El-Naggar AK. Gene expression profiling of differentiated thyroid neoplasms: diagnostic and clinical implications. Clin Cancer Res. 2004;10(19):6586–97.
5. Chevillard S, Lebeau J, Pouillart P, de Toma C, Beldjord C, Asselain B, Klijanienko J, Fourquet A, Magdelénat H, Vielh P. Biological and clinical significance of concurrent p53 gene alterations, MDR1 gene expression, and S-phase fraction analyses in breast cancer patients treated with primary chemotherapy or radiotherapy. Clin Cancer Res. 1997;3(12):2471–8.
6. Rodriguez C, Suciu V, Poterie A, Lacroix L, Miran I, Boichard A, Delaloge S, Deneuve J, Azoulay S, Mathieu MC, Valent A, Michiels S, Arnedos M, Vielh P. Concordance between HER-2 status determined by qPCR in fine needle aspiration cytology (FNAC) samples compared with IHC and FISH in core needle biopsy (CNB) or surgical specimens in breast cancer patients. Mol Oncol. 2016;10(9):1430–6. https://doi.org/10.1016/j.molonc.2016.07.009.

7. Uzan C, Andre F, Scott V, Laurent I, Azria E, Suciu V, Balleyguier C, Lacroix L, Delaloge S, Vielh P. Fine-needle aspiration for nucleic acid-based molecular analyses in breast cancer. Cancer. 2009;117(1):32–9.

8. Ferlicot S, Coué O, Gilbert E, Beuzeboc P, Servois V, Klijanienko J, Delattre O, Vielh P. Intraabdominal desmoplastic small round cell tumor: report of a case with fine needle aspiration, cytologic diagnosis and molecular confirmation. Acta Cytol. 2001;45(4):617–21.

9. Voit C, Schoengen A, Schwürzer M, Weber L, Mayer T, Proebstle TM. Detection of regional melanoma metastases by ultrasound B-scan, cytology or tyrosinase RT-PCR of fine-needle aspirates. Br J Cancer. 1999;80(10):1672–7.

10. Marzioni M, Germani U, Agostinelli L, Bedogni G, Saccomanno S, Marini F, Bellentani S, Barbera C, De Minicis S, Rychlicki C, Santinelli A, Ferretti M, Di Maira PV, Baroni GS, Benedetti A, Caletti G, Lorenzini I, Fusaroli P. PDX-1 mRNA expression in endoscopic ultrasound-guided fine needle cytoaspirate: perspectives in the diagnosis of pancreatic cancer. Dig Liver Dis. 2015;47(2):138–43.

11. Peter M, Michon J, Vielh P, Neuenschwander S, Nakamura Y, Sonsino E, Zucker JM, Vergnaud G, Thomas G, Delattre O. PCR assay for chromosome 1p deletion in small neuroblastoma samples. Int J Cancer. 1992;52(4):544–8.

12. Pfaffl MW, Tichopad A, Prgomet C, Neuvians TP. Determination of stable housekeeping genes, differentially regulated target genes and sample integrity: BestKeeper–excel-based tool using pair-wise correlations. Biotechnol Lett. 2004;26(6):509–15.

13. Carr AC, Moore SD. Robust quantification of polymerase chain reactions using global fitting. PLoS One. 2012;7(5):e37640.

14. Dhanasekaran S, Doherty TM, Kenneth J, TB Trials Study Group. Comparison of different standards for real-time PCR-based absolute quantification. J Immunol Methods. 2010;354(1–2):34–9.

15. Schefe JH, Lehmann KE, Buschmann IR, Unger T, Funke-Kaiser H. Quantitative real-time RT-PCR data analysis: current concepts and the novel "gene expression's CT difference" formula. J Mol Med. 2006;84(11):901–10.

16. Kozera B, Rapacz M. Reference genes in real-time PCR. J Appl Genet. 2013;54(4):391–406.

17. Halling KC, Kipp BR. Fluorescence in situ hybridization in diagnostic cytology. Hum Pathol. 2007;38(8):1137–44.

18. Bauman JG, Wiegant J, Bors P, van Duijn P. A new method for fluorescence microscopical localization of specific DNA sequences by in situ hybridization of fluorochromelabelled RNA. Exp Cell Res. 1980;128(2):485–90.

19. Klijanienko J, Couturier J, Galut M, El-Naggar AK, Maciorowski Z, Padoy E, Mosseri V, Vielh P. Detection and quantitation by fluorescence in situ hybridization (FISH) and image analysis of HER-2/neu gene amplification in breast cancer fine-needle samples. Cancer. 1999;87(5):312–8.

20. Layfield LJ, Ehya H, Filie AC, Hruban RH, Jhala N, Joseph L, Vielh P, Pitman MB, Papanicolaou Society of Cytopathology. Utilization of ancillary studies in the cytologic diagnosis of biliary and pancreatic lesions: the Papanicolaou society of cytopathology guidelines for pancreatobiliary cytology. Diagn Cytopathol. 2014;42(4):351–62.

21. Savic S, Bubendorf L. Common fluorescence in situ hybridization applications in cytology. Arch Pathol Lab Med. 2016;140(12):1323–30. https://doi.org/10.5858/arpa.2016-0202-RA.

22. Young R, Pailler E, Billiot F, Drusch F, Barthelemy A, Oulhen M, Besse B, Soria JC, Farace F, Vielh P. Circulating tumor cells in lung cancer. Acta Cytol. 2012;56(6):655–60.

23. Truong K, Guilly MN, Gerbault-Seureau M, Malfoy B, Vielh P, Bourgeois CA, Dutrillaux B. Quantitative FISH by image cytometry for the detection of chromosome 1 imbalances in breast cancer: a novel approach analyzing chromosome rearrangements within interphase nuclei. Lab Investig. 1998;78(12):1607–13.

24. Kieleczawa J, Mazaika E. Optimization of protocol for sequencing of difficult templates. J Biomol Tech. 2010;21(2):97–102.

25. Maher CA, Kumar-Sinha C, Cao X, Kalyana-Sundaram S, Han B, Jing X, Sam L, Barrette T, Palanisamy N, Chinnaiyan AM. Transcriptome sequencing to detect gene fusions in cancer. Nature. 2009;458(7234):97–101.

26. Ingolia NT, Brar GA, Rouskin S, McGeachy AM, Weissman JS. The ribosome profiling strategy for monitoring translation in vivo by deep sequencing of ribosome-protected mRNA fragments. Nat Protoc. 2012;7(8):1534–50.
27. Liu D, Graber JH. Quantitative comparison of EST libraries requires compensation for systematic biases in cDNA generation. BMC Bioinformatics. 2006;7:77.
28. Teixeira MR. Recurrent fusion oncogenes in carcinomas. Crit Rev Oncog. 2006;12(3–4):257–71.
29. de Magalhães JP, Finch CE, Janssens G. Next-generation sequencing in aging research: emerging applications, problems, pitfalls and possible solutions. Ageing Res Rev. 2010;9(3):315–23.
30. Farazi TA, Spitzer JI, Morozov P, Tuschl T. miRNAs in human cancer. J Pathol. 2011;223(2):102–15.
31. Sandhu S, Garzon R. Potential applications of microRNAs in cancer diagnosis, prognosis, and treatment. Semin Oncol. 2011;38(6):781–7.
32. Beca F, Schmitt F. MicroRNA signatures in cytopathology: are they ready for prime time? Cancer Cytopathol. 2016;124(9):613–5.
33. Vigliar E, Malapelle U, de Luca C, Bellevicine C, Troncone G. Challenges and opportunities of next-generation sequencing: a cytopathologist's perspective. Cytopathology. 2015;26(5):271–83.
34. Shao K, Ding W, Wang F, Li H, Ma D, Wang H. Emulsion PCR: a high efficient way of PCR amplification of random DNA libraries in aptamer selection. PLoS One. 2011;6(9):e24910.
35. Williams R, Peisajovich SG, Miller OJ, Magdassi S, Tawfik DS, Griffiths AD. Amplification of complex gene libraries by emulsion PCR. Nat Methods. 2006;3(7):545–50.
36. Bentley DR, et al. Accurate whole human genome sequencing using reversible terminator chemistry. Nature. 2008;456(7218):53–9.
37. Churko JM, Mantalas GL, Snyder MP, Wu JC. Overview of high throughput sequencing technologies to elucidate molecular pathways in cardiovascular diseases. Circ Res. 2013;112(12):1613–23.
38. Huang YF, Chen SC, Chiang YS, Chen TH, Chiu KP. Palindromic sequence impedes sequencing-by-ligation mechanism. BMC Syst Biol. 2012;6(Suppl 2):S10.
39. Rusk N. Torrents of sequence. Nat Methods. 2011;8(1):44.
40. Gleeson FC, Kerr SE, Kipp BR, Voss JS, Minot DM, Tu ZJ, Henry MR, Graham RP, Vasmatzis G, Cheville JC, Lazaridis KN, Levy MJ. Targeted next generation sequencing of endoscopic ultrasound acquired cytology from ampullary and pancreatic adenocarcinoma has the potential to aid patient stratification for optimal therapy selection. Oncotarget. 2016;7(34):54526–36. https://doi.org/10.18632/oncotarget.9440.
41. Nishino M. Molecular cytopathology for thyroid nodules: a review of methodology and test performance. Cancer Cytopathol. 2016;124(1):14–27.
42. Roy-Chowdhuri S, Chow CW, Kane MK, Yao H, Wistuba II, Krishnamurthy S, Stewart J, Staerkel G. Optimizing the DNA yield for molecular analysis from cytologic preparations. Cancer Cytopathol. 2016;124(4):254–60.
43. Piqueret-Stephan L, Marcaillou C, Reyes C, Honoré A, Letexier M, Gentien D, Droin N, Lacroix L, Scoazec JY, Vielh P. Massively parallel DNA sequencing from routinely processed cytological smears. Cancer Cytopathol. 2016;124(4):241–53.
44. Beca F, Schmitt F. Growing indication for FNA to study and analyze tumor heterogeneity at metastatic sites. Cancer Cytopathol. 2014;122(7):504–11.
45. Ashley EA. Towards precision medicine. Nat Rev Genet. 2016;17(9):507–22.
46. Layfield LJ, Roy-Chowdhuri S, Baloch Z, Ehya H, Geisinger K, Hsiao SJ, Lin O, Lindeman NI, Roh M, Schmitt F, Sidiropoulos N, VanderLaan PA. Utilization of ancillary studies in the cytologic diagnosis of respiratory lesions: the papanicolaou society of cytopathology consensus recommendations for respiratory cytology. Diagn Cytopathol. 2016;44(12):1000–9. https://doi.org/10.1002/dc.23549.
47. Macintyre G, Ylstra B, Brenton JD. Sequencing structural variants in cancer for precision therapeutics. Trends Genet. 2016;32(9):530–42.

48. Kallioniemi A, Kallioniemi OP, Sudar D, Rutovitz D, Gray JW, Waldman F, Pinkel D. Comparative genomic hybridization for molecular cytogenetic analysis of solid tumors. Science. 1992;258(5083):818–21.
49. Weiss MM, Hermsen MA, Meijer GA, van Grieken NC, Baak JP, Kuipers EJ, van Diest PJ. Comparative genomic hybridization. Mol Pathol. 1999;52(5):243–51.
50. de Ravel TJ, Devriendt K, Fryns JP, Vermeesch JR. What's new in karyotyping? The move towards array comparative genomic hybridisation (CGH). Eur J Pediatr. 2007;166(7):637–43.
51. Wiszniewska J, Bi W, Shaw C, Stankiewicz P, Kang SH, Pursley AN, Lalani S, Hixson P, Gambin T, Tsai CH, Bock HG, Descartes M, Probst FJ, Scaglia F, Beaudet AL, Lupski JR, Eng C, Cheung SW, Bacino C, Patel A. Combined array CGH plus SNP genome analyses in a single assay for optimized clinical testing. Eur J Hum Genet. 2014;22(1):79–87.
52. Kulkarni MM. Digital multiplexed gene expression analysis using the NanoString nCounter system. Curr Protoc Mol Biol. 2011;25:25B.10.
53. Clark DP. Seize the opportunity. Underutilization of fine-needle aspiration biopsy to informed targeted cancer therapy. Cancer. 2009;117(5):289–97.
54. Gonzalez-Angulo AM, Hennessy BTJ, Mills GB. Future of personalized medicine in oncology: a systems biology approach. J Clin Oncol. 2010;28(16):2777–83.
55. Haspel RL, Arnaout R, Briere L, Kantarci S, Marchand K, Tonellato P, Connolly J, Boguski MS, Saffitz JE. A call to action: training pathology residents in genomics and personalized medicine. Am J Clin Pathol. 2010;133(6):832–4.
56. Malapelle U, de Luca C, Vigliar E, Ambrosio F, Rocco D, Pisapia P, Bellevicine C, Troncone G. EGFR mutation detection on routine cytological smears of non-small cell lung cancer by digital PCR: a validation study. J Clin Pathol. 2016;69(5):454–7.

Molecular Cytology Applications on Head and Neck

4

Marc P. Pusztaszeri, Joaquín J. García,
and William C. Faquin

4.1 Molecular Cytology Applications in the Salivary Gland

4.1.1 Background

Salivary gland FNA is one of the most challenging areas of cytopathology due to (1) the extraordinary diversity of both benign and malignant salivary gland tumors (SGT), particularly with the recognition of several new entities during the past decade; (2) the cytomorphologic overlap between many benign and malignant SGT; (3) the spectrum and heterogeneity of microscopic features within the same tumor; and (4) the rarity of many SGT [1]. Nonetheless, FNA can play an important role in the evaluation of salivary gland lesions, and is reported to have a relatively high sensitivity (86–98%) for detecting carcinoma, and high specificity (>90%) for differentiating benign and malignant tumors [1–4]. The overall high diagnostic accuracy is linked to the fact that the majority of SGT are pleomorphic adenoma (PA), Warthin tumor (WT), or high grade (HG) carcinomas including metastatic carcinoma to intra- and peri-parotid lymph nodes, for which the cytologic diagnosis is usually straightforward. However, the accuracy is more variable when cytology is used to specifically subtype a neoplasm (48–94%) and to determine its grade [1–4]. Even in the hands of an experienced cytopathologist and despite cellular adequacy, indeterminate diagnoses with descriptive reports are given in about 1/3 of parotid

M. P. Pusztaszeri (✉)
Department of Pathology, McGill University, Montreal, Canada
e-mail: Marc.Pusztaszeri@mcgill.ca

J. J. García
Department of Laboratory Medicine and Pathology, Mayo Clinic, Rochester, NY, USA

W. C. Faquin
Department of Pathology, Massachusetts General Hospital, Boston, MA, USA

Harvard Medical School, Boston, MA, USA

© Springer International Publishing AG, part of Springer Nature 2018
F. C. Schmitt (ed.), *Molecular Applications in Cytology*,
https://doi.org/10.1007/978-3-319-74942-6_4

gland FNAs [5]. This creates a clinical dilemma for patient counseling, risk stratification, and surgical planning (i.e., type and extent of surgery), and highlights the role of ancillary studies as a possible alternative to repeat FNA. It is important to keep in mind that the most important role of salivary gland FNA is to distinguish neoplastic from non-neoplastic lesions, and when neoplastic, benign and LG SGT from HG SGT and metastases, in order to guide the clinical management efficiently. Thus, ancillary studies for salivary gland FNAs must be used judiciously in this context. Traditionally, immunohistochemical markers were of limited value for solving diagnostic problems in SGT, primarily because they lacked specificity as many SGT have a similar composition of epithelial and myoepithelial cells with overlapping immunochemical profiles. However, the discovery of several novel immunohistochemical markers and specific translocations for SGT has resulted in greater diagnostic usefulness [6–8].

4.1.2　Ancillary Studies in Salivary Gland Cytology

Different methods (described in Chap. 3) including immunocytochemistry (ICC), fluorescence in situ hybridization (FISH), reverse transcription-polymerase chain reaction (RT-PCR), and next generation sequencing (NGS) can be successfully applied to FNA material to improve the diagnostic accuracy for SGT [6–12]. Most of these methods can be readily integrated into the diagnostic workflow particularly as they become more widely available, cost-effective, and efficient with respect to turnaround time. While many of the immunocytochemical and molecular techniques can be applied to a variety of cytologic preparations including alcohol-fixed and/or air-dried smears, cytospins, and liquid-based preparations, their application to formalin-fixed paraffin-embedded cell block material is probably most reliable [12]. Cell blocks also have an advantage for selected cases where a panel of ancillary studies will be anticipated (see below) [12]. Rapid on-site evaluation of a salivary gland FNA can be very useful to ensure that adequate material is collected and processed appropriately for the purposes of performing ancillary studies. This may require separate dedicated FNA pass(es).

4.1.3　Translocations and Fusion Oncogenes in Salivary Gland Tumors

Over the past decade, new SGT have been recognized and new molecular alterations and immunoprofiles have been described for some tumors [6–8, 13–15]. The SGT currently known to harbor recurrent genetic alterations are summarized in Table 4.1. With advances in molecular diagnostics including whole-genome sequencing, it is certain that other SGT as well as additional molecular alterations will join this list in the near future. Although some of these gene rearrangements can be found in tumors and tumor analogues from other organs, they are highly specific in the spectrum of SGT, representing powerful diagnostic markers in surgical specimens as

Table 4.1 Benign and malignant salivary gland tumors associated with characteristic chromosomal alterations

Salivary gland tumor	Most common recurrent chromosomal alteration	Most common genes involved	Prevalence (%)
Benign			
Pleomorphic adenoma	t(3;8)(p21;q12)	*PLAG1, CTNNB1, LIFR, others*	50–60
	12q14–15	*HMGA2*	10
Basal cell adenoma nonmembranous type	LOH/mutation 8q12	*CTNNB1*	52
Basal cell adenoma membranous type	LOH/mutation 16q12–13	*CYLD*	75–80
Malignant			
Mucoepidermoid carcinoma	t(11;19)(q21–22;p13) or t(11;15)(q21;q26)	*MAML2, CRTC1, CRTC3*	60–80
Adenoid cystic carcinoma	t(6;9)(q22–23;p23–24)	*MYB, NFIB*	28–86
Mammary analogue secretory carcinoma	t(12;15)(p13;q25)	*ETV6, NTRK3*	90–100
Hyalinizing clear cell carcinoma	t(12;22)(q13;q12)	*EWSR1, ATF1*	85
Carcinoma ex pleomorphic adenoma	Same as pleomorphic adenoma	Same as pleomorphic adenoma	
Basal cell adenocarcinoma	Same as basal cell adenoma	Same as basal cell adenoma	
Polymorphous low-grade adenocarcinoma	*PRKD1* mutation	*PRKD1*	73
	PRKD gene family rearrangements	*PRKD1, PRKD2, PRKD3, ARID1A or DDX3X*	10
Cribriform adenocarcinoma of minor salivary glands	*PRKD* gene family rearrangements	*PRKD1, PRKD2, PRKD3, ARID1A or DDX3X*	80

well as FNA material [6–15]. The absence of a given rearrangement, however, may not exclude a particular SGT as its prevalence varies significantly between different entities and studies (Table 4.1). Although an understanding of their precise role in the carcinogenesis of certain SGT is still evolving, these translocations and resulting fusion oncoproteins typically target transcription factors involved in various growth factor signaling pathways and cell cycle regulation [14, 15]. Therefore, in addition to their diagnostic role, they may also represent prognostic markers and therapeutic targets [14, 15].

4.1.3.1 Pleomorphic Adenoma and Carcinoma Ex Pleomorphic Adenoma

PA the most common SGT of all sites in both adults and children, representing about 60% of all SGT and up to 75–80% of parotid gland tumors [16]. About 3–4% of PA, especially when recurrent or left untreated, transform over time into a malignant tumor known as carcinoma ex pleomorphic adenoma (Ca-ex-PA). FNA is highly accurate in diagnosing PA, but diagnostic difficulties may arise in: (1) cellular specimens with sparse or absent matrix; (2) lesions with hyaline globules or adenoid cystic-like areas; (3) lesions with squamous and/or mucinous metaplasia; and (4) lesions with focal cytologic atypia [1, 8]. Cytogenetically, 50–60% of PA have a translocation t(3;8)(p21;q12) involving *PLAG1* and one of several other fusion partners, the most common being *CTNNB1*, the gene encoding β-catenin [17–20]. Besides PLAG1, approximately 10% of PA have rearrangements in 12q13–15 involving *HMGA2* [16, 21, 22]. *HMGA2* can be amplified or rearranged with fusion of *WIF1* or other gene partners [21, 22]. This phenomenon is often accompanied by *MDM2* amplification, which may contribute to the malignant transformation of PA [16, 22]. Within SGT, the *PLAG1* and *HMGA2* gene rearrangements are present only in PA and Ca-ex-PA and have not been found in any other SGT. A subset of Ca-ex-PA also shows mutations of *p53* gene (TP53) and amplification of *HER2/neu* gene which may also play an important role in the progression of Ca-ex-PA, especially of ductal type, and may represent a prognostic and predictive marker [23–25].

4.1.3.2 Mucoepidermoid Carcinoma

MEC is the most common malignant SGT, in both adults and children, representing approximately 5–10% of SGT [16]. The cytology of MEC is variable cytology depending upon the grade of the tumor [1]. It is important to distinguish between LG-MEC and HG-MEC due to major differences in the management and in the prognosis with 90% and 40% five-year survivals, respectively. LG-MEC accounts for about 80% of all MEC and is the most common cause of a false negative cytologic diagnosis, being often wrongly diagnosed as a retention cyst (mucocele) [1, 4, 26]. This is due to the fact that LG-MEC is often cystic, aspirates are hypocellular, and may yield only cyst contents with scant epidermoid cells and isolated mucinous cells that can be misinterpreted as histiocytes or muciphages. Therefore, any residual solid mass following initial aspiration of a cystic lesion should be reaspirated, and a cell block preparation can be very valuable as it may provide diagnostic elements and/or material for ancillary techniques. The presence of lymphocytes and/or oncocytic cells is also a common feature in MEC that can mimic several other SGT such as WT [1]. An oncocytic variant of MEC has been described and may be difficult to distinguish from other SGT with oncocytic features such as WT, oncocytoma, and AciCC (see below). In contrast to LG-MEC, HG-MEC is characterized by more markedly atypical cells, usually with a predominance of epidermoid cells and intermediate cells and with scant mucinous cells, making it potentially difficult to distinguish from other HG carcinomas [1].

A specific translocation t(11;19) (q14–21;p12–13), involving *MECT1* (mucoepidermoid carcinoma translocated-1 or CRTC1) gene at 19p13 and *MAML2* (mastermind-like 2) gene at 11q21, has been reported in approximately 60–70% of MEC [27–31]. The fusion transcript was found to disrupt the Notch signaling pathway [27]. Expression of the fusion transcript is preferentially found in LG-MEC as well as in a few cases of LG-MEC that have progressed to HG-MEC [32]. The presence of this translocation is also associated with fewer recurrences, metastases, and tumor-related mortality [27–31]. The translocation is considered to be a reliable diagnostic and prognostic biomarker for MEC (Fig. 4.1). Nevertheless, a subset of WT with mucinous or squamoid metaplasia have been found to harbor the

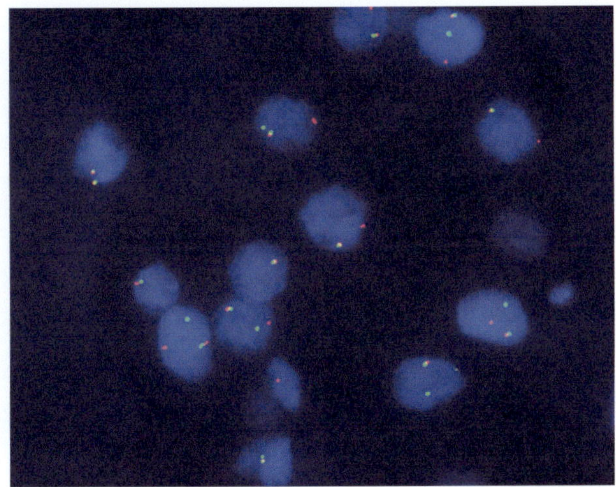

Fig. 4.1 Mucoepidermoid carcinoma. Fluorescent in situ hybridization (FISH) showing rearrangement of the *MAML2* locus (separation of red and green signals)

CRTC1-MAML2 fusion and may thus represent MEC or MEC arising in a background of WT (so-called "Warthin-like MEC") [33]. CRTC3, another member of the CRTC gene family, may also be fused to MAML2 in approximately 6% of MEC, and is also associated with a favorable prognosis [34, 35].

4.1.3.3 Adenoid Cystic Carcinoma

Adenoid cystic carcinoma (AdCC) represents approximately 10% of all SGT, and most frequently involves middle-aged women [16]. It typically has a relentless clinical course but with frequent recurrences, late onset of metastasis, and usually a fatal outcome [16]. AdCC can be divided into three histological subtypes, tubular, cribriform, and solid, and most tumors display features of more than one of these morphologic patterns [16]. Tumors with a predominantly cribriform and tubular growth pattern have a better prognosis than those with a more solid growth pattern [16]. Cytologically, a subset of AdCC, especially the solid subtype, can be difficult to distinguish from other basaloid or matrix producing tumors such as PA, basal cell adenoma (BCA), basal cell adenocarcinoma (BCAd), epithelial-myoepithelial carcinoma, and polymorphous low-grade adenocarcinoma (PLGA), due to the lack of characteristic matrix (see below) [1, 36, 37].

AdCC is characterized by the specific translocation t(6;9), involving *MYB* and *NFIB*, in approximately 64% of cases (28–86%) (Fig. 4.2a) [38–43]. Furthermore, both MYB and NFIB overexpression occurs in most AdCCs including those without the *MYB-NFIB* fusion, suggesting that other molecular mechanisms may be involved. *MYB* is a transcription factor with well-known oncogenic capabilities, involved in proliferation, survival, and differentiation, with many target genes such as *MYC, Bcl2,* and *c-KIT.* Several other cytogenetic changes and frequent alterations of genes involved in chromatin regulation, Notch, Rho, and several other signaling pathways have been reported in AdCC [44]. Interestingly, genomic deletions in chromosome 6 (6q24.1q25.1), containing several genes such as *PLAG1*, have been found in up to 57% of AdCC [45].

Fig. 4.2 Adenoid cystic carcinoma. Fluorescent in situ hybridization (FISH) showing rearrangement of the *MYB* locus (separation of the red and green signals) (**a**). MYB immunostaining showing strong expression in the tumor cells in a cytologic smear (**b**). CD117 immunostaining showing strong expression in the tumor cells in a cytologic smear (**c**)

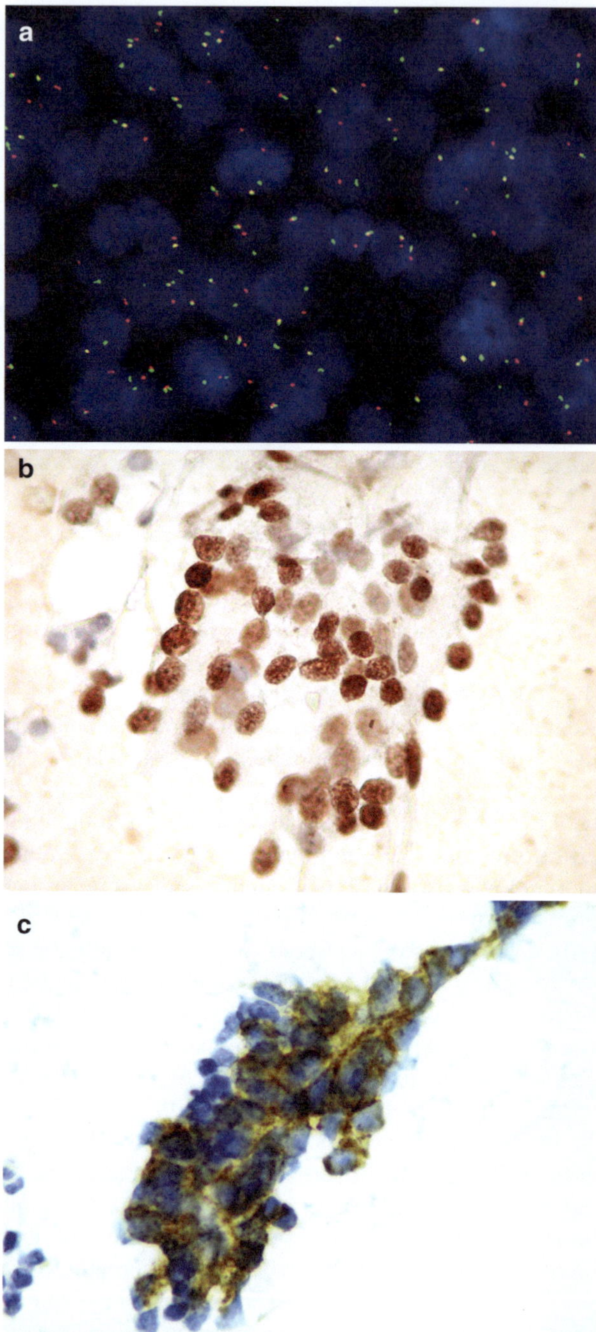

4.1.3.4 Polymorphous Low Grade Adenocarcinoma

PLGA is the second most common intraoral malignant SGT, preferentially involving the minor salivary glands of the palate (60% of cases) [16, 46, 47]. Most patients are 50–70 years old. PLGA has a relatively indolent clinical course, with lymph node metastasis in up to 25% of cases and distant metastasis in up to 7.5% of cases [16, 46, 47]. It is characterized by a monomorphic population of cuboidal to columnar cells with oval nuclei and open chromatin and small indistinct nucleoli, arranged as the name implies in various cytomorphological patterns. Extracellular matrix, usually scant or absent in PLGA, can mimic both the PA (i.e., fibrillar) and AdCC (i.e., hyaline globules) types of matrix [1]. Although *MYB* aberrations including monosomy or deletion can be seen in PLGA, the *MYB* rearrangement of AdCC is not found in PLGA. The vast majority of PLGA harbor a *PRKD1* E710D mutation (73%) or PRKD gene family (*PRKD1, PRKD2* or *PRKD3)* rearrangements, which have not been found in other SGT besides cribriform adenocarcinoma of the salivary glands (CASG), a neoplastic entity closely related to PLGA [47–49]. Moreover, PLGA with and without *PRKD1* mutation have been found to overexpress the PRKD1 protein, a serine-threonine kinase involved in cell adhesion, cell migration, and cell survival. The presence of the *PRKD1* mutation was significantly associated with metastasis-free survival [47]. Therefore, *PRKD1* mutations may have diagnostic and prognostic utility, helping to distinguish indolent PLGA from more aggressive SGT such as AdCC. Additional studies are required to investigate whether ICC for PRKD1 will prove to be helpful as well.

4.1.3.5 Mammary Analogue Secretory Carcinoma

MASC was first described in 2010 by Skalova et al. in a report of 16 cases [50]. MASC occurs more commonly in males, both at parotid and extra-parotid sites [50, 51]. The cytomorphology, immunochemical and molecular profiles of MASC are identical to secretory carcinoma of the breast. The prognosis of patients with MASC appears to be similar to other LG carcinomas, including acinic cell carcinoma (AciCC), although there may be a higher trend towards lymph node metastasis, but studies are limited [52]. MASC is characterized by the specific translocation t(12;15)(p13;q25), leading to fusion between *ETV6* and *NTRK3*. The latter is an essential feature of MASC since it is found in nearly 100% of cases and has not been reported in any other SGT, besides one case of SDC so far [50–53]. Prior to its recognition as a separate entity, MASC was classified either as AciCC (zymogen granule poor), adenocarcinoma NOS, or as MEC [54]. On cytology, MASC can be confused with other oncocytic SGT such as PA, MEC, AciCC, and WT (see below). Demonstration of an *ETV6* rearrangement is useful to make the diagnosis of MASC in difficult cases and to rule out the other SGT (Fig. 4.3a) [55]. However, the impact of a correct diagnosis of MASC is only marginal, because the initial management of these LG neoplasms is usually the same.

Fig. 4.3 Mammary analogue secretory carcinoma of salivary glands. Fluorescent in situ hybridization (FISH) showing rearrangement of the *ETV6* locus (separation of red and green signals) (**a**). Mammaglobin immunostaining showing strong expression in the tumor cells (Cellblock) (**b**)

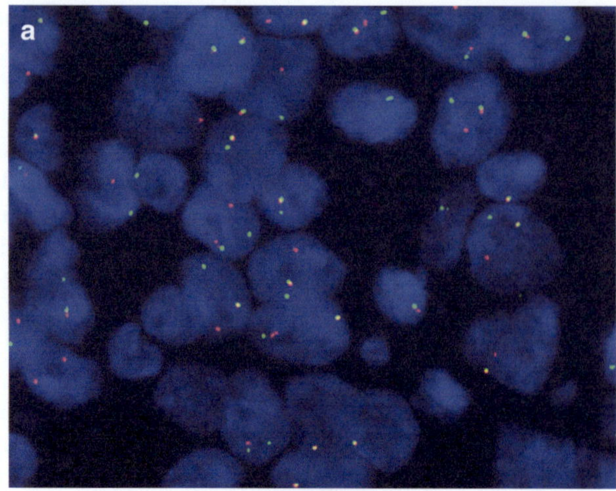

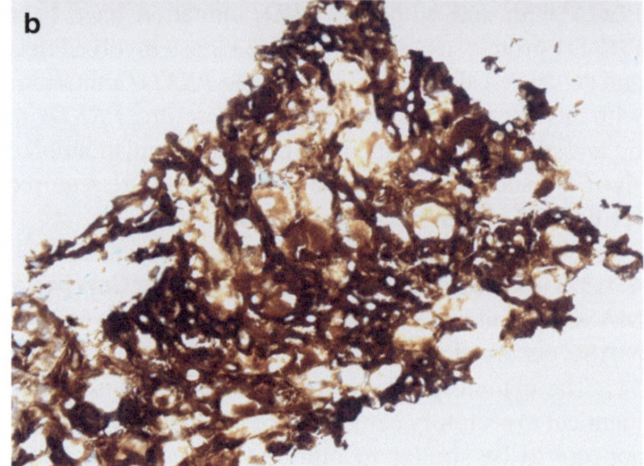

4.1.3.6 Hyalinizing Clear Cell Carcinoma

Hyalinizing clear cell carcinoma (HCCC) is a rare LG carcinoma that typically arises from the minor salivary glands of the oral cavity with the potential for local recurrence [16, 56, 57]. Histologically, HCCC is composed of trabeculae, cords, nests, and solid sheets of epithelial cells with clear cytoplasm, owing to large amounts of glycogen [16, 56]. The differential diagnosis of HCCC on cytology is broad and includes other SGT with clear cell features such as clear cell oncocytoma, LG-MEC, epithelial-myoepithelial carcinoma, clear cell myoepithelioma/myoepithelial carcinoma, AciCC, metastatic renal clear cell carcinoma (RCC), SCC clear-cell variant, and melanoma [1, 11, 57]. HCCC is characterized by the specific translocation t(12;22)(q13;q12) generating an *EWSR1-ATF1* fusion gene, which is present in approximately 85% of cases (Fig. 4.4) [58–61]. ICC is of limited value for the diagnosis of HCCC. Therefore, a definite diagnosis of HCCC relies on the

Fig. 4.4 Hyalinizing clear cell carcinoma. Fluorescent in situ hybridization (FISH) showing rearrangement of the *EWSR1* locus (separation of the red and green signals)

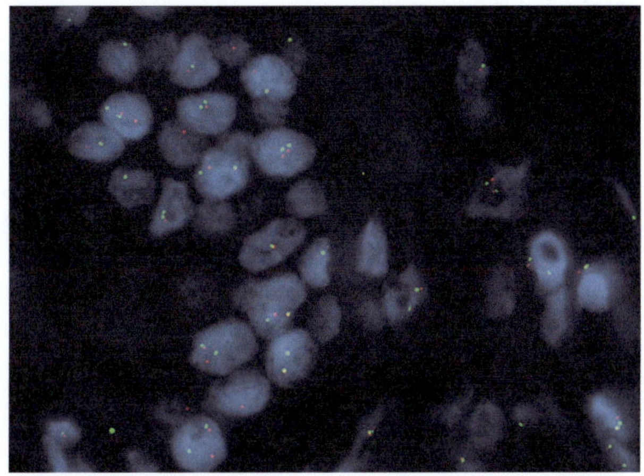

demonstration of the specific *EWSR-1* rearrangement which is not present in other clear cell tumors within the differential diagnosis [11, 57].

4.1.3.7 NUT (Nuclear Protein in Testis) Midline Carcinoma (NMC)

NMC is an uncommon form of poorly differentiated SCC characterized by rearrangement of the *NUT* gene on chromosome 15q14, typically with the *BRD4* gene on chromosome 19p13, resulting in a BRD4-NUT fusion gene [62]. Since the first reported case of NMC in 1991, more than 70 cases have been reported in children and adults of all ages. Although NMC has a predilection for midline structures including the nose, mouth, sinuses, and upper airways, tumors occurring outside the midline including the salivary gland have been reported. NMC is refractory to conventional chemotherapy and radiotherapy, and is rapidly fatal with an average survival from the time of diagnosis of <1 year. However, clinical trials investigating specific drugs targeting BRD4-NUT are underway. Therefore, an accurate and early diagnosis of NMC may become even more critical in the future. Cytologically, NMC has non-specific features, and mimics other "small round cell" tumors and basaloid neoplasms [62]. Squamous or glandular differentiation is typically absent in NMC. The main differential diagnosis in adults is with poorly differentiated SCC, undifferentiated (nasopharyngeal) carcinoma, and small cell carcinoma, while in children other pediatric small cell tumors such as Ewing sarcoma must also be considered [62]. Almost all NMC show immunoreactivity to p63 reflecting the squamous nature of this tumor. NMC can also express p16 even though there is no known association with HPV. In order to confirm the diagnosis of NMC, demonstration of a rearranged *NUT* gene using one of the methods described earlier is necessary. Alternatively, ICC using NUT antibodies can be used successfully on cytologic material with a very high sensitivity (87%) and specificity (100%) [62]. Any poorly differentiated carcinoma in the head and neck (HN) should be considered for NUT immunostaining and/or rearrangement testing.

4.1.4 Selected Immunohistochemical Stains in the FNA Diagnosis of Salivary Gland Tumors

Because the required molecular diagnostic techniques for detecting genetic abnormalities described above are not routinely available in some laboratories, the overexpression of translocation-associated proteins and/or other proteins may serve as a diagnostic surrogate in salivary gland FNAs. This can be essentially helpful in the context of basaloid neoplasms and oncocytic lesions, which are two of the most common diagnostically challenging areas. In addition, a panel of immunostains can be very helpful for HG carcinomas to distinguish a primary SGT from a metastasis; the work-up of metastases is discussed in Chap. 13.

4.1.4.1 Basaloid Neoplasms

Among basaloid neoplasms of the salivary gland, the distinction between AdCC and PA is crucial as it carries significant clinical implications. The translocation in PA typically leads to an overexpression of PLAG1 that can be assessed using ICC; most PA (94%) with or without of *PLAG1* rearrangement are immunoreactive for PLAG1 [63–65]. In contrast, PLAG1 is negative in the most common salivary gland carcinomas, including AdCC, MEC, and AciCC, although a subset of PLGA may be positive for PLAG1 [64]. The translocation in AdCC typically leads to an overexpression of MYB that can be assessed using ICC (Fig. 4.2a, b); most AdCC (55–82%), with or without the *MYB-NFIB* fusion transcript, are positive for MYB, compared with 14% of non-AdCC neoplasms [41–43]. On cytology, a majority of AdCC also shows strong immunoreactivity for MYB (Fig. 4.2b), while PA and other SGT are negative or focally positive [9, 12, 66]. MYB immunostaining appears to be more effective in alcohol-fixed cytological smears than in corresponding FFPE tissue from surgical resections or cell blocks, because of the presence of more faint peripheral staining (zonal staining) on FFPE [9, 12]. This can be attributed to different fixation methods affecting the degradation and immunoreactivity of the MYB protein. In addition to MYB overexpression, most (90%) AdCC show strong and diffuse expression of c-KIT (CD117) (Fig. 4.2c) [1, 6, 7, 12]. In order to increase the sensitivity and specificity in distinguishing AdCC and PA from each other and from other SGT, an immunopanel of MYB, c-KIT, PLAG1, and HMGA2 on FNA cell blocks is probably the most useful [12].

PLGA is also in the differential diagnosis of PA and AdCC. PLGA has a consistent p63+/p40− immunophenotype, reflecting the lack of a myoepithelial cell component, that helps distinguish it from AdCC and cellular PA that characteristically demonstrate concordant p63 and p40 immunostaining patterns [67, 68]. In contrast to AdCC, Ki-67 labeling index is typically low in PLGA [69], although its assessment on cytologic material may not be reliable.

BCA and BCAdc represent two other basaloid neoplasms that show cytomorphologic similarity but differ at the histologic level by their invasive qualities. Nuclear β-catenin immunoexpression has been found to have a relatively high sensitivity (82%) and a high specificity (96%) for BCA in comparison with other basaloid neoplasms [70]. A *CTNNB1* gene mutation can also be found in about 1/3–1/2 of BCA. BCAdc also frequently harbors nuclear β-catenin expression, with or without the corresponding gene mutation, as well as aberrations in genes affecting different signaling pathways such as PIK3CA [70, 71].

4.1.4.2 Salivary Gland Tumors with Oncocytic Features

SGT with oncocytic features represent a common diagnostic challenge for FNA. They include mostly WT, oncocytoma, and oncocytic carcinoma, AciCC, MEC, MASC, and metastasis (e.g., RCC) [1]. WT and oncocytoma are common causes of false-positive cytology interpretations, while AciCC and MEC are among the most common causes of false-negative cytology interpretations [1]. A limited ICC panel consisting of DOG-1, SOX-10, and p63 can be very helpful in separating AciCC from WT, MEC, and oncocytoma [72]. DOG-1 and SOX-10, which are markers of salivary acinar and intercalated duct differentiation, are strongly positive in AciCC and are predominantly negative in WT, oncocytoma and oncocytic carcinoma, MASC and MEC [73]. Conversely, p63 typically shows diffuse expression in MEC, including its oncocytic variant, and is negative in AciCC and metastatic RCC. P63 expression in WT and in oncocytoma/oncocytic carcinoma is usually more focal and restricted to basal or peripheral cells than in MEC [74], a feature that is not readily appreciated in cytologic material [72]. S100 and mammaglobin are very useful to support the diagnosis of MASC since other oncocytic neoplasms in the differential diagnosis are usually negative for the latter (Fig. 4.3b). Recently, overexpression of signal transducer and activator of transcription 5a (STAT5a), which may be related to the *ETV6-NTRK3* translocation, has been found in MASC, and can be assessed on cytological material using ICC [75]. STAT5a may thus represent a useful additional marker for MASC. Nevertheless, the most definitive diagnostic markers of MASC and MEC (including its oncocytic variant) are the presence of the specific translocations as described previously.

4.2 HPV-Associated Head and Neck Squamous Cell Carcinoma

4.2.1 Background

There are several characteristic clinico-pathological features of HPV-associated HN SCC (HPV-SCC) which makes it a truly a distinct variant of HN SCC [76, 77]. In contrast to patients with conventional HN SCC, patients with sexually transmitted HPV-SCC of the oropharynx are often younger, typically nonsmokers and nondrinkers, and of higher socioeconomic status [76]. HPV type 16 is the most common genotype, accounting for 90–95% of HPV-SCC in the oropharynx [76, 78]. HPV-SCC arises most commonly in the lingual and palatine tonsils within the deep crypt lining epithelium; a dysplastic precursor lesion is not currently recognized. This may explain why certain screening methods, including both oral rinses and oral brushing specimens, have not been very successful at detecting HPV-SCC precursor lesions [79, 80]. Oropharyngeal HPV-SCC commonly present with occult or small (T1/T2) primary tumors but with advanced loco-regional disease (N2/N3), with cervical lymphadenopathy often being the presenting clinical finding [76, 81, 82]. The prognosis of patients with HPV-SCC is often better than conventional HN-SCC, due in part to increased chemo- and radiosensitivity [76, 81]. Accordingly, several clinical trials investigating less intensive treatment regimens ("treatment de-escalation") with less morbidity, or new tailored immunotherapies ("therapeutic vaccines") are ongoing in patients with HPV-SCC [83].

4.2.1.1 Cytologic Evaluation of HPV-Related HNSCC

Many of the primary tumors that are identified among patients with HN SCC of unknown primary are located within the oropharynx, and up to 80–90% of oropharyngeal SCC are caused by oncogenic high risk (HR) HPV [76, 78]. In contrast, only a small percentage of SCC arising from non-oropharyngeal HN sites is positive for HR-HPV. Therefore, the detection of transcriptionally active HR-HPV in FNA specimens from metastatic SCC in cervical lymph nodes strongly implicates the ipsilateral oropharynx as the site of origin [84]. In addition, determining HPV status is prognostically relevant and can give a patient eligibility for clinical trials investigating novel treatment options for this tumor type (e.g., radiotherapy de-escalation or vaccine-based therapies) [83]. While HPV DNA may be detected in a significant subset of non-oropharyngeal HN cancers, it is usually not transcriptionally active virus and its presence is not believed to be clinically or biologically relevant [85–88]. One exception appears to be the sinonasal tract, where 20–30% of SCC can harbor transcriptionally active HPV, but the clinical significance of HPV-SCC in this site is not yet clear [89, 90]. Therefore, routine HR-HPV testing should be currently limited to SCC of the oropharynx and metastatic carcinomas of unknown primary in lymph nodes that may have arisen from the oropharynx. This recommendation has recently been endorsed by the College of American Pathologists, the Royal College of Pathologists, and Cancer Care Ontario [91–93]. There is no role for the routine testing of HN cancers for the "low-risk" types of HPV (i.e., types 6 and 11). These HPV types cause squamous and respiratory papillomas in the upper and lower aerodigestive tracts, but do not cause oropharyngeal HPV-SCC.

Metastatic HPV-SCC has a fairly typical cytologic appearance characterized by cohesive clusters of oval to somewhat elongate basaloid epithelial cells often in a cystic background of macrophages and cellular debris (Fig. 4.5a). The basaloid appearance reflects the non-keratinizing nature of these cancers which are thought to derive from the specialized reticulated epithelium of the tonsils. This cytologic pattern differs from conventional HN SCC which is frequently keratinizing and easier to diagnose. The differential diagnosis of metastatic HPV-SCC on cytology includes other metastatic carcinomas with basaloid features such as basaloid SCC, nasopharyngeal carcinoma (EBV-associated), small cell neuroendocrine carcinoma, and AdCC [84]. In addition to testing for HR-HPV, cytology and ICC can usually distinguish between these entities [84]. Cervical metastases from HPV-SCC are often large and cystic, and this can make the distinction with branchial cleft cyst (BrCC) difficult clinically, radiologically and cytologically as well [84]. Due to several factors including limited cellularity (e.g., cyst contents only) and cellular degeneration, a definite diagnosis on FNA may not be possible. Since cystic metastases of HN-SCC usually harbor HR-HPV, p16 ICC in conjunction with specific

Fig. 4.5 FNA of HPV-related HNSCC showing a cohesive group of non-keratinizing squamous cells with a basaloid appearance (**a**). HPV-related HNSCC showing strong diffuse cytoplasmic and nuclear positivity for p16 (**b**). In situ hybridization for high-risk HPV DNA in an HPV-related HNSCC of the oropharynx (**c**)

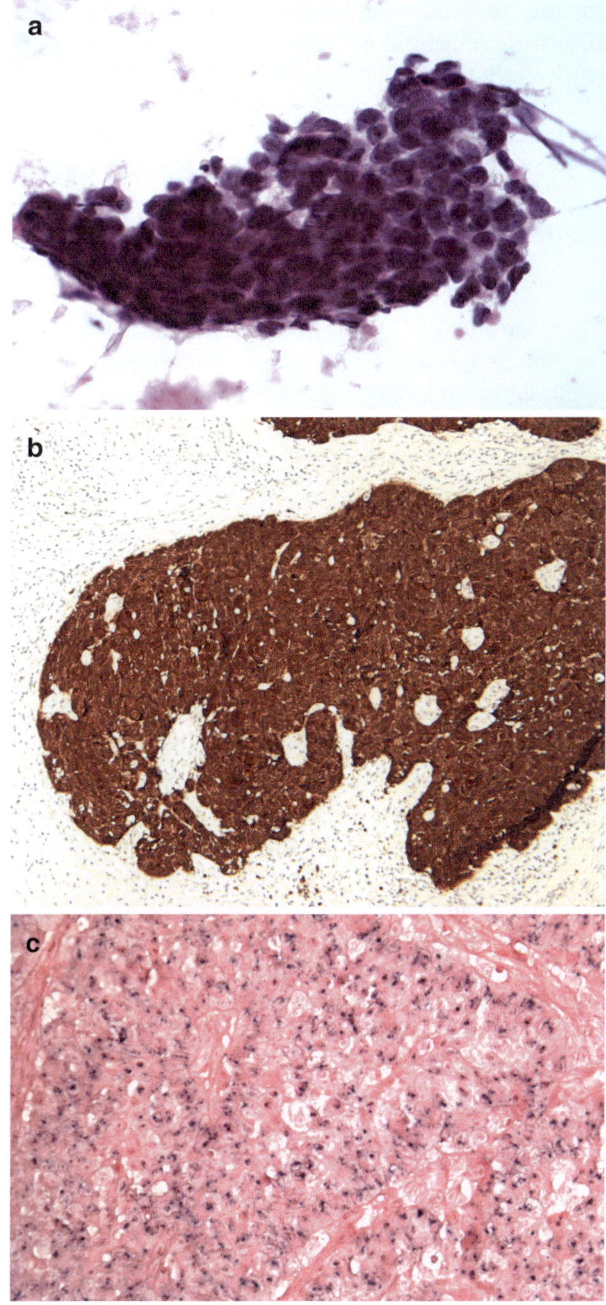

testing for HR-HPV (see below) can be useful when the distinction between BrCC and a cystic metastasis of an HPV-SCC remains unclear based on cytological and clinico-radiological grounds (Fig. 4.5b, c). Caution is warranted, however, in interpreting p16 ICC alone since focal strong p16 immunoreactivity can be seen in the superficial lining cells of BrCC [94]. Although ancillary studies for detecting HR-HPV are helpful when positive, a negative result does not exclude malignancy, particularly those not associated with HR-HPV.

4.3 Detection Methods for HPV in Cytologic Material

4.3.1 Conventional Methods for HPV Testing Using FFPE Material

There are many different methods available for HPV testing of HN cancers, but none of them is absolutely optimal with respect to sensitivity, specificity, cost, and applicability to a diagnostic laboratory in routine practice. P16 appears to be the best stand-alone test for specific selected scenarios involving tissue biopsies, but the best HPV detection method for cytologic preparations of metastatic carcinoma is less clear.

4.3.2 p16 Immunohistochemistry

The simplest and most accessible type of HPV testing involves using a surrogate marker, p16. In biopsies of the oropharynx of a squamous cell carcinoma with non-keratinizing morphology, a p16 positive result is sufficient to conclude that the carcinoma is HPV-associated. The HPV viral oncoprotein E7 binds to and degrades the retinoblastoma protein, which leads to the accumulation of p16, which in turn can easily be detected by IHC (Fig. 4.5b) [95]. There are many advantages to using p16 IHC for HPV testing: it is widely available, can be performed on cell blocks, and is very sensitive (up to 100%) for the presence of transcriptionally active HPV [96, 97]. On the other hand, p16 is not entirely specific for HR-HPV since other molecular mechanisms may cause p16 overexpression in cancer [96, 97]. As a result, the use and interpretation of p16 alone should be done with care and in the context of a carcinoma with the appropriate non-keratinizing morphology. In addition, p16 should only be used as a surrogate marker for high risk HPV in the oropharynx and in non-keratinizing metastases (from the oropharynx) to level 2–3 cervical lymph nodes, because outside of these locations the specificity of p16 for high risk HPV is reduced [87, 88, 98]. Finally, to be considered as positive in tissue, p16 immunoexpression must be seen in at least 70% of tumor cells in a nuclear and cytoplasmic distribution. The problem for cytology, however, is that quantifying p16 positivity in dispersed cytologic material can be difficult, especially in a background of necrosis and/or degenerating tumor cells. In addition, the percentage of p16 positivity in cell block material compared with tissue biopsy samples may be lower for a positive result [99]. When in doubt in cytologic samples which are usually for metastatic disease, p16 can be used initially as a sensitive screening method followed by confirmation using a more specific HPV detection technique.

4.3.3 Polymerase Chain Reaction-Based Techniques

PCR-based techniques are commonly utilized to identify HPV DNA in tissue. These methods are very sensitive because PCR can amplify even very small amounts of HPV DNA. This sensitivity comes at the expense of specificity because the mere presence of HPV does not convey whether the virus is transcriptionally active or simply a bystander. Detection of the HPV E6 and E7 mRNA transcripts by PCR is clinically more relevant because it confirms that HPV is both present and transcriptionally active. Unfortunately, PCR for E6/E7 mRNA is technically challenging and is currently not available in most diagnostic laboratories.

4.3.4 DNA and RNA In Situ Hybridization

DNA ISH allows the direct visualization of the viral DNA in the context of the tumor histology, and is relatively simple to integrate into the diagnostic pathology workflow. The presence of punctate ISH signals in tumor nuclei is a very specific pattern for integration of HPV DNA into the host genome (Fig. 4.5c). On the other hand, at low copy levels HPV DNA can be undetectable by ISH, limiting the sensitivity of this method. Moreover, the interpretation of HPV DNA ISH can be challenging in cases with scant, focal, or unusually faint signals. In addition, akin to HPV DNA PCR, this method does not directly inform the reader about the transcriptional activity of the virus. The recent introduction of ISH for HPV E6/E7 mRNA is an important advance because this method combines the direct visualization of DNA ISH in the cells with the specificity for transcriptionally active HPV of mRNA PCR [87, 100]. In addition, RNA ISH using advanced technology appears to be more sensitive than DNA ISH because at low viral copy numbers where DNA ISH signals are absent or equivocal, RNA ISH signals are consistently robust [87]. Widespread implementation of this promising HPV detection method may be imminent.

4.3.5 Combination of Different Testing Methods

With the recognition that no HPV detection method is entirely optimal particularly for cytologic samples, some centers have turned to multimodality HPV detection strategies applied to FNA. One strategy employs the very high sensitivity of p16 IHC with a more specific ISH or PCR-based test on cell block material. The two tests can be done simultaneously or in an algorithmic manner where only a p16-positive result leads to the second test. The addition of p16 IHC to a DNA-based HPV detection strategy is also useful because it offers insight into the significance of any HPV DNA that is present. For example, if p16 is negative but HPV DNA is present, it is unlikely that the HPV is transcriptionally active and biologically significant. On the other hand, if p16 is positive but HPV DNA is absent by one method in a SCC that has the non-keratinizing morphology of an HPV-SCC, it might be appropriate to use yet another method to confirm the presence or absence of HPV. It is not yet clear how the introduction of newer mRNA-based HPV detection strategies will affect these multimodal HPV testing algorithms, or whether they will be useful for cytologic preparations.

Finally, techniques already in use for HPV detection in liquid-based cervical cytology such as the Roche cobas platform [101], Cervista [102], and Hybrid Capture [103] can also be applied for HPV detection in FNAs of metastatic HN SCC, and may in fact be the best option. The advantage of these liquid-based techniques is that several of them are already approved by the US Food and Drug Administration, they are economical, some are automated, and they are widely implemented and validated in laboratories.

References

1. Faquin WC, Powers CN. Salivary gland cytopathology. Essentials in cytopathology series, vol. 5. New York: Springer; 2008.
2. Colella G, Cannavale R, Flamminio F, et al. Fine-needle aspiration cytology of salivary gland lesions: a systematic review. J Oral Maxillofac Surg. 2010;68:2146–53.
3. Schmidt RL, Hall BJ, Wilson AR, et al. A systematic review and meta-analysis of the diagnostic accuracy of fine-needle aspiration cytology for parotid gland lesions. Am J Clin Pathol. 2011;136:45–59.
4. Hughes JH, Volk EE, Wilbur DC. Pitfalls in salivary gland fine-needle aspiration cytology: lessons from the College of American Pathologists Interlaboratory Comparison Program in nongynecologic cytology. Arch Pathol Lab Med. 2005;129:26–31.
5. Fundakowski C, Castaño J, Abouyared M, et al. The role of indeterminate fine-needle biopsy in the diagnosis of parotid malignancy. Laryngoscope. 2014;124:678–81.
6. Pusztaszeri MP, García JJ, Faquin WC. Salivary gland FNA: new markers and new opportunities for improved diagnosis. Cancer Cytopathol. 2016;124:307–16.
7. Pusztaszeri MP, Faquin WC. Update in salivary gland cytopathology: recent molecular advances and diagnostic applications. Semin Diagn Pathol. 2015;32:264–74.
8. Wang H, Fundakowski C, Khurana JS, Jhala N. Fine-needle aspiration biopsy of salivary gland lesions. Arch Pathol Lab Med. 2015;139:1491–7.
9. Pusztaszeri MP, Sadow PM, Ushiku A, et al. MYB immunostaining is a useful ancillary test for distinguishing adenoid cystic carcinoma from pleomorphic adenoma in fine-needle aspiration biopsy specimens. Cancer Cytopathol. 2014;122:257–65.
10. Hudson JB, Collins BT. MYB gene abnormalities t(6;9) in adenoid cystic carcinoma fine-needle aspiration biopsy using fluorescence in situ hybridization. Arch Pathol Lab Med. 2014;138:403–9.
11. Fulciniti F, Pia Curcio M, Liguori G, et al. Hyalinizing clear cell carcinoma of the parotid gland: report of a recurrent case with aggressive cytomorphology and behavior diagnosed on fine-needle cytology sample. Diagn Cytopathol. 2014;42:63–8.
12. Foo WC, Jo VY, Krane JF. Usefulness of translocation-associated immunohistochemical stains in the fine-needle aspiration diagnosis of salivary gland neoplasms. Cancer Cytopathol. 2016;124:397–405.
13. Weinreb I. Translocation-associated salivary gland tumors: a review and update. Adv Anat Pathol. 2013;20:367–77.
14. Stenman G, Persson F, Andersson MK. Diagnostic and therapeutic implications of new molecular biomarkers in salivary gland cancers. Oral Oncol. 2014;50:683–90.
15. Andersson MK, Stenman G. The landscape of gene fusions and somatic mutations in salivary gland neoplasms–implications for diagnosis and therapy. Oral Oncol. 2016;57:63–9.

16. El-Naggar AK, Huvos AG. Tumours of the salivary glands. In: Barnes L, Eveson JW, Reichart P, Sidransky D, editors. World health organization classification of tumours. Pathology and genetics of head and neck tumours. Lyon: IARC Press; 2005. p. 209–81.

17. Voz ML, Aström AK, Kas K, et al. The recurrent translocation t(5;8)(p13;q12) in pleomorphic adenomas results in upregulation of PLAG1 gene expression under control of the LIFR promoter. Oncogene. 1998;16:1409–16.

18. Kas K, Voz ML, Röijer E, et al. Promoter swapping between the genes for a novel zinc finger protein and beta-catenin in pleiomorphic adenomas with t(3;8)(p21;q12) translocations. Nat Genet. 1997;15:170–4.

19. Aström AK, Voz ML, Kas K, et al. Conserved mechanism of PLAG1 activation in salivary gland tumors with and without chromosome 8q12 abnormalities: identification of SII as a new fusion partner gene. Cancer Res. 2009;59:918–23.

20. Debiec-Rychter M, Van Valckenborgh I, Van den Broeck C, et al. Histologic localization of PLAG1 (pleomorphic adenoma gene 1) in pleomorphic adenoma of the salivary gland: cytogenetic evidence of common origin of phenotypically diverse cells. Lab Investig. 2001;81:1289–97.

21. Queimado L, Lopes CS, Reis AM. WIF1, an inhibitor of the Wnt pathway, is rearranged in salivary gland tumors. Genes Chromosomes Cancer. 2007;46:215–25.

22. Persson F, Andrén Y, Winnes M, et al. High-resolution genomic profiling of adenomas and carcinomas of the salivary glands reveals amplification, rearrangement, and fusion of HMGA2. Genes Chromosomes Cancer. 2009;48:69–82.

23. Röijer E, Nordkvist A, Ström AK, et al. Translocation, deletion/amplification, and expression of HMGIC and MDM2 in a carcinoma ex pleomorphic adenoma. Am J Pathol. 2002;160:433–40.

24. Hashimoto K, Yamamoto H, Shiratsuchi H, et al. HER-2/neu gene amplification in carcinoma ex pleomorphic adenoma in relation to progression and prognosis: a chromogenic in-situ hybridization study. Histopathology. 2012;60:E131–42.

25. Nishijima T, Yamamoto H, Nakano T, et al. Dual gain of HER2 and EGFR gene copy numbers impacts the prognosis of carcinoma ex pleomorphic adenoma. Hum Pathol. 2015;46:1730–43.

26. Joseph TP, Joseph CP, Jayalakshmy PS, Poothiode U. Diagnostic challenges in cytology of mucoepidermoid carcinoma: report of 6 cases with histopathological correlation. J Cytol. 2015;32:21–4.

27. Tonon G, Modi S, Wu L, et al. t(11;19)(q21;p13) translocation in mucoepidermoid carcinoma creates a novel fusion product that disrupts a notch signaling pathway. Nat Genet. 2003;33:208–13.

28. Behboudi A, Enlund F, Winnes M, et al. Molecular classification of mucoepidermoid carcinomas-prognostic significance of the MECT1-MAML2 fusion oncogene. Genes Chromosomes Cancer. 2006;45:470–81.

29. Seethala RR, Dacic S, Cieply K, et al. A reappraisal of the MECT1/MAML2 translocation in salivary mucoepidermoid carcinomas. Am J Surg Pathol. 2010;34:1106–21.

30. Okabe M, Miyabe S, Nagatsuka H, et al. MECT1-MAML2 fusion transcript defines a favorable subset of mucoepidermoid carcinoma. Clin Cancer Res. 2006;12:3902–7.

31. Okumura Y, Miyabe S, Nakayama T, et al. Impact of CRTC1/3–MAML2 fusions on histological classification and prognosis of mucoepidermoid carcinoma. Histopathology. 2011;59:90–7.

32. Nagao T, Gaffey TA, Kay PA, et al. Dedifferentiation in low-grade mucoepidermoid carcinoma of the parotid gland. Hum Pathol. 2003;34:1068–72.

33. Ishibashi K, Ito Y, Masaki A, et al. Warthin-like mucoepidermoid carcinoma: a combined study of fluorescence in situ hybridization and whole-slide imaging. Am J Surg Pathol. 2015;39:1479–87.

34. Nakayama T, Miyabe S, Okabe M, et al. Clinicopathological significance of the CRTC3-MAML2 fusion transcript in mucoepidermoid carcinoma. Mod Pathol. 2009;22(12):1575–81.

35. Fehr A, Röser K, Heidorn K, Hallas C, Löning T, Bullerdiek J. A new type of MAML2 fusion in mucoepidermoid carcinoma. Genes Chromosomes Cancer. 2008;47:203–6.

36. Stanley MW, Horwitz CA, Rollins SD, et al. Basal cell (monomorphic) and minimally pleomorphic adenomas of the salivary glands. Distinction from the solid (anaplastic) type of adenoid cystic carcinoma in fine-needle aspiration. Am J Clin Pathol. 1996;106:35–41.
37. Lee SS, Cho KJ, Jang JJ, et al. Differential diagnosis of adenoid cystic carcinoma from pleomorphic adenoma of the salivary gland on fine needle aspiration cytology. Acta Cytol. 1996;40:1246–52.
38. Persson M, Andrén Y, Mark J, et al. Recurrent fusion of MYB and NFIB transcription factor genes in carcinomas of the breast and head and neck. Proc Natl Acad Sci U S A. 2009;106:18740–1874.
39. Persson M, Andrén Y, Moskaluk CA, et al. Clinically significant copy number alterations and complex rearrangements of MYB and NFIB in head and neck adenoid cystic carcinoma. Genes Chromosomes Cancer. 2012;51:805–17.
40. Nordkvist A, Mark J, Gustafsson H, et al. Non-random chromosome rearrangements in adenoid cystic carcinoma of the salivary glands. Genes Chromosomes Cancer. 1994;10:115–21.
41. Brill LB 2nd, Kanner WA, Fehr A, et al. Analysis of MYB expression and MYB-NFIB gene fusions in adenoid cystic carcinoma and other salivary neoplasms. Mod Pathol. 2011;24:1169–76.
42. Mitani Y, Li J, Rao PH, et al. Comprehensive analysis of the MYB-NFIB gene fusion in salivary adenoid cystic carcinoma: incidence, variability, and clinicopathologic significance. Clin Cancer Res. 2010;16:4722–31.
43. Mitani Y, Rao PH, Futreal PA, et al. Novel chromosomal rearrangements and break points at the t(6;9) in salivary adenoid cystic carcinoma: association with MYB-NFIB chimeric fusion, MYB expression, and clinical outcome. Clin Cancer Res. 2011;17:7003–14.
44. Rettig EM, Talbot CC Jr, Sausen M, et al. Whole-genome sequencing of salivary gland adenoid cystic carcinoma. Cancer Prev Res (Phila). 2016;9:265–74.
45. Rutherford S, Yu Y, Rumpel CA, Frierson HF Jr, Moskaluk CA. Chromosome 6 deletion and candidate tumor suppressor genes in adenoid cystic carcinoma. Cancer Lett. 2006;18(236):309–17.
46. Patel TD, Vazquez A, Marchiano E, Park RC, Baredes S, Eloy JA. Polymorphous low-grade adenocarcinoma of the head and neck: a population-based study of 460 cases. Laryngoscope. 2015;125:1644–9.
47. Weinreb I, Piscuoglio S, Martelotto LG, et al. Hotspot activating PRKD1 somatic mutations in polymorphous low-grade adenocarcinomas of the salivary glands. Nat Genet. 2014;46:1166–9.
48. Weinreb I, Zhang L, Tirunagari LM, et al. Novel PRKD gene rearrangements and variant fusions in cribriform adenocarcinoma of salivary gland origin. Genes Chromosomes Cancer. 2014;53:845–56.
49. Piscuoglio S, Fusco N, Ng CK, et al. Lack of PRKD2 and PRKD3 kinase domain somatic mutations in PRKD1 wild-type classic polymorphous low-grade adenocarcinomas of the salivary gland. Histopathology. 2016;68:1055–62.
50. Skalova A, Vanecek T, Sima R, et al. Mammary analogue secretory carcinoma of salivary glands, containing the ETV6-NTRK3 fusion gene: a hitherto undescribed salivary gland tumor entity. Am J Surg Pathol. 2010;34:599–608.
51. Connor A, Perez-Ordoñez B, Shago M, et al. Mammary analog secretory carcinoma of salivary gland origin with the ETV6 gene rearrangement by FISH: expanded morphologic and immunohistochemical spectrum of a recently described entity. Am J Surg Pathol. 2012;36:27–34.
52. Chiosea SI, Griffith C, Assaad A, et al. Clinicopathological characterization of mammary analogue secretory carcinoma of salivary glands. Histopathology. 2012;61:387–94.
53. Dalin MG, Desrichard A, Katabi N, et al. Comprehensive molecular characterization of salivary duct carcinoma reveals actionable targets and similarity to apocrine breast cancer. Clin Cancer Res. 2016;22(18):4623–33.
54. Bishop JA, Yonescu R, Batista D, et al. Most nonparotid "acinic cell carcinomas" represent mammary analog secretory carcinomas. Am J Surg Pathol. 2013;37:1053–7.

55. Oza N, Sanghvi K, Shet T, et al. Mammary analogue secretory carcinoma of parotid: is preoperative cytological diagnosis possible? Diagn Cytopathol. 2016;44:519–25.
56. Milchgrub S, Gnepp DR, Vuitch F, et al. Hyalinizing clear cell carcinoma of salivary gland. Am J Surg Pathol. 1994;18:74–82.
57. Milchgrub S, Vuitch F, Saboorian MH, et al. Hyalinizing clear cell carcinoma of salivary glands in fine needle aspiration. Diagn Cytopathol. 2000;23:333–7.
58. Antonescu CR, Katabi N, Zhang L, et al. EWSR1-ATF1 fusion is a novel and consistent finding in hyalinizing clear-cell carcinoma of salivary gland. Genes Chromosomes Cancer. 2011;50:559–70.
59. Bilodeau EA, Weinreb I, Antonescu CR, et al. Clear cell odontogenic carcinomas show EWSR1 rearrangements: a novel finding and a biological link to salivary clear cell carcinomas. Am J Surg Pathol. 2013;37:1001–5.
60. Shah AA, LeGallo RD, van Zante A, et al. EWSR1 genetic rearrangements in salivary gland tumors: a specific and very common feature of hyalinizing clear cell carcinoma. Am J Surg Pathol. 2013;37:571–8.
61. Thway K, Fisher C. Tumors with EWSR1-CREB1 and EWSR1-ATF1 fusions: the current status. Am J Surg Pathol. 2012;36:e1-e11.
62. Bishop JA, French CA, Ali SZ. Cytopathologic features of NUT midline carcinoma: a series of 26 specimens from 13 patients. Cancer Cytopathol. 2016;124(12):901–8.
63. Matsuyama A, Hisaoka M, Nagao Y, et al. Aberrant PLAG1 expression in pleomorphic adenomas of the salivary gland: a molecular genetic and immunohistochemical study. Virchows Arch. 2011;458:583–92.
64. Rotellini M, Palomba A, Baroni G, Franchi A. Diagnostic utility of PLAG1 immunohistochemical determination in salivary gland tumors. Appl Immunohistochem Mol Morphol. 2014;22:390–4.
65. Bahrami A, Dalton JD, Shivakumar B, et al. PLAG1 alteration in carcinoma ex pleomorphic adenoma: immunohistochemical and fluorescence in situ hybridization studies of 22 cases. Head Neck Pathol. 2012;6:328–35.
66. Moon A, Cohen C, Siddiqui MT. MYB expression: potential role in separating adenoid cystic carcinoma (ACC) from pleomorphic adenoma (PA). Diagn Cytopathol. 2016;44(10):799–804.
67. Rooper L, Sharma R, Bishop JA. Polymorphous low grade adenocarcinoma has a consistent p63+/p40− immunophenotype that helps distinguish it from adenoid cystic carcinoma and cellular pleomorphic adenoma. Head Neck Pathol. 2015;9:79–84.
68. Argyris PP, Wetzel SL, Greipp P, et al. Clinical utility of myb rearrangement detection and p63/p40 immunophenotyping in the diagnosis of adenoid cystic carcinoma of minor salivary glands: a pilot study. Oral Surg Oral Med Oral Pathol Oral Radiol. 2016;121:282–9.
69. Skálová A, Simpson RH, Lehtonen H, Leivo I. Assessment of proliferative activity using the MIB1 antibody help to distinguish polymorphous low grade adenocarcinoma from adenoid cystic carcinoma of salivary glands. Pathol Res Pract. 1997;193:695–703.
70. Jo VY, Sholl LM, Krane JF. Distinctive patterns of CTNNB1 (β-catenin) alterations in salivary gland basal cell adenoma and basal cell adenocarcinoma. Am J Surg Pathol. 2016;40:1143–50.
71. Wilson TC, Ma D, Tilak A, Tesdahl B, Robinson RA. Next-generation sequencing in salivary gland basal cell adenocarcinoma and basal cell adenoma. Head Neck Pathol. 2016;10(4):494–500.
72. Schmitt AC, McCormick R, Cohen C, Siddiqui MT. DOG1, p63, and S100 protein: a novel immunohistochemical panel in the differential diagnosis of oncocytic salivary gland neoplasms in fine-needle aspiration cell blocks. J Am Soc Cytopathol. 2014;3:303–8.
73. Hsieh MS, Lee YH, Chang YL. SOX10-positive salivary gland tumors: a growing list, including mammary analogue secretory carcinoma of the salivary gland, sialoblastoma, low-grade salivary duct carcinoma, basal cell adenoma/adenocarcinoma, and a subgroup of mucoepidermoid carcinoma. Hum Pathol. 2016;56:134–42.
74. Weinreb I, Seethala RR, Perez-Ordoñez B, Chetty R, Hoschar AP, Hunt JL. Oncocytic mucoepidermoid carcinoma: clinicopathologic description in a series of 12 cases. Am J Surg Pathol. 2009;33:409–16.

75. Kawahara A, Taira T, Abe H, et al. Diagnostic utility of phosphorylated signal transducer and activator of transcription 5 immunostaining in the diagnosis of mammary analogue secretory carcinoma of the salivary gland: a comparative study of salivary gland cancers. Cancer Cytopathol. 2015;123:603–11.

76. Marur S, D'Souza G, Westra WH, et al. HPV-associated head and neck cancer: a virus-related cancer epidemic. Lancet Oncol. 2010;11:781–9.

77. Rautava J, Syrjänen S. Biology of human papillomavirus infections in head and neck carcinogenesis. Head Neck Pathol. 2012;6:S3–15.

78. Paz IB, Cook N, Odom-Maryon T, et al. Human papillomavirus (HPV) in head and neck cancer. An association of HPV 16 with squamous cell carcinoma of Waldeyer's tonsillar ring. Cancer. 1997;79:595–604.

79. Fakhry C, Rosenthal BT, Clark DP, et al. Associations between oral HPV16 infection and cytopathology: evaluation of an oropharyngeal 'Pap-test equivalent' in high-risk populations. Cancer Prev Res. 2011;4:1378–84.

80. Jarboe EA, Willis M, Bentz B, et al. Detection of human papillomavirus using hybrid capture II in oral brushings from patients with oropharyngeal squamous cell carcinoma. Am J Clin Pathol. 2011;135:766–9.

81. Hafkamp HC, Manni JJ, Haesevoets A, et al. Marked differences in survival rate between smokers and nonsmokers with HPV 16-associated tonsillar carcinomas. Int J Cancer. 2008;122:2656–64.

82. Kobayashi K, Saito Y, Omura G, et al. Clinical features of human papilloma virus-related head and neck squamous cell carcinoma of an unknown primary site. ORL J Otorhinolaryngol Relat Spec. 2014;76:137–46.

83. Mirghani H, Amen F, Blanchard P, et al. Treatment de-escalation in HPV-positive oropharyngeal carcinoma: ongoing trials, critical issues and perspectives. Int J Cancer. 2015;136:1494–503.

84. Pusztaszeri MP, Faquin WC. Cytologic evaluation of cervical lymph node metastases from cancers of unknown primary origin. Semin Diagn Pathol. 2015;32:32–41.

85. Lewis JS Jr, Ukpo OC, Ma XJ, et al. Transcriptionally-active high-risk human papillomavirus is rare in oral cavity and laryngeal/hypopharyngeal squamous cell carcinomas–a tissue microarray study utilizing E6/E7 mRNA in situ hybridization. Histopathology. 2012;60:982–91.

86. Poling JS, Ma XJ, Bui S, et al. Human papillomavirus (HPV) status of non-tobacco related squamous cell carcinomas of the lateral tongue. Oral Oncol. 2014;50:306–10.

87. Bishop JA, Ma XJ, Wang H, et al. Detection of transcriptionally active high-risk HPV in patients with head and neck squamous cell carcinoma as visualized by a novel E6/E7 mRNA in situ hybridization method. Am J Surg Pathol. 2012;36:1874–82.

88. Chernock RD, Wang X, Gao G, et al. Detection and significance of human papillomavirus, CDKN2A(p16) and CDKN1A(p21) expression in squamous cell carcinoma of the larynx. Mod Pathol. 2013;26:223–31.

89. Robinson M, Suh YE, Paleri V, et al. Oncogenic human papillomavirus-associated nasopharyngeal carcinoma: an observational study of correlation with ethnicity, histological subtype and outcome in a UK population. Infect Agents Cancer. 2013;8:30.

90. Bishop JA, Guo TW, Smith DF, et al. Human papillomavirus-related carcinomas of the sinonasal tract. Am J Surg Pathol. 2013;37:185–92.

91. Protocol for the examination of specimens from patients with carcinomas of the pharynx. 2013. Accessed at http://www.cap.org/ShowProperty?nodePath=/UCMCon/Contribution%20Folders/WebContent/pdf/larynx-13protocol-3300.pdf.

92. Routine HPV Testing in head and neck squamous cell carcinoma. 2013. Accessed at https://www.cancercare.on.ca/common/pages/UserFile.aspx?fileId=279838.

93. Dataset for histopathology reporting of mucosal malignancies of the pharynx. 2013. Accessed at https://www.rcpath.org/resourceLibrary/g111_pharynxmucosaldataset_nov13-pdf.html.

94. Pai RK, Erickson J, Pourmand N, Kong CS. p16(INK4A) immunohistochemical staining may be helpful in distinguishing branchial cleft cysts from cystic squamous cell carcinomas originating in the oropharynx. Cancer. 2009;117:108–19.

95. Munger K, Baldwin A, Edwards KM, et al. Mechanisms of human papillomavirus-induced oncogenesis. J Virol. 2004;78:11451–60.
96. Schache AG, Liloglou T, Risk JM, et al. Evaluation of human papilloma virus diagnostic testing in oropharyngeal squamous cell carcinoma: sensitivity, specificity, and prognostic discrimination. Clin Cancer Res. 2011;17:6262–71.
97. Jordan RC, Lingen MW, Perez-Ordonez B, et al. Validation of methods for oropharyngeal cancer HPV status determination in US cooperative group trials. Am J Surg Pathol. 2012;36:945–54.
98. Lingen MW, Xiao W, Schmitt A, et al. Low etiologic fraction for high-risk human papillomavirus in oral cavity squamous cell carcinomas. Oral Oncol. 2013;49:1–8.
99. Begum S, Gillison ML, Nicol TL, Westra WH. Detection of human papillomavirus-16 in fine-needle aspirates to determine tumor origin in patients with metastatic squamous cell carcinoma of the head and neck. Clin Cancer Res. 2007;13:1186–91.
100. Ukpo OC, Flanagan JJ, Ma XJ, et al. High-risk human papillomavirus E6/E7 mRNA detection by a novel in situ hybridization assay strongly correlates with p16 expression and patient outcomes in oropharyngeal squamous cell carcinoma. Am J Surg Pathol. 2011;35:1343–150.
101. Kerr DA, Pitman MB, Sweeney B, et al. Performance of the Roche cobas 4800 high-risk human papillomavirus test in cytologic preparations of squamous cell carcinoma of the head and neck. Cancer Cytopathol. 2014;122:167–74.
102. Guo M, Khanna A, Dhillon J, et al. Cervista HPV assays for fine-needle aspiration specimens are a valid option for human papillomavirus testing in patients with oropharyngeal carcinoma. Cancer Cytopathol. 2014;122:96–103.
103. Bishop JA, Maleki Z, Valsamakis A, et al. Application of the hybrid capture II assay to squamous cell carcinomas of the head and neck: a convenient liquid-phase approach for the reliable determination of human papillomavirus status. Cancer Cytopathol. 2012;120:18–25.

Molecular Cytology Applications on the Lung

Alessia Di Lorito, Daniel Stieber, and Fernando C. Schmitt

5.1 Diagnosis

Lung cancer is the leading cause of cancer death among males in both more and less developed countries and has surpassed breast cancer as the leading cause of cancer death among females in more developed countries. According to the global cancer statistics, an estimated 1.8 million new lung cancer cases occurred in 2012, accounting for about 13% of total cancer diagnoses [1].

Lung carcinoma is generally categorized into non-small cell lung carcinoma (NSCLC) and small-cell carcinoma. Approximately 85% of lung cancers are of NSCLC type. NSCLCs include squamous cell carcinoma (SCC), adenocarcinoma (ADC), and large-cell carcinoma that is a combination of poorly differentiated ADC and other uncommon cell types. Historically, all subtypes of NSCLCs were given similar chemotherapy, so further categorization of NSCLC into ADC and SCC in the past was not important [2]. However, during the last years, the discovery of molecular alterations and the development of targeted therapies in NSCLC have pointed out the role of the classification of NSCLC into adenocarcinoma and squamous cell carcinomas. Recent advances in the treatment of lung cancer have

A. Di Lorito (✉)
Department of Medicine and Science of Aging, G. d'Annunzio University Chieti, Pescara, Italy

D. Stieber
National Health Laboratory, Dudelange, Luxembourg

F. C. Schmitt
Medical Faculty of Porto University, Porto, Portugal

I3S, Instituto de Investigação e Inovação em Saúde, Universidade do Porto, Porto, Portugal

IPATIMUP, Institute of Molecular Pathology and Immunology of Porto University, Porto, Portugal
e-mail: fschmitt@ipatimup.pt

demonstrated the efficacy of new drugs designed to block specific molecules and pathways involved in the tumor cell growth and survival [3–5].

In 2011, the International Association for the Study of Lung Cancer/American Thoracic Society/European Respiratory Society developed a new classification providing criteria and a standard terminology for the diagnosis of lung cancer in histology, in cytology, and in small biopsies. According to this classification, if clear squamous or adenocarcinoma differentiation is seen on morphology, a tumor can be diagnosed as SCC or ADC. In the cases in which morphology alone is not able to make a diagnosis, a panel of immunohistochemistry is mandatory [6, 7].

In fact, in the present era, lung cancer treatment is based on the subtype of lung cancer (ADC vs. SCC) and on the molecular status, that is, epidermal growth factor receptor (EGFR) or Kirsten rat sarcoma viral oncogene (KRAS) mutations or anaplastic lymphoma kinase (ALK) or proto-oncogene 1 receptor tyrosine kinase ROS1 rearrangements. An accurate diagnosis of NSCLC into ADC and SCC and the identification of the molecular status are necessary for the appropriate therapy [6–8].

5.2 Sampling

In NSCLCs, clinical trials have shown dramatic responses to targeted therapies [3–5, 9, 10]. Resected tumors were considered for a long time the only type of material for molecular tests. However, less than 30% of patients with NSCLC are eligible for surgical treatment, limiting the availability of neoplastic tissue for molecular tests [11, 12]. In fact, at the time of diagnosis, more than 60% of NSCLCs show unresectable stage IIIB or IV disease, where the only pathologic material accessible to make diagnosis and to determine therapy are small biopsy or cytology specimens [2, 13]. It is well demonstrated that cytology is a powerful tool in the diagnosis of lung cancer, in particular in the distinction of ADC from SCC. A previous study considered 192 preoperative cytology diagnoses: 88% were definitive, 8% favored, and 4% unclassified. When compared with the resection specimens, the accuracy of cytologic diagnosis was 93%, and for definitive diagnoses, it was 96%. For the ADC and SCC cases, only 3% of cases were unclassified, and the overall accuracy was 96%. When immunohistochemistry was used in 9% of these cases, the accuracy was 100% [2, 5].

The most frequently used techniques to obtain cytological material are bronchoscopy and fine-needle aspiration performed under imaging guidance (FNA). Other cytological samples comprise sputum and body cavity fluids/effusions, along with other minimally invasive aspirations of distant, deep-seated, or superficial metastatic lesions [14, 15].

Bronchoscopy specimens include bronchial brush, bronchial wash and aspirate, and bronchoalveolar lavage. In the bronchial brush, the material is collected by brushing the specific area identified with a little brush, which is inserted into smaller bronchi. The material can be immediately fixed in alcohol if a direct smear is performed or can be placed in a physiological solution and immediately sent to the laboratory. In the bronchial wash, aspirates of bronchial secretions and washes are performed with normal saline solution. The bronchoalveolar lavage is made by placing the bronchoscope into the selected segment of bronchus, inducing normal saline solution, and aspirating 20–50 mL aliquots in order to collect cells from bronchioles and alveoli [14, 15].

Fine-needle aspiration (transbronchial or transthoracic) is a simple, relatively safe, and rapid and reliable technique, which is performed under imaging guidance by ultrasounds or computed tomography, frequently coupled with core needle biopsies. It is a minimally painful and nonoperative procedure as compared to biopsy that is associated with higher risk of pneumothorax. Previous studies reported that the sensitivity of FNA for lung carcinoma diagnosis ranged from 50% to more than 90% and specificity was approximately 100%. The overall positive predictive value was nearly 99% with false-negative rate of around 10%. The false-negative rate is due to the failure of sampling [12, 16].

Transbronchial or transtracheal FNAs obtain samples by a flexible needle into a channel of a flexible bronchoscope placed through the tracheal or bronchial wall until reaching the area to be analyzed. The lesion is aspirated and the needle withdrawn [14, 15].

Percutaneous FNA is made under ultrasound or CT assistance, using a needle of 22 gauge or less, in order to obtain a core biopsy or a needle aspiration. The core biopsy is fixed in formalin solution and processed as are histological samples. If direct smears are performed, the slides, in general two, are immediately fixed, stained with Diff-Quik stains, and analyzed on site, the "ROSE" (rapid on-site evaluation) method. The other material obtained is sent to the laboratory in a physiological solution and processed according to the laboratory's procedures [14, 16].

During the on-site assessment, cytopathologist or experienced cytotechnologist prepares direct smears, using the contents expelled from the needle, at the location of the procedure. In this way, each needle pass can be examined to determine tumor cell adequacy; there is an opportunity to engage the clinical care provider in a conversation regarding the preliminary diagnosis and relevant molecular diagnostic tests; and the cytopathologist can help ensure that the specimen is processed in a manner that optimizes triage for ancillary tests, including molecular studies. Many works have demonstrated that the ROSE performed by a cytopathologist or experienced cytotechnologist has the potential to improve patient care by reducing the nondiagnostic and the false-negative rates, shortening procedure times, and preserving material for ancillary studies [12, 17, 18]. The main goal of ROSE is to prevent unnecessary repeat procedures to obtain additional tissue just for molecular studies, which can lead to delays in treatment. The ROSE reporting evaluates the on-site adequacy of the sampling, indicating, when it is possible, the diagnostic category [12].

Other technique largely used is the endobronchial ultrasound-guided transbronchial needle aspiration (EBUS-TBNA), considered as a major tool in the diagnosis of mediastinal abnormalities and used to stage lung cancer by the sampling of lymph node stations. Fluid samples are another important type of samples routinely sent to the cytopathology laboratory. The cytological evaluation of effusion samples determines the presence or the absence of malignant cells and if the lesion is primitive or metastasis. In many cases, samples show high cellularity, and applying an immunocytochemical panel is possible to correctly establish the primary site. The cell block preparation can be also obtained [14, 15].

5.3 Pre-Analytical Phase

Samples from aspirations are typically smeared directly onto glass slides, air-dried, or fixed in alcohol and stained using Diff-Quik or Papanicolaou stain. Hematoxylin-eosin (H&E) is the standard stain for histological material such as cell blocks and core biopsies [15].

Lung cytological samples can be also processed as liquid-based cytology (LBC), analogous to the processing of cervical cytology specimens, performed by collecting the needle rinse in an alcohol-based fixative and preparing a cell monolayer slide. LBC preparations include ThinPrep (Hologic, Bedford, MA, USA), SurePath (Becton Dickinson, Franklin Lakes, NJ, USA), thin-layer advanced cytology assay system (TACAS, MBL, Tokyo, Japan), and Liqui-PREP (LGM International Inc., Ft. Lauderdale, FL, USA). It is also possible to adopt both methods: smears and LBC [12]. The remaining LBC fixative fluid or the residual needle rinse from the aspiration can be also used for a paraffin-embedded, cellblock preparation. Body cavity fluids, bronchial brushings, bronchial washings, bronchoalveolar lavages, and sputum samples can be processed as cytospin preparations or as LBC, with or without cellblock preparations. Material derived from aspirates or effusions may have more tumor cells than a small biopsy obtained at the same time, so any positive cytology samples should be preserved as cellblocks. It is highly recommendable to preserve as much material as possible for potential molecular studies [5, 6].

Cellblocks are the most used lung cytological samples for molecular techniques [19–21]. The main advantages are that the majority of ancillary tests are validated for formalin-fixed paraffin-embedded (FFPE) sections. FFPE cellblocks are treated similarly to traditional surgical pathology FFPE blocks. Furthermore, multiple serial sections from cellblocks can be utilized to perform a battery of ancillary studies. However, in the institutions in which ROSE is performed, the cellblock preparation is based on the cellularity of the direct smears that not means the adequacy of the cellblocks for performing ancillary studies. In fact, it is possible, in some cases, that cellblock preparation can be paucicellular and inadequate for molecular testing, especially for techniques that require relatively large amounts of DNA. Indeed, not in all institutions, the rapid on-site evaluation is possible, and the preparation of the cellblock is variable across laboratories. In addition, the standard 4- to 5-micron cellblock sections do not represent the entire nuclei from the cell and are likely to have lower nucleic acid yields for molecula testing per cell compared to the whole sections utilized when only smears samples are available. Other important point is that cellblock is fixed in formalin, as the histological sections. For this reason, the nucleic acid extracted can be affected by sequencing artifacts, leading to possible false-negative and false-positive results in molecular reports, due to the cross-linking of nucleic acids and proteins [20, 21].

Regarding the possibility to use the cytology smears to perform the molecular analysis, in the past, cytopathologists were not agreeing to use them in order to save the slides for archival purpose. However, many studies have demonstrated how ancillary techniques as immunocytochemistry and molecular assays can be directly applied on smears and cytospin with the same results as observed for histological samples. Indeed, smears from FNA and cytospin provide a high-quality of nucleic acids, due to the use of air-dried and/or alcohol fixatives, as compared to formaldehyde-based fixatives used in histology [12, 22, 23].

Furthermore, recent reports have observed and demonstrated that cellularity on the order of 100–500 cells is sufficient for DNA sequencing-based assays while for fluorescence in situ hybridization (FISH) assays, 100 analyzable tumor cell nuclei are generally sufficient [12, 24]. In this point of view, FNA smears offer a suitable material to apply molecular tests, considering also the absence of stromal cells.

Following that, updated College of American Pathologists (CAP) guidelines reported that if other material is not available or sufficient to perform molecular tests, it is allowed to sacrifice the smears in order to make a molecular diagnosis. In cases in which the diagnostic material is on a single smear or cytospin sample, the slide can be scanned, or it is suggested to make a picture of the neoplastic cells for archival purpose and medicolegal reasons [25].

Regarding the liquid-based cytology (LBC), it is easy to obtain because it does not require a technical support for specimen adequacy as the ROSE method. In fact, the specimen is put into a cell preservative solution to be processed subsequently in the cytology laboratory as a cell monolayer slide. It is also possible to obtain a cell-block from this material. The advantages of LBC specimens are the optimal preservation of cells, the ease of specimen transportation because of the stability of cells at room temperature, and the minimal amount of background debris and blood on the slide. Many studies have well-performed molecular techniques on LBC samples or by scraping off cells from the slides or using directly the rinse solution for the DNA extraction. Indeed, LBC is largely used for FISH, while only few reports have demonstrated the possibility to apply FISH on direct smears [26].

5.4 Sequencing

Sequencing is routinely used in order to study EGFR and KRAS mutations in lung cancer cytology. It has been demonstrated that approximately 10–15% of NSCLC show sensitizing mutations in the EGFR gene and 30–40% harbor KRAS mutations, predominantly in lung adenocarcinomas [12].

The *epidermal growth factor receptor* (EGFR) gene encodes a transmembrane growth factor receptor that exhibits tyrosine kinase activity. Upon activation, intracellular signaling is mediated by cytoplasmic effectors in the RAS-RAF-MEK-ERK, PI3K, AKT, and STAT pathways [20, 21].

The presence of mutations in exons 18–21, the L858R missense mutation in exon 21, and deletions in exon 19 are the most commonly observed mutations and account for up to 90% of all EGFR mutations in this setting [27]. These mutations are more commonly associated with East Asian ethnicity, female gender, and nonsmoking history. However, these features are not a rule and should not be used to exclude lung cancer patients from mutation testing [5, 7].

Lung adenocarcinomas, harboring these sensitizing mutations in EGFR, have been shown to have relevant clinical responses to EGFR tyrosine kinase inhibitors

(TKIs) such as gefitinib (Iressa; AstraZeneca) or erlotinib (Tarceva;Genentech/ Roche). Clinical trials have shown that about 75–80% of patients with lung cancer carrying EGFR mutations obtained important radiographic responses to TKI treatment. In addition, progression-free survival (PFS) and overall survival (OS) were significantly better for EGFR-TKI-treated patients with EGFR mutations than those with EGFR wild type. Moreover, EGFR-mutated patients treated in the maintenance setting had a large benefit in terms of PFS [28].

However, several mechanisms of TKI resistance have been described. The most common are the presence of secondary mutation (T790M, C797S), the activation of alternative pathway of signaling (Tyrosine-protein kinase (MET), HGF, AXL, ERBB2, IGF-1R), the aberrance of the downstream pathways (AKT mutations, loss of phosphatase and tensin homolog (PTEN)), and the histological transformation [29].

Resistance is divided into intrinsic and secondary or acquired. Intrinsic resistance is usually defined as an immediate inefficacy of EGFR-TKIs, due to the presence of a nonsensitive EGFR mutation. The most important and frequent drug-resistant EGFR mutations are represented by an exon 20 insertion and the T790M mutation. Exon 20 insertion frequency ranges from 1% to 10% of the total number of EGFR mutations. This alteration causes reduced affinity for EGFR-TKIs. The T790M point mutation increases the affinity of EGFR for ATP and consequently attenuates the binding efficacy of EGFR-TKIs. The reported frequency of baseline EGFR T790M mutations varies in the literature mainly as a consequence of the detection method used. It seems that the presence of the baseline EGFR T790M mutation is associated with poor clinical outcomes in patients treated with EGFR-TKIs. The impact on responsiveness to EGFR-TKI therapy of the preexisting T790M mutation may depend on the proportion of pretreatment EGFR T790M-mutant alleles within a tumor that may range from a small subclone to one clonally dominant [29].

Secondary or acquired resistance typically occurs after prolonged treatment, and several molecular mechanisms have been suggested to contribute to the resistance phenotype. The most common are development of secondary mutations in the EGFR, phenotypic transformation, and the activation of alternative pathways. The most common secondary mutation responsible for acquisition of resistance occurs in exon 20 (T790M). The presence of the T790M mutation was observed in approximately 50% of the cases in which biopsy was obtained at the time of relapse following gefitinib or erlotinib treatment in patients with the exon 19 deletion or the L858R EGFR mutation.

The natural history of tumors harboring the T790M mutation could be indolent or with a rapid clinical decline and short survival. However in 2015, FDA has approved the use of AZD9291 (osimertinib, AstraZeneca) for the treatment of patients with metastatic EGFR-T790M mutation-positive NSCLCs, whose disease has progressed on or after EGFR-TKI therapy. On March 30, 2017, FDA granted regular approval to osimertinib, based on AURA3 (NCT012151981) trial, for patients with metastatic EGFR T790M mutation-positive NSCLC who had progressive disease following first-line EGFR-TKI therapy. All patients were required to have EGFR T790M mutation-positive NSCLC identified by the Cobas EGFR mutation assay (Roche), performed in a central laboratory. This assay was also FDA-approved as companion diagnostic kit.

Another resistant mechanism is the histological transformation from adenocarcinoma to small cell carcinoma (SCLC) and the epithelial-mesenchymal transformation (EMT). The histological transformation is possible probably because the cell of origin between adenocarcinoma and SCLC could be the same. Probably, SCLC cells originate from the minor preexistent cell clone under the selection pressure of EGFR-TKIs, or transdifferentiate from the adenocarcinoma cells, or arise from the multipotent stem cells. Instead, the EMT process is linked to the loss of polarity and cell-cell contacts by the epithelial cell layers, which undergo a dramatic remodeling of their cytoskeleton. In this way, cells acquire expression of mesenchymal components, with the loss of E-cadherin expression and the upregulation of mesenchymal proteins such as vimentin, fibronectin, and N-cadherin.

This knowledge has led to identify the molecular mechanism driving disease progression. Repeat biopsy or cytological sampling and molecular testing to identify EGFR T790M or MET amplification or histological transformation are now required.

However, repeating biopsy or cytology sampling is limited by its invasive nature, risk of complications, and potential for delaying subsequent therapy. Indeed, it could be possible that biopsy of a single metastatic site may not be representative of the resistance mechanism in other metastatic sites. Increasing data have demonstrated that plasma genotyping of cell-free DNA (cfDNA) allows for the rapid and noninvasive detection of EGFR mutations, in particular the T790M point mutation. Various platforms for plasma genotyping exist with variable levels of validation. Plasma genotyping may be particularly useful for patients in which repeating tissue sampling is not feasible while also having the potential to detect EGFR T790M mutations that are missed by standard tissue genotyping. If the positive result of the test is considered "actionable," a negative plasma result may mean the absence of a mutation or that a patient's tumor is not shedding cfDNA at detectable levels. In these cases, it is necessary to confirm the result on tissue biopsy to rule out a false-negative plasma result [29, 30].

RAS (*rat sarcoma viral oncogene homolog*) genes are members of the guanidine triphosphatase (GTPase) gene superfamily. *KRAS, HRAS (Harvey rat sarcoma viral oncogene homologue)*, and *NRAS (Neuroblastoma RAS viral oncogene homolog)* encode for 21-kd proteins that share considerable sequence homology and have common intrinsic GTPase activity to hydrolyze guanidine triphosphate to guanidine diphosphate. Ras transduces the EGFR activation signal to multiple downstream pathways, and activated Ras-guanidine triphosphate is switched off by the intrinsic GTPase activity of Ras protein. *RAS* mutations on codons 12, 13, and 61 result in inhibition of GTPase activity, thus leading to the constitutive activation of Ras protein, which may render tumor cells independent of EGFR signaling and thereby resistant to EGFR-TKI therapy.

Many trials reported that lung adenocarcinoma patients with *KRAS* mutations are not responsive to gefitinib or erlotinib. Studies demonstrated KRAS mutation frequency of 26% in current/former smokers and 6% in never-smoker patients [5, 7, 31].

The clinical relevance of EGFR and KRAS mutational status has been deeply discussed in recent years, and testing for these mutations has rapidly become a standard practice. EGFR and KRAS mutations are commonly checked via polymerase chain reaction (PCR) and sequencing-based approaches. Direct Sanger sequencing is considered the gold standard due to the acquisition of direct DNA sequence. Using this method, the presence of all potential mutations including common, known mutations and novel mutations is demonstrated. However, the analytic sensitivity of Sanger sequencing is 20–25% mutant allele that means the presence of at least 40–50% of cancer cells due to the heterozygous nature of mutations, without any amplification [7, 32–34]. In fact, this method requires a higher enrichment of tumor cell DNA content in samples [14]. However, the enrichment could be a problem in small biopsy and cytological samples, including cellblocks in which the background with benign cells such as inflammatory cells, normal epithelial cells, and stromal cells is prominent in many cases. This means that if a sample is negative for mutations, this result can be due to the real absence of the mutation in the tumor cells or to the percentage of tumor content that is not sufficient to reach the analytic sensitivity threshold, resulting in the failure to detect the mutation even, despite the presence of the mutation [12, 23, 33]. Furthermore, in these cases, a possible strategy is to enrich the tumor content by manual or laser capture microdissection before DNA extraction and sequencing by demarcating tumor-rich areas directly on the slide. For cellblock sections, the circled hematoxylin-eosin-stained slide can be used to guide tissue extraction from unstained sections, whereas for smear/cytospin/LBC preparations, the de-coverslipped slide is scraped on the bottom using a diamond-tip pen for tissue extraction from designated tumor-rich areas.

However, this procedure is time-consuming and not suitable for all routine diagnosis. In addition, cross contaminations and artifactual genomic changes could be encountered with working with low amount of DNA [33]. Indeed, Sanger sequencing is relatively more labor-intensive and time-consuming and can lead to longer turnaround times [34].

Other PCR-based techniques, such as peptide nucleic acid (PNA)-locked PCR clamping [27], allele-specific quantitative real-time PCR [35], and scorpion ARMS (amplification refractory mutation system) [36], have been developed for sensitive detection of somatic mutations. Several commercial kits have been developed and extensively clinically validated based on these methods especially for the detection of mutations in the EGFR and KRAS and NRAS genes. New developments are underway in order to automatize and streamline the whole genotyping procedure. An example of this is the Idylla system from Biocartis which automatizes nucleic acid extraction and multiplex target detection in cartridge-based design.

These techniques can check the mutations for which they have been developed (known mutation), and the sensitivity obtained does not exceed 1:100. The main limitation of these techniques is that they require multiple PCRs and therefore an adequate amount of gDNA, not always available when working with cytological samples. The advantages of these approaches include their improved analytic sensitivity and less time-consuming nature leading to reduced turnaround times [11].

Several studies of comparison between Sanger sequencing and these techniques have demonstrated a higher sensitivity and greater ease of use for assessing the mutation status of these techniques in samples with low amount of gDNA (as cytology specimens) or prestained NSCLC clinical samples [37].

Non-sequencing-based procedures for mutation detection, more sensitive than Sanger sequencing, such as high-resolution melting (HRM) and restriction fragment length polymorphism (RFLP), have also been used on cytological samples. However, these procedures are screening tests that give indirect evidence of the mutation status, requiring sequencing to accurately identify the type of mutation revealed [38].

Depending on the methods used, previous studies reported the detection of these mutations in cytology samples containing 0.1–10% of tumor cells or in specimens containing at least 100 tumor cells. The failure rate of EGFR and KRAS molecular testing reported in the literature on cytology samples ranges from 2 to 8%. This value depends on the technique utilized and on the quality (especially low tumor content and high content of nonneoplastic cells) of the material used [39].

Although the choice of platform used for the detection of EGFR/KRAS mutations remains a decision of the individual molecular laboratories performing the assay, the 2013 CAP/IASLC/AMP guidelines recommended that the technique utilized detect mutations in samples with at least 50% tumor component. Furthermore, more sensitive platforms that are able to detect mutations in specimens with as little as 10% tumor are strongly encouraged. It is also recommended that the platform utilized to check alterations should be able to detect all mutations reported in the literature with a frequency of at least 1% [7].

In 2018, CAP/IASLC/AMP have published the update of the 2013 molecular NSCLC testing guidelines, recommended to test EGFR/ALK/ROS1 gene alterations before treatment. Multiplexed genetic sequencing panels (e.g., NGS testing) are preferred over multiple single-gene tests to identify other treatment options beyond EGFR, ALK, and ROS1, however single gene assays are still acceptable. Several other genes are also reported as important to be tested – BRAF, ERBB2, MET, RET, and KRAS. However, these genes are not essential when only single gene tests are performed and could be tested in EGFR/ALK/ROS1 negative carcinomas. Indeed in these updated guidelines as expert consensus opinion suggestion, "laboratories should use, or have available at an external reference laboratory, clinical lung cancer biomarker molecular testing assays that are able to detect molecular alterations in specimens with as little as 20% cancer cells". Expert recommended also to pathologists to use either cell blocks or other cytologic preparations as suitable specimens for lung cancer biomarker molecular testing [40].

5.5 FISH

Fluorescence in situ hybridization (FISH) is considered gold standard method to detect rearrangements in NSCLCs. It can be applied on all lung cytology specimens such as smears, cytospin, LBC, cellblocks, and stained slides, also after immunocytochemistry [41].

Recently, preclinical and clinical data have demonstrated the efficacy of the kinase inhibitor crizotinib to treat a subset of NSCLCs harboring ALK and ROS1 gene rearrangements and MET amplification. Indeed, the clinical importance of other genes such as REarranged during Transfection (RET) is currently under investigations in NSCLCs [42].

The *anaplastic lymphoma kinase* (ALK) gene encodes a receptor tyrosine kinase that is normally not expressed in lung cells. Approximately 3–5% of unselected NSCLCs show *ALK* gene rearrangements, enriched by testing only EGFR and KRAS wild-type carcinomas. ALK rearrangements as oncogenic drivers in NSCLC were discovered in 2007 by Soda et al. [43]. The most common rearrangement is a small intrachromosomal inversion, inv(2)(p21;p23), resulting in the fusion of *ALK* with echinoderm microtubule-associated protein-like 4 gene. The *ALK*/echinoderm microtubule-associated protein-like 4 fusion (EML4) produces an abnormal, constitutively active chimeric protein kinase which leads to aberrant ALK expression and constitutive activation of downstream signaling pathways involved in tumor cell survival [43].

The ALK breakpoint is located at exon 20, while EML4 shows different breakpoints in the amino terminal that means different EML4-ALK fusion variants, comprising different EML4-ALK protein isoforms. Other ALK fusion partners have been also reported, as FHIT and KBI47. All ALK fusion variants maintain the kinase domain that is predictive for crizotinib responsiveness. Targeted ALK tyrosine kinase inhibitors have proven anticancer activity, with crizotinib showing a good clinical response in advanced NSCLC patients harboring *ALK* rearrangements. Second-generation ALK inhibitors, such as alectinib and ceritinib, are effective not only in crizotinib-naïve patients but also in those patients with acquired resistance to crizotinib [44]. The US Food and Drug Administration approved an in vitro diagnostic class fluorescence in situ hybridization (FISH) test as a companion diagnostic tool for crizotinib-based treatment eligibility (Abbott Molecular Vysis [AMV], Des Plaines, IL). As a consequence, FISH is currently considered the definitive standard for *ALK* status testing. The commercial break-apart FISH format is made up of two probes labeled with SpectrumOrange and SpectrumGreen that flank the highly conserved translocation breakpoint within *ALK* gene. The SpectrumOrange-labeled probe includes the tyrosine kinase domain at the 3′ end, so it is able to detect all ALK rearrangements irrespective of the fusion partner, and it has been validated in clinical trials [45, 46].

Normal cells exhibit red and green signals, which are immediately adjacent to each other or fused (yellow) (Fig. 5.1a). If there is the ALK rearrangement caused by intrachromosomal inversion, there is a break-apart signal (single red and single green signal with a signal separation distance of at least 2 signal diameters). Another cytogenetic rearrangement pattern occurring in approximately 30% of all ALK-rearranged NSCLCs is intrachromosomal inversion followed by deletion of the 5′ end of the chromosome, leading to a single red signal without presence of a corresponding green signal. The presence of a single green signal pattern without presence of a corresponding red signal is not indicative of rearrangement, because the 5′ green signal does not include the kinase domain, and therefore the drug target is not

Fig. 5.1 (**a**) Lung adenocarcinoma FNA and FISH of ALK-negative case. FISH image shows signals adjacent and less than two signal diameters apart. (**b**) Lung adenocarcinoma FNA and FISH of ALK-positive case. FISH image shows broken-apart signals more than two signal diameters apart

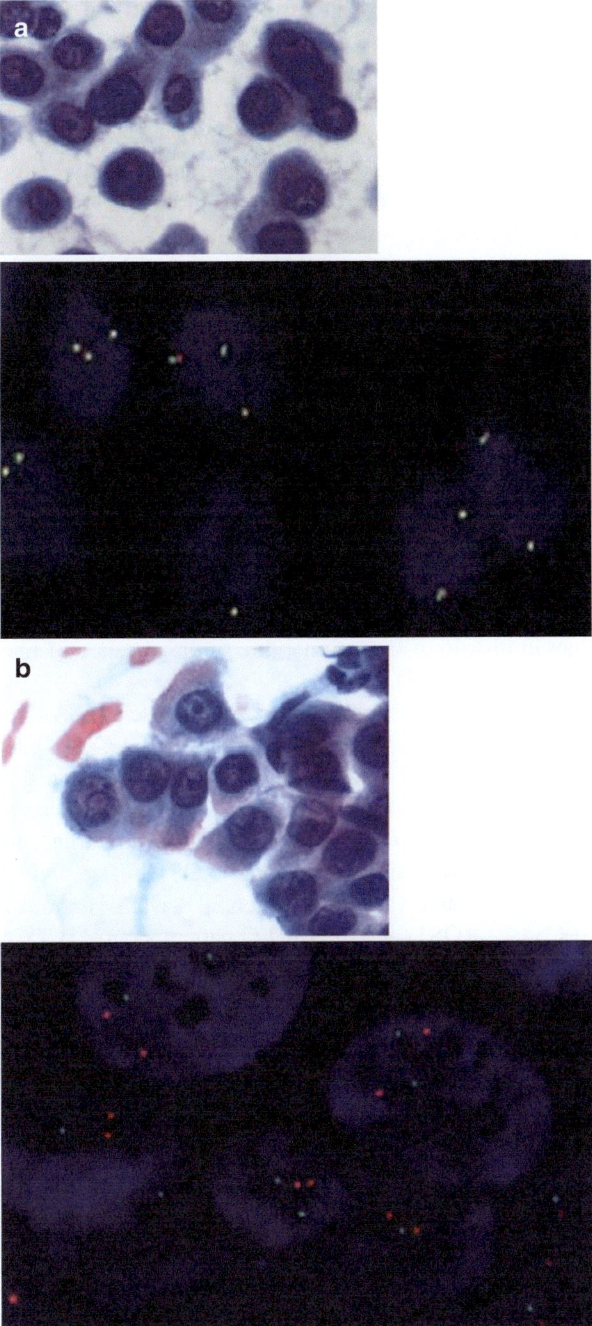

present. In summary, a case is defined as positive for ALK rearrangement if neoplastic cells show a break-apart signal or a single red signal. It is necessary to score at least 50 cancer cell nuclei, and a case is interpreted as *ALK*-positive by FISH when 15% or more tumor cell nuclei demonstrate isolated green and red signals or isolated red signals, among 50 tumor nuclei scored [46, 47] (Fig. 5.1b). It is also common an increased copy number of native ALK signals due to chromosome 2 polysomy, due to the overall aneuploidy of NSCLC. Recently, FISH platforms including imaging and capturing software have been developed; the imaging system makes the evaluation of these multiple FISH signals much easier on z-stacked images on a computer screen. In literature, it is reported that cytological specimens are suitable for FISH assessment, reporting feasibility of ALK FISH on cytology ranging from 79% to 97%. In several studies, FISH makes a diagnosis in at least 80–90% of samples. Some studies comparing FISH results between cytology (direct smears and cell blocks) and small biopsies as well as between direct cytological smear and cell blocks indicate that FISH analysis is more adequate when conducted on cytology and that insufficient cellularity occurs more frequently in cell blocks than in direct smears. Some authors suggest that direct smears represent the elective material for FISH assay, allowing to immediately verify the adequacy of the sample and avoiding the delay of FFPE procedure and related technical problems as fixation artifacts. Moreover, direct smear allows a more accurate signal enumeration than in histological sections, due to the absence of overlapping nuclei and nuclear truncation [47, 48].

Other oncogenic receptor tyrosine kinase (RTK) gene rearrangements with a clinical significance have been reported in NSCLCs. In particular, recent advances have identified the *ROS1* (c-ros oncogene 1, located at 6q22) gene rearrangements in NSCLC. The ROS1 gene encodes a receptor tyrosine kinase of the insulin receptor family. To date, no ROS1 ligand has been identified, but cellular attachment via its extracellular domain could trigger ROS1 kinase activation. Rikova et al. identified two ROS1 fusion variants as potential driver mutations in NSCLC cell line (HCC78; SLC34A2-ROS1) and in NSCLC patient sample (CD74-ROS1) [49]. All these rearrangements have a highly conserved breakpoint region in the RTK gene with a retained kinase domain and various breakpoints in the fusion partner, leading to different fusion variants. More recently, five additional fusion partners (TPM3, SDC4, EZR, LRIG3, FIG) to ROS1 have been identified, representing 12 ROS1 fusion variants in NSCLC. ROS1 kinase modifications lead to a constitutive activation of the kinase and of the downstream signaling of several oncogenic pathways, controlling cell proliferation and survival and cell cycling such as STAT3, PI3K/AKT/mTOR, and RAS-MAPK/ERK pathways. The first two major works described ROS1 rearrangements in 0.9–1.7% NSCLC cases and, remarkably, only in wild-type EGFR, KRAS, and ALK lung adenocarcinomas. Recently, the phase 1 trial results showed that ROS1 fusions in NSCLC are associated with sensitivity to the ALK/MET inhibitor crizotinib. In fact, the amino acid sequence of ROS1 and ALK is similar within the tyrosine kinase domains, and the crizotinib-binding site is nearly identical. So that, ROS1 has emerged as a new molecular subtype and now comprises a distinct molecular classification. Bergethon et al. identified ROS1 rearrangements in 18 (1.7%) of 1073 patients with NSCLC using FISH and suggested that ROS1

Fig. 5.2 Lung adenocarcinoma FNA and FISH of ROS1-positive case. FISH image shows signals adjacent and broken-apart signals (more than two signal diameters apart)

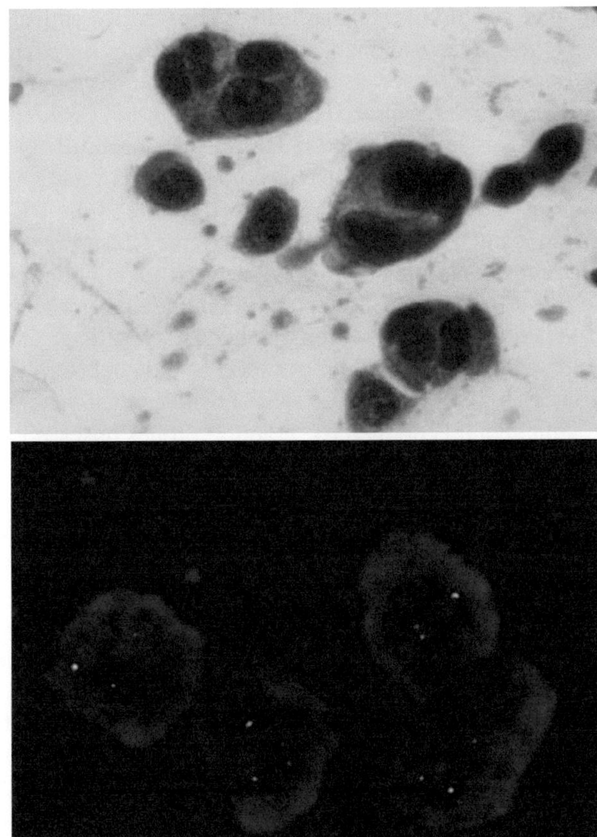

rearrangements define a unique molecular subset of lung cancer with distinct clinical features [50]. These clinicopathologic characteristics included younger patient age (median age, approximately 50 years), adenocarcinoma subtype, and never smokers, also associated with both EGFR mutations and ALK rearrangements [49, 50]. ROS1 rearrangements are evaluated also by FISH, using a break-apart FISH assay, commercially available. Regarding the probe mix, the distal (5′) ROS1 region probe is direct-labeled with SpectrumOrange, while the proximal (3′) ROS1 region probe is direct-labeled with SpectrumGreen. Tumor tissues are considered as ROS1 FISH positive (ROS1-rearranged) if >15% tumor cells show split red and green signals (signals separated by ≥1 signal diameter) and/or single 3′ signals. Otherwise, the samples are considered as FISH negative (80) (Fig. 5.2).

Recently, rearrangements in the rearranged during transfection proto-oncogene RET have been described also in NSCLCs. RET gene encodes a receptor tyrosine kinase for members of the glial cell line-derived neurotrophic factor family of extracellular signaling molecules. The gene is located on chromosome 10q11.2. Chromosomal rearrangements generate a fusion gene consisting of the juxtaposition of the C-terminal region of the RET protein with the N-terminal portion of another protein. It can also lead to constitutive activation of the RET kinase. The RET gene rearrangements, as represented by papillary thyroid carcinoma, were most often observed as coiled-coil domain-containing 6 (CCDC6)-RET (PTC1) and nuclear receptor coactivator 4 (NCOA4)-RET (PTC3) fusion genes. Rearrangements involving RET are most commonly interchromosomal. Several studies have simultaneously reported a novel fusion gene comprising parts of the kinesin family member 5B gene (KIF5B) and the RET gene in lung carcinomas. Subsequently, other fusion partners of the RET genes CCDC6, NCOA4, and tripartite motif containing 33 (TRIM33) were identified in NSCLCs. These fusion transcripts were detected in 0.6–10% of lung adenocarcinomas. The RET rearrangements have been observed in younger patients, patients with no smoking history, and solid and papillary. These fusion genes did not coexist with EGFR and ALK alterations. Sample is considered FISH positive when there's a break-apart (split) signal. A split signal is defined by 5′ and 3′ probes observed at a distance of greater than onefold the signal size. A FISH positive case is defined as more than 15% of tumor cells have any split signals or any isolated 3′ (green) signals [41]. Several RET inhibitors (sunitinib, sorafenib, and vandetanib) are currently studied in clinical trials in RET-rearranged NSCLCs. The first reports published show very promising results [51, 52].

FISH is utilized also to study MET amplification. *MET* gene amplification has been reported in many primary human tumors, and it acts as primary "oncogenic driver" in TKI-naïve lung adenocarcinomas [53, 54]. The rate of MET amplification in NSCLC remains controversial and ranges from 3% to up to 10% depending on the detection technique and cutoff criteria. Furthermore, MET overexpression in NSCLC is variable, ranging from 5% to 75% [53, 54]. *MET* amplification has also been described as a secondary event, both in preclinical and clinical studies, in EGFR-TKI-resistant NSCLC after treatment with gefitinib or erlotinib with a frequency ranging from 5% to 25%. In this NSCLC population, TKI treatment specifically selects preexisting *MET*-amplified clones in which the ERBB3/PI3K/AKT signaling pathway is active, suggesting the potential impact of a concomitant blockade of MET for overcoming EGFR-TKI resistance [55]. Crizotinib at the beginning was developed as a MET inhibitor; in fact in the presence of MET amplification, NSCLCs respond also to this targeted drug. The commercial FISH kit is made up of probes labeled with SpectrumRed that recognize MET gene and SpectrumGreen direct against the centromere of the chromosome 7. The presence of MET gene amplification is defined by the presence of tight gene clusters and a ratio of *MET* to chromosome 7 of 2 or more than 5 copies of *MET* per cell in 10% of cells, according to the criteria reported in literature [54].

5.6   RT-PCR

Reverse transcriptase polymerase chain reaction (RT-PCR) and quantitative reverse transcription-polymerase chain reaction (qRT-PCR) are alternative diagnostic assays used to improve the sensitivity and accuracy of sequencing to study molecular alterations in NSCLCs. Studies have demonstrated the feasibility of LBC preparations and the utility of fresh and archival cytology specimens (including slides prepared from liquid-based cytology platforms) as useful templates for RT-PCR/qRT-PCR analysis [55]. RT-PCR or qRT-PCR analysis can be successfully performed with limited amounts of material such as FNA cytology (1–2 µg) because they are extremely sensitive techniques and amplification results can be obtained with total RNA template levels in the range of 10 pg–1 µg per reaction. There is also clinical utility for the performance of RT-PCR on archival FNA cytology material with the slide-scrape-lysate procedure. Tumor cell enrichment is not usually necessary for the detection of fusion mRNA transcripts by RT-PCR or qRT-PCR analysis because of the high analytic sensitivity of the procedure (1 tumor cell in 104–105 total mononuclear cells) [56].

The mutations of EGFR and KRAS gene can be studied by sensitive methods with real-time quantitative PCR, using specific probes or amplification refractory mutation system (ARMS) technology. Scorpion ARMS technology is based on the preferential amplification of the excess mutant allele. Because it can detect 1% of mutated *EGFR* in a wild-type DNA background, this method requires only a few neoplastic cells even in heterogeneous samples such as cytological specimens [57]. Studies of comparison between FFPE and cytological samples have demonstrated the applicability of RT-PCR on cytological samples, showing high concordance rates between histological and cytological samples. The possibility to detect EGFR mutations even in bronchial washing fluid or pleural and ascitic fluids with a few neoplastic cells against a wide background of normal cells has been also reported. It has successfully been applied by some authors on RNA obtained by scraping cells from diagnostic glass slides by manual microdissection with a surgical blade [24, 48]. The minimum tumor cell percentage and tumor cell count required for EGFR mutation testing in cytological materials depend on the platform used. This minimum was published as 10% and 16 cells for RT-PCR [24, 58]. Tumor cell enrichment will increase this sensitivity if tumor cells are <10% of the sample cell population. The adequacy of the samples in terms of tumor cell content can be established by a pathologist revision of cytology slides [59].

Several studies have utilized a multiplex RT-PCR system to check ALK and ROS1 rearrangements, demonstrating that there is a high concordance between the RT-PCR results with FISH, and it has been confirmed that RT-PCR is a reliable technique for the diagnosis of EML4-ALK [60, 61]. The EML4/ALK fusion has been detected by qRT-PCR with RNA isolated from either Diff-Quik- and Papanicolaou-stained smears obtained from lung adenocarcinomas, demonstrating the detection of EML4/ALK fusion with 1% molecular alteration rate [62].

However, some limitations avoid its full implementation in the clinical setting. RT-PCR is the most sensitive method (compared to FISH, immunocytochemistry (ICC), and sequencing) and can identify different variants or rearrangement partners. However, it cannot cover the unknown rearrangements. In fact, multiplex RT-PCR assays for the detection of all the different *ALK* rearrangements require continuous optimization, given the increasing numbers of fusion variants and partners identified. Secondly, more recent reverse transcription quantitative real-time

PCR (RT-qPCR) assays based on the unbalanced expression of the 5′ and 3′ portions of the *ALK* transcript, which occurs when *ALK* is rearranged, require significant amounts of RNA (50–100 ng per PCR reaction) [63].

5.7 Next-Generation Sequencing (NGS)

Fast technologic advances have made next-generation sequencing (NGS) platforms affordable, and those are increasingly becoming available in routine pathology laboratories. The two most widely used benchtop instruments in pathology laboratories are the IonTorrent phosphoglucomutase-1 (PGM) and the Illumina MiSeq. Both machines have their distinct advantages and pitfalls, mainly linked to the different sequencing chemistries used. Several other benchtop instruments formed by these vendors have also been recently released (Illumina NextSeq and MiniSeq and IonTorrent S5) addressing different throughput needs. With the advent of these platforms, there are no main limitations for the application of NGS in clinical practice. The complete sequencing protocol from nucleic extraction to sequencing data analysis is typically performed in 2–3 working days with multiple samples sequenced in parallel in one sequencing run. This makes the technology affordable; typical reagents costs per sample are now in the range of 200–300€ if five to ten samples are batched. The costs are thus comparable to other CE-IVD marked kits for the interrogation of hotspot mutations in the EGFR gene alone. The major advantage of NGS over these methods is its ability to produce an important amount of data per sample which allows the parallel interrogation of multiple genes (by panel-based sequencing) with significantly lower cost and sample requirements than multiple single-gene analysis [64].

Ultradeep massively parallel sequencing allows reaching a sensitivity of 1:10,000 in dilution experiments, meaning the method is about 100 times more sensitive than RT-PCR and PNA-LNA clamp and 1000 times more sensitive than Sanger sequencing. In clinical practice, a detection limit of 1–3% is normally applied owing to the intrinsic error rate of the sequencing methods and the ability to bioinformatically delineate true variants from sequencing artifacts. It is important to note that the actual detection limit correlates with the average sequencing depth per base that is used in a given sequencing run. For somatic mutations, a good starting point is to have a minimum coverage of 1000×. This means that for a 1% variant, the actual molecular event is observed ten times.

Whole- genome and whole exome sequencing approaches are not yet economically feasible on a regular basis in a clinical setting for most laboratories. Thus, in a current clinical diagnostic setting, the primary application of NGS in molecular pathology is in gene panel sequencing. Several commercially available panels have been developed which allow for the sequencing of multiple genes or cancer-relevant hotspot regions in parallel. This panel is intended to identify somatic variants in genes linked to diagnostic, prognostic, or theranostic features in solid tumors. Some of these panels are specifically aimed at the detection of mutations and/or gene fusions relevant to NSCLCs. Different panel sizes are available from 15 to >200 genes. The gene content of the panels varies by manufacturer. Typically, it is based on a list of genes compiled, for the relevant cancer type(s), from curated databases such as the Cancer Gene Census or COSMIC (Catalogue of Somatic Mutations in Cancer) and whole genome/exome sequencing studies from scientific networks including the Cancer Genome Atlas.

For NSCLC, a useful set of genes would include AKT1, ALK, APC, ATM, BAI3, BAP1, BRAF, CDKN2A, EGFR, EPHA5, ERBB2, ERBB4, FBXW7, FGFR1, FGFR2, GRM8, KDR, KEAP1, KIT, KMT2D, KRAS, LRP1B, MDM2, MET, MLH1, MUC16, MYC, NF1, NFE2L2, NOTCH1, PDGFRA, PIK3CA, PIK3CG, PKHD1, PTEN, RARB, RB1, RET, ROS1, RUNX1T1, SMAD4, SMARCA4, SOX2, STK11, and TP53 (Human Lung Cancer GeneRead DNAseq Targeted Panel V2 from Qiagen), but many other options exist, and it is up to the molecular pathology laboratory to decide which panel should be implemented. In general, these panels rely either on liquid-phase capture or on PCR amplification for target enrichment. Capture-based enrichment is based on the use of nucleic acid baits (DNA or RNA depending on the technology) to capture the parts of the genome which are intended to be sequenced. The probes are designed to overlap partially which allows for a tilling coverage of the region of interest. The main advantages of this method are a higher specificity and the avoidance of sequencing artifacts or PCR-induced errors, as multiple independent individual molecules cover each base (tilling). A major drawback of this method, especially about lung cytopathology, is the substantial amount of high-quality DNA (100 ng or more) which is typically needed for capture strategies. Amplicon-based enrichment on the other hand relies on the specific amplification of the regions of interest, typically using multiplex PCR reactions. One advantage of the amplicon method is that very little starting material is required (typically 20 ng of DNA or less); the main pitfalls of this strategy are the nonhomogeneity of sequencing coverage among different amplicons and the risk of allelic dropouts. In both technologies, the samples are individually indexed and subsequently pooled for sequencing.

As most currently available NGS panels do not have a CE-IVD marking yet, in accredited laboratories, these have to be validated before being used for diagnostic purposes. Guidelines for clinical validation of NGS panels were recently published [65]. In that regard, the inclusion of reference materials in the validation process and in the routine clinical practice can be helpful as it allows to establish the specificity, the sensitivity, and the limit of detection of the method. In routine use, the utilization of reference samples in each run allows to monitor the stability of the reagents and the reproducibility of the downstream analysis platform. Reference materials (e.g., from Horizon Discovery) are typically composed of cell lines which have been engineered to harbor specific mutations. Different cell lines having distinct mutations are then mixed together in different proportions to have mutations at distinct allele frequencies and are treated as would be clinical samples, for instance, by formalin fixation and paraffin embedding. Recently in an interlaboratory ring trial study it has been demonstrated that the next-generation sequencing and other multigene mutational assays are robust and accurate in cytological samples. In particular, the performance of laboratories using next-generation sequencing is excellent, regardless of the platform or gene panel type [66].

Furthermore, careful selection, optimization, and validation of the bioinformatics pipeline are important as the analytical settings and the filtering strategy greatly influence the list of variants reported from NGS data. Many variant calling tools have been developed and most are freely available, and some of those are specifically aimed at the analysis of somatic samples (e.g., MuTect, Strelka, VarScan2, and others). It is important to note that bioinformatically trained users should use these tools as small changes in the software setting can result in the reporting of false positives and/or false negatives. This is especially acute for tumor-poor or genetically heterogeneous samples as these often contain mutations at a low allele frequency where it is crucial to reliably delineate true mutations from sequencing artifacts. Most sequencing kit vendors now address this problem by bundling their products with a dedicated analytical pipeline, which is accessible to their customers.

Regarding the sample type, FFPE samples have long been considered to be optimal for molecular studies; however, studies recently published have demonstrated the applicability of NGS on lung cytology specimens [66–68]. Protocol optimization for enrichment methods has led to the possibility to use NGS even with limited amount of starting material. Some library preparation methods, mainly based on multiplex PCR, can be used with as little as 10 ng of DNA. It is important to note that this is a best-case scenario for good-quality DNA. In practice, the amount a starting material to be used depends also on the quality of the extracted DNA. Several methods exist to describe the amount of "amplifiable" DNA in a sample (e.g., by qPCR), and the laboratory then has to adjust the input quantity accordingly. This is an important problem for formalin-fixed samples as fixation inevitably leads to a degradation of nucleic acids, the DNA extracted from FFPE samples is rarely of the best quality, and thus the input quantity has to be adjusted. Cytological samples typically fare better in that regard.

Several studies have recently highlighted the possibility to effectively use panel-based NGS in lung cancer cytology. Buttitta et al. [69] analyzed 48 samples (Bronchoalveolar lavage (BAL) and pleural fluid) from patients with EGFR mutations in resected tumors. These samples included 36 cases with 0.3–9% of neoplastic cells (series A) and 12 cases without evidence of tumor (series B). All samples were analyzed by Sanger sequencing and NGS on the Roche 454 platform. Interestingly, EGFR mutations were found in 42% of the samples without cytopathologic evidence of neoplastic cells. The EGFR mutations discovered in the cytology samples were exactly corresponding to those detected in tumor tissue. Most of the specimens analyzed were bronchial washing and pleural effusions, particularly dirty, with large and thick cell conglomerates that obscured morphology in many areas. These findings indicated the high sensitivity of the NGS diagnostic approach to detect somatic mutations of frequently mutated genes in lung tumors (i.e., p53, KRAS, EGFR) [69].

More recently, others analyzed a large series of gene mutations applying the IonTorrent platform in order to screen for mutations in 89 cases of lung adenocarcinoma metastatic lymph node specimens obtained by fine-needle aspiration cytology (FNAC) [70]. They found mutations in known and unknown genes, with the possibility to promote the development of new targeted therapies. Furthermore, other authors have demonstrated the feasibility of using NGS-based methods to perform gene mutation analysis in routine cytological specimens obtained by FNA, including stained smears and cell blocks demonstrating that mutational profiling of multiple genes is possible using an extremely low quantity of DNA, which can be extracted from specimens obtained by FNA, thereby enhancing the utility of the FNA approach [65].

The success of the NGS approach in detecting single nucleotide variants (SNV) and indels from DNA will most likely be replicated with new applications on RNA. Several panels have now been developed which allow to interrogate small amounts of RNA extracted from tumor samples for the presence of structural genomic events including gene fusions and rearrangements. This is very important in NSCLC where it is mandatory, from a theranostic perspective, to identify tumors harboring activating translocations implicating the ALK and Proto-oncogene tyrosine-protein kinase (ROS) genes. The unbiased RNA sequencing approach has several advantages over FISH or Immunohistochemistry (IHC). FISH does not provide single-nucleotide resolution of the breakpoint and may be confounded by complex rearrangements. Further, although FISH is inexpensive as a single assay, in NSCLC, a FISH panel composed of several probes should be performed. This does result in high costs per sample. NGS-based translocation detection is capable of examining multiple loci for gene rearrangements in parallel and can be combined with NGS testing for mutations, thus yielding a comprehensive molecular portrait of a given tumor in one assay [71]. In addition to reducing testing costs by combining translocation detection with gene mutation analysis, additional prognostic information can be obtained from the elucidation of exact rearrangement loci. For the ALK inhibitor crizotinib, the clinical response generally increased progression-free survival in *ALK*-rearranged lung cancers, but considerable heterogeneity in response depending on the exact genomic event has been described [42]. Furthermore, it has been demonstrated that knowledge of the somatically acquired breakpoint sequence may allow for the monitoring of minimal residual disease from plasma-derived cell-free DNA using patient- and breakpoint-specific quantitative PCR [72].

5.8 Immunotherapy

The immune surveillance theory involves a set of cells and immune system molecules that play a role in the active elimination of immunogenic tumor cells. However, it seems that cancer immunosurveillance is just one step of the cancer immunoediting. This concept recognizes that even after the phase of elimination when the tumor escapes immunosurveillance, the fate of the tumor is built by immunity and follow two subsequent phases: the equilibrium phase, during which the tumor may either be silent or be immunologically built by immune "editors" to produce new variants that carry more mutations, which would increase resistance to immune attack, and the escape phase, in which the tumor becomes clinically detectable [73].

Programmed cell death 1 (PD-1) is a negative costimulatory receptor expressed primarily on the surface of activated T cells. The binding of PD-1 to one of its ligands, PD-L1 or PD-L2, can inhibit a cytotoxic T-cell response. Tumors can use this pathway to escape T cell-induced antitumor activity. In this background, biomarkers are needed to guide patient selection and to provide indicators of response, based on evolving understanding of the biological mechanisms of the PD-1/PD-L1 pathway. In NSCLCs in particular, testing of PD-1/PD-L1 inhibitors in early-phase trials has been accompanied by the parallel development of companion diagnostic assays to evaluate immunohistochemical staining of PD-L1 on immune cells and/or tumor cells detected on tumor tissue samples. In almost all cases, the expression of PD-L1 is evaluated on bronchial or transthoracic biopsies. The main problem is how to define a threshold for positive PD-L1 labeling on biopsy tissue samples, considering that some patients respond to treatment targeting PD-L1/PD-1, despite low or absent immunoreactivity of this biomarker. It is also well demonstrated that NSCLC tumors show significant intra-tumor heterogeneity for PD-L1 expression, with poor association of the PD-L1 expression between lung biopsies and corresponding resected tumors. There is heterogeneous PD-L1 expression in different regions of the same tumor specimen and in various sections of the same tumor. So it is very important to establish the minimal number of bronchial biopsies to obtain from patients (four or more) and the duration of fixation for bronchial biopsies between 6 and 24 h. Recently, pathology recommendations on the use of PDL1 as biomarker in clinical setting have been published. This report recommended to evaluate tumor cell as well as immune cell staining; to consider PD-L1 results in a global tumor context (mutational load, hypoxia, etc.); to perform combined immunohistochemistry for PD-L1, PD-1, and CD8; and to associate a complex immunohistochemical analysis that evaluates biomarkers of different populations of immune cells. Regarding the possibility to use cytological material, currently, cytological samples do not allow correct evaluation of the immune cells labeled with anti-PD-L1 antibodies [74]. Since recently pembrolizumab was approved for the treatment of patients with unresectable or metastatic, microsatellite instability-high, or mismatch repair-deficient tumors after prior treatment and genomic instability can be studied in cytological material, this opens a possibility to use (especially cell block) to guide immunotherapy [75].

References

1. Torre LA, Bray F, Siegel RL, et al. Global cancer statistics, 2012. CA Cancer J Clin. 2015;65:87–108.
2. Rekhtman N, Brandt SM, Sigel CS, et al. Suitability of thoracic cytology for new therapeutic paradigms in non-small cell lung carcinoma high accuracy of tumor subtyping and feasibility of EGFR and KRAS molecular testing. J Thorac Oncol. 2011;6:451–8.
3. Martini M, Vecchione L, Siena S, et al. Targeted therapies: how personal should we go? Nat Rev Clin Oncol. 2011;9:87–97.
4. Mitsudomi T. Erlotinib, gefitinib, or chemotherapy for EGFR mutation positive lung cancer? Lancet Oncol. 2011;12:710–1.
5. Travis WD, Brambilla E, Noguchi M, et al. International association for the study of lung cancer/American thoracic society/European respiratory society international multidisciplinary classification of lung adenocarcinoma. J Thorac Oncol. 2011;6:244–85.

6. Travis WD, Rekhtman N, Riley GJ, et al. Pathologic diagnosis of advanced lung cancer based on small biopsies and cytology: a paradigm shift. J Thorac Oncol. 2010;5(4):411.
7. Lindeman NI, Cagle PT, Beasley MB, et al. Molecular testing guideline for selection of lung cancer patients for EGFR and ALK tyrosine kinase inhibitors: guideline from the College of American Pathologists, international association for the study of lung cancer, and association for molecular pathology. J Mol Diagn. 2013;15:415–53.
8. Mitsudomi T, Yatabe Y. Mutations of the epidermal growth factor receptor gene and related genes as determinants of epidermal growth factor receptor tyrosine kinase inhibitors sensitivity in lung cancer. Cancer Sci. 2007;98:1817–24.
9. Shepherd FA, Rodrigues Pereira J, et al. Erlotinib in previously treated non-small-cell lung cancer. N Engl J Med. 2005;353:123–32.
10. Mok TS, Wu YL, Thongprasert S, et al. Gefitinib or carboplatinpaclitaxel in pulmonary adeno-carcinoma. N Engl J Med. 2009;361:947–57.
11. da Cunha Santos G, Saieg MA, Geddie W, et al. EGFR gene status in cytological samples of non small cell lung carcinoma: controversies and opportunities. Cancer Cytopathol. 2011;119:80–91.
12. Roh MH. The utilization of cytologic fine-needle aspirates of lung cancer for molecular diagnostic testing. J Pathol Transl Med. 2015;49:300–9.
13. Schrump DS, Altorki NK, Henschke CL, et al. Non-small cell lung cancer. In: DeVita VT, Hellman S, Rosenberg SA, editors. Cancer: principles and practices of oncology. Philadelphia: Lippincott Williams & Wilkins; 2005. p. 753–810.
14. Erozan YS, Ramzy I. Specimen collection and processing in pulmonary cytopathology. In: Essentials in cytopathology, vol. 6. Berlin: Springer; 2009. p. 1–7. https://doi.org/10.1007/978-0-387-88888-01.
15. Koss LG. Koss' diagnostic cytology and its histopathologic bases, vol. 1. 5th ed. Philadelphia: Lippincott Williams & Wilkins; 2006. p. 4–18.
16. Gupta N, Sekar A, Rajwanshi A. Role of FNAC, fluid specimens, and cell blocks for cytological diagnosis of lung cancer in the present era. J Cytol. 2015;32:217–22.
17. da Cunha Santos G, Ko HM, Saieg MA, et al. "The petals and thorns" of ROSE (rapid on-site evaluation). Cancer Cytopathol. 2013;121:4–8.
18. Steinfort DP, Leong TL, Laska IF, et al. Diagnostic utility and accuracy of rapid on site evaluation of bronchoscopic brushings. Eur Respir J. 2015;45:1653–60.
19. Crapanzano JP, Heymann JJ, Monaco S, et al. The state of cell block variation and satisfaction in the era of molecular diagnostics and personalized medicine. CytoJournal. 2014;11:7.
20. da Cunha Santos G, Shepherd FA, Tsao MS. *EGFR* mutations and lung cancer. Annu Rev Pathol. 2011;6:49–69.
21. Marchetti A, Martella C, Felicioni L, et al. *EGFR* mutations in non-small-cell lung cancer: analysis of a large series of cases and development of a rapid and sensitive method for diagnostic screening with potential implications on pharmacologic treatment. J Clin Oncol. 2005;23:857–65.
22. Roh MH. Triage of cytologic direct smears for ancillary studies: a case-based illustration and review. Arch Pathol Lab Med. 2013;137:1185–90.
23. Betz BL, Roh MH, Weigelin HC, et al. The application of molecular diagnostic studies interrogating EGFR and KRAS mutations to stained cytologic smears of lung carcinoma. Am J Clin Pathol. 2011;136:564–71.
24. Allegrini S, Antona J, Mezzapelle R, et al. Epidermal growth factor receptor gene analysis with a highly sensitive molecular assay in routine cytologic specimens of lung adenocarcinoma. Am J Clin Pathol. 2012;138(3):377–81.
25. da Cunha Santos G, Saieg MA. Preanalytic parameters in epidermal growth factor receptor mutation testing for non-small cell lung carcinoma: a review of cytologic series. Cancer Cytopathol. 2015;123:633–43.
26. Abedi-Ardekani B, Vielh P. Is liquid-based cytology the magic bullet for performing molecular techniques? Acta Cytol. 2014;58:574–81.

27. Kawahara A, Azuma K, Sumi A, et al. Identification of non-small-cell lung cancer with activating EGFR mutations in malignant effusion and cerebrospinal fluid: rapid and sensitive detection of exon 19 deletion E746-A750 and exon 21 L858R mutation by immunocytochemistry. Lung Cancer. 2011;74:35–40.

28. Pirker R, Herth FJ, Kerr KM, et al. Consensus for EGFR mutation testing in non-small cell lung cancer: results from a European workshop. J Thorac Oncol. 2010;5:1706–13.

29. Haung L, Fu L. Mechanisms of resistance to EGFR tyrosine kinase inhibitors. Acta Pharm Sin B. 2015;5:390–401.

30. Sacher AG, Oxnard GR. Personalizing therapy for acquired resistance to EGFR kinase inhibitors in advanced NSCLC. AJHO. 2016;12:5–8.

31. Aviel-Ronen S, Blackhall FH, Shepherd SA, et al. K-ras mutations in non-small-cell lung carcinoma: a review. Clin Lung Cancer. 2006;8:30–8.

32. Lozano MD, Zulueta JJ, Echeveste JI, et al. Assessment of epidermal growth factor receptor and K-ras mutation status in cytological stained smears of non-small cell lung cancer patients: correlation with clinical outcomes. Oncologist. 2011;16:877–85.

33. Aisner DL, Sams SB. The role of cytology specimens in molecular testing of solid tumors: techniques, limitations, and opportunities. Diagn Cytopathol. 2012;40:511–24.

34. Thunnissen E, Kerr KM, Herth FJ, et al. The challenge of NSCLC diagnosis and predictive analysis on small samples. Practical approach of a working group. Lung Cancer. 2012;76:1–18.

35. van Eijk R, Licht J, Schrumpf M, et al. Rapid KRAS, EGFR, BRAF and PIK3CA mutation analysis of fine needle aspirates from non-small-cell lung cancer using allele-specific qPCR. PLoS One. 2011;6:e17791.

36. Horiike A, Kimura H, Nishio K, et al. Detection of epidermal growth factor receptor mutation in transbronchial needle aspirates of non-small cell lung cancer. Chest. 2007;131:1628–34.

37. Lozano MD, Labiano T, Echeveste J, et al. Assessment of EGFR and KRAS mutation status from FNAs and core-needle biopsies of non-small cell lung cancer. Cancer Cytopathol. 2015;123:230.

38. Fassina A, Gazziero A, Zardo D, et al. Detection of EGFR and KRAS mutations on transthoracic needle aspiration of lung nodules by high resolution melting analysis. J Clin Pathol. 2009;62:1096–102.

39. Moreira AL, Hasanovic A. Molecular characterization by immunocytochemistry of lung adenocarcinoma on cytology specimens. Acta Cytol. 2012;56:603–10.

40. Lindeman NI, Cagle PT, Aisner DL, et al. Updated molecular testing guideline for the selection of lung cancer patients for treatment with targeted tyrosine kinase inhibitors: guideline from the College of American Pathologists, the International Association for the Study of Lung Cancer, and the Association for Molecular Pathology. J Mol Diagn. 2018;20(2):129–59.

41. Savic S, Bubendorf L. Common fluorescence in situ hybridization applications in cytology. Arch Pathol Lab Med. 2016;140(12):1323–30. https://doi.org/10.5858/arpa.2016-0202-RA.

42. Shaw AT, Kim DW, Nakagawa K, et al. Crizotinib versus chemotherapy in advanced ALK-positive lung cancer. N Engl J Med. 2013;368:2385–94.

43. Soda M, Choi YL, Enomoto M, et al. Identification of the transforming EML4-ALK fusion gene in non-small-cell lung cancer. Nature. 2007;448:561–6.

44. Rossi A. Alectinib for ALK-positive non-small-cell lung cancer. Expert Rev Clin Pharmacol. 2016;9:1005–13.

45. National Cancer Institute. FDA approval for crizotinib. https://www.cancer.gov/cancertopics/druginfo/fda-crizotinib. Accessed June 18 2014.

46. Abbott Laboratories. Vysis ALK break apart FISH probe kit [package insert]. Abbott Park: Abbott Laboratories; 2011.

47. Bubendorf L, Savic S, Ruiz C. Molecular techniques. In: Bibbo M, Wibur D, editors. Comprehensive cytopathology. 4th ed. London: Elsevier Saunders; 2015. p. 912–25.

48. Betz BL, Dixon CA, Weigelin HC, et al. The use of stained cytologic direct smears for ALK gene rearrangement analysis of lung adenocarcinoma. Cancer Cytopathol. 2013;121:489–99.

49. Rikova K, Guo A, Zeng Q, et al. Global survey of phosphotyrosine signaling identifies onco-genic kinases in lung cancer. Cell. 2007;131:1190–203.
50. Bergethon K, Shaw AT, Ou SH, et al. ROS1 rearrangements define a unique molecular class of lung cancers. J Clin Oncol. 2012;30:863–70.
51. Kohno T, Ichikawa H, Totoki Y, et al. KIF5B-RET fusions in lung adenocarcinoma. Nat Med. 2012;18:375–7.
52. Lee JS, Hirsh V, Park K, et al. Vandetanib versus placebo in patients with advanced non-small-cell lung cancer after prior therapy with an epidermal growth factor receptor tyro-sine kinase inhibitor: a randomized, double-blind phase III trial (ZEPHYR). J Clin Oncol. 2012;30:1114–21.
53. Gelsomino F, Facchinetti F, Haspinger ER, et al. Targeting the MET gene for the treatment of non-small-cell lung cancer. Crit Rev Oncol Hematol. 2014;89:284–99.
54. Cappuzzo F, Janne PA, Skokan M, et al. MET increased gene copy number and primary resis-tance to gefitinib therapy in non-small-cell lung cancer patients. Ann Oncol. 2009;20:298–304.
55. Sequist LV, Waltman BA, Dias-Santagata D, et al. Genotypic and histological evolution of lung cancers acquiring resistance to EGFR inhibitors. Sci Transl Med. 2011;3:75ra26.
56. Malami SA. Fine-needle aspiration cytology is an alternative source of high quality archival samples in biobanking. ISRN Pathol. 2011;2011:129785.
57. Ellison G, Donald E, McWalter G, et al. A comparison of ARMS and DNA sequencing for mutation analysis in clinical biopsy samples. J Exp Clin Cancer Res. 2010;29:132.
58. Aisner DL, Deshpande C, Baloch Z, et al. Evaluation of EGFR mutation status in cytology specimens: an institutional experience. Diagn Cytopathol. 2013;41:316–23.
59. Wang S, Yu B, Ng CC, et al. The suitability of small biopsy and cytology specimens for EGFR and other mutation testing in non-small cell lung cancer. Transl Lung Cancer Res. 2015;4:119–25.
60. Wang Y, Zhang J, Gao G, et al. EML4-ALK fusion detected by RT-PCR confers similar response to crizotinib as detected by FISH in patients with advanced NSCLC. J Thorac Oncol. 2015;10:1546–52.
61. Demidova I, Barinov A, Savelov N, et al. Immunohistochemistry, fluorescence in situ hybrid-ization, and reverse transcription-polymerase chain reaction for the detection of anaplastic lymphoma kinase gene rearrangements in patients with non-small cell lung cancer: potential advantages and methodologic pitfalls. Arch Pathol Lab Med. 2014;138:794–802.
62. Oktay MH, Adler E, Hakima L, et al. The application of molecular diagnostics to stained cytol-ogy smears. J Mol Diagn. 2016;18:407–15.
63. Dama E, Tillhon M, Bertallot G, et al. Sensitive and affordable diagnostic assay for the quan-titative detection of anaplastic lymphoma kinase (*ALK*) alterations in patients with non-small cell lung cancer. Oncotarget. 2016;7:37160–76.
64. Di Lorito A, Schmitt FC. (Cyto)pathology and sequencing: next (or last) generation? Diagn Cytopathol. 2012;40:459–61.
65. Kanagal-Shamanna R, Portier BP, Singh RR, et al. Next-generation sequencing-based multi-gene mutation profiling of solid tumors using fine needle aspiration samples: promises and challenges for routine clinical diagnostics. Mod Pathol. 2014;27:314–27.
66. Malapelle U, Mayo-de-Las Casas C, Molina-Vila M, et al. Consistency and reproducibil-ity of next-generation sequencing and other multigene mutational assays: a worldwide ring trial study on quantitative cytological molecular reference specimens. Cancer Cytopathol. 2017;125(8):615–26. https://doi.org/10.1002/cncy.21868.
67. Krøigård AB, Thomassen M, Lænkholm A-V, Kruse TA, Larsen MJ. Evaluation of nine somatic variant callers for detection of somatic mutations in exome and targeted deep sequenc-ing data. PLoS One. 2016;11(3):e0151664. https://doi.org/10.1371/journal.pone.0151664.
68. Velizheva NP, Rechsteiner MP, Wong CE, et al. Cytology smears as excellent starting material for next-generation sequencing-based molecular testing of patients with adenocarcinoma of the lung. Cancer Cytopathol. 2016;125(1):30–40. https://doi.org/10.1002/cncy.21771.
69. Buttitta F, Felicioni L, Del Grammastro M, et al. Effective assessment of egfr mutation status in bronchoalveolar lavage and pleural fluids by next-generation sequencing. Clin Cancer Res. 2013;19:691–8.

70. Qiu T, Guo H, Zhao H, et al. Next-generation sequencing for molecular diagnosis of lung adenocarcinoma specimens obtained by fine needle aspiration cytology. Sci Rep. 2015;5:11317.
71. Abel HJ, Al-Kateb H, Cottrell CE, et al. Detection of gene rearrangements in targeted clinical next-generation sequencing. J Mol Diagn. 2014;16:405–17.
72. Leary RJ, Sausen M, Kinde I, et al. Detection of chromosomal alterations in the circulation of cancer patients with whole-genome sequencing. Sci Transl Med. 2012;4:162ra54.
73. Topalian SL, Taube JM, Anders RA, Pardoll DM. Mechanism driven biomarkers to guide immune checkpoint blockade in cancer therapy. Nat Rev Cancer. 2016;16:275–87.
74. Ilie M, Hofman V, Dietel M, Soria JC, Hofman P. Assessment of the PD-L1 status by immunohistochemistry: challenges and perspectives for therapeutic strategies in lung cancer patients. Virchows Arch. 2016;468:511–25.
75. Bubendorf L, Lantuejoul S, de Langen AJ, et al. Nonsmall cell lung carcinoma: diagnostic difficulties in small biopsies and cytological specimens. Eur Respir Rev. 2017;26:170007.

Molecular Cytology of Serous Effusions

6

Ben Davidson

6.1 Introduction

Metastasis is a decisive event in tumor progression and the presence of cancer cells outside the organ of origin dictates in the majority of cases a need to explore treatment modalities beyond surgery. This is particularly true for malignant effusions, since tumor cells within the peritoneal, pleural, and pericardial spaces cannot be surgically removed. Chemotherapy and radiotherapy, while highly effective in many cancers, are usually unable to eliminate all tumor cells.

Among the primary cancers of the serosal cavities are malignant mesothelioma (MM), primary peritoneal carcinoma (PPC), primary effusion lymphoma, and other, rarer entities. The majority of tumors affecting the serosal cavities are nevertheless metastatic, constituting in adults most often adenocarcinomas of the breast, lung, ovary, or gastrointestinal tract. Other carcinomas and hematological cancers, as well as sarcomas, germ cell tumors, and malignant melanomas, are less frequently encountered but have all been described at this anatomic site [1].

Molecular techniques have become central in cancer management in recent years and are used as aids in the diagnostic setting, as well as in assessing therapeutic options, in predicting treatment response, and in prognostication. Effusions are ideal specimens for molecular analysis, as they often contain large numbers of viable cells in suspension, often dissociated or in small groups. Effusion supernatants are also informative, as they contain DNA, RNA, microRNA, or protein from tumor, as well as host cells. Virtually any molecular technique, including high-throughput analyses, has been applied to effusion specimens, and considerable knowledge has

B. Davidson
Department of Pathology, Oslo University Hospital, Norwegian Radium Hospital,
Oslo, Norway

University of Oslo, Faculty of Medicine, Institute of Clinical Medicine, Oslo, Norway
e-mail: bend@medisin.uio.no

© Springer International Publishing AG, part of Springer Nature 2018
F. C. Schmitt (ed.), *Molecular Applications in Cytology*,
https://doi.org/10.1007/978-3-319-74942-6_6

been gained in these studies [2]. Translation of these studies into clinical practice has, as in many other settings, nevertheless been slower and of more limited scope, and many of these publications represent single studies that have not been reproduced by other investigators. Others, e.g., telomerase assays, have been studied by several groups and yet have failed to become standard practice. This chapter focuses on diagnostic and therapy-related tests which constitute current practice, at least in tertiary cancer centers. The use of these tests is dictated by the origin of the tumor diagnosed in the effusion specimen and thereby does not represent an assay specific for cancers at this anatomic site. Rather, effusions are one of several types of specimens, including fine-needle aspirates and biopsies, which may be studied using the same technology. Hematological cancers are not discussed in this chapter.

6.2   Molecular Tests Applied to Effusion Diagnosis

The two main molecular assays applied to effusion diagnosis are in situ hybridization (ISH) and polymerase chain reaction (PCR).

ISH is a commonly used method which has the advantage of combining molecular analysis with morphological assessment. Visualization may be achieved using a colorimetric assay (chromogenic ISH, CISH), silver staining (SISH), or fluorescence (FISH). Within the diagnostic context, FISH is the most frequently applied test.

Han et al. analyzed 72 malignant effusions from patients with different cancers, of which the majority were lung carcinomas, and 21 benign effusions using probes for chromosomes 7, 11, and 17. The observed sensitivity and specificity combining morphology and FISH were 88% and 94.5%, respectively [3]. Rosolen and co-workers studied 200 effusions, including 82 cytologically malignant specimens, 67 suspicious ones, and 51 cases diagnosed as benign, applying FISH probes for chromosomes 7 and 17. FISH confirmed the cytological diagnosis in malignant and benign specimens and aided in detecting malignant cells in cases with inconclusive cytology [4]. FISH analysis using probes for chromosomes 11 and 17 was found to be useful in differentiating malignant from benign effusions in another series [5].

FISH has been used as a tool for diagnosing MM in several studies, applying probes detecting chromosomal aberrations which frequently occur in this cancer, in particular the homozygous deletion of the *CDKN2A* gene, encoding the tumor suppressor proteins p14 and p16 at chromosome 9p21. Deletion at this chromosomal site was shown to be a common event in MM and effectively differentiated this tumor from benign effusions in three studies [6–8]. The presence of homozygous *CDKN2A* deletion was shown to be closely similar in effusion specimens and patient-matched biopsies in two recent studies, of which one showed the same agreement for BAP1 immunohistochemistry (IHC) [9, 10]. Combination of *CDKN2A* by FISH and BAP1 by IHC was reported to be useful in a recent study of 67 effusions (32 MM, 35 atypical mesothelial proliferations), of which 38 were analyzed using both methods [11].

The UroVysion™ kit, containing centromeric probes for chromosomes 3, 7, and 17 and a probe for chromosome 9p21, has been applied to effusion diagnosis, with focus on MM.

Analysis of 68 effusions, including 21 MM, 29 metastatic tumors, mainly of lung and breast origin, and 18 reactive specimens, showed 9p21 deletions in 12/21 MM and 3/29 metastases and none of the reactive specimens. Gains at 9p21 were more common in metastases, while gains in chromosomes 3, 7, and 17 were frequent in both MM and metastases [12].

In another study, in which 52 MM and 28 reactive effusions were analyzed, positive FISH analysis, most frequently 9p21 deletion, was found in 41/52 (79%) MM compared to 0/28 reactive specimens [13]. FISH analysis using centromeric probes for chromosomes 7 and 9 was found to be useful in differentiating MM from benign effusions in another study [14].

Example of the 9p21 FISH assay is shown in Fig. 6.1.

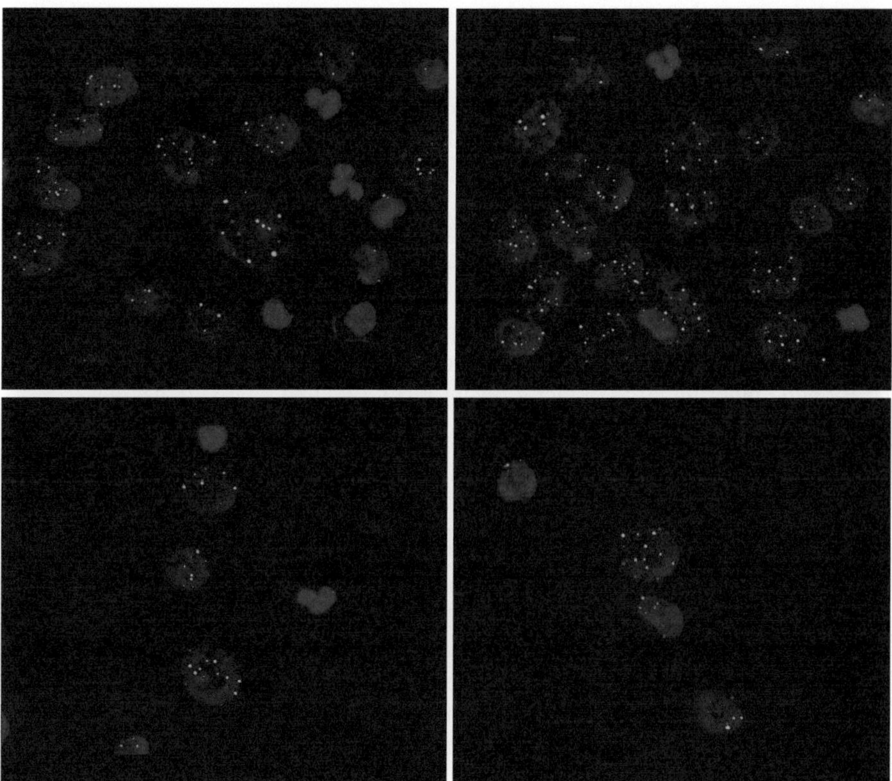

Fig. 6.1 Chromosome 9p21 deletion by fluorescent in situ hybridization (FISH). Malignant mesothelioma (MM) pleural effusion analyzed using a probe for chromosome 9p21 (UroVysion™ kit). MM cells lack yellow dots, corresponding to homozygous chromosome 9p21 deletion. (Courtesy Prof. Anders Hjerpe, Karolinska Institute, Stockholm, Sweden)

Several other groups have reported on ISH- or PCR-based assays as adjuncts to morphology in effusion diagnosis. However, these have been single reports which are yet to be validated. In two studies using ISH, [35S]UTP-labeled probes against *MUC2* and *MUC5AC* were applied to pseudomyxoma peritonei specimens [15], and thyroid transcription factor-1 (*TTF1*) gene amplification by FISH was analyzed in lung carcinoma [16].

Quantitative RT-PCR (qRT-PCR) assay analyzing the expression of the mucin genes *MUC1*, *MUC2*, and *MUC5AC* in 112 pleural effusions found *MUC1* and *MUC5AC* to be sensitive and specific in the diagnosis of malignancy [17]. Similar results were reported for an RT-PCR assay detecting *EGP2* (*EPCAM*) [18] and for the melanoma-associated antigen (MAGE) family members *MAGE1* and *MAGE3* and the related genes *BAGE* and *GAGE1-2* [19]. An RT-PCR assay for prepro-gastrin-releasing peptide (prepro-GRP) detected small cell lung carcinoma in effusion specimens [20], while an assay detecting the mammaglobin and mammaglobin B genes *hMAM* and *hMAMB* was positive in effusions from patients with breast carcinoma, as well as other gynecologic carcinomas and lung carcinoma [21]. The combined use of *CLDN4*, *EPCAM*, and *CK20* PCR was suggested as adjunct to cytology in another study [22].

Analysis of effusion supernatants for cyclin E gene copy number by qPCR [23] or *BIRC5* mRNA levels [24] was similarly reported to effectively differentiate malignant from benign effusions.

6.3 Molecular Tests Applied to Effusions as Predictive Test

ISH and PCR have in recent years been applied to evaluate the presence and expression level of molecules which may be targeted in different cancers, particularly HER2 and epidermal growth factor receptor (EGFR) and related molecules.

6.3.1 HER2 Status

HER2 amplification is present in 20–25% of breast carcinomas and is associated with aggressive disease. HER2 is targeted by the monoclonal antibodies trastuzumab (Herceptin®) and pertuzumab (PERJETA™) and by the tyrosine kinase inhibitors (TKIs) lapatinib (Tykerb®), afatinib, and neratinib (HKI-272) [25]. Trastuzumab is additionally used in treating gastroesophageal carcinomas that overexpress HER2 [26], as well as in a subgroup of patients with HER2-overexpressing colorectal carcinoma [27]. HER2 status is evaluated at the protein level using IHC or at the gene level using CISH, SISH, or FISH (Figs. 6.2 and 6.3).

A comprehensive review of 47 studies in which 3384 patient-matched primary breast carcinomas and metastases were compared, with focus on solid lesions, showed that HER2, as well as hormone receptor expression, is not infrequently discordant between primary and metastatic breast carcinoma, highlighting the

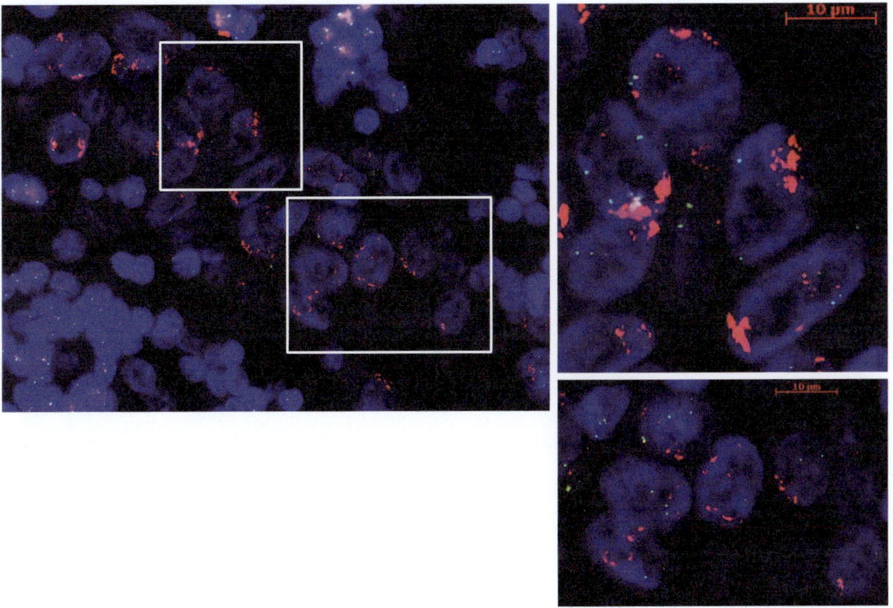

Fig. 6.2 HER2 amplification by FISH. Left: two clusters of tumor cells (marked by frame), in which cells have HER2 copy number >20 (pink clusters), while the CEP17 centrosomal probe detects 1–2 copies (green dots) per cell, evidence of HER2 amplification. High-power detail is shown to the right. (Courtesy Dr. Hege Russnes, Oslo University Hospital)

relevance of testing metastases for HER2 status [28]. Several studies have focused on effusion specimens in this context.

Shabaik et al. compared HER2 status by IHC in cell blocks from cytological specimens ($n = 42$), including 15 effusions, and 40 patient-matched core biopsies, and found good agreement between these specimens, suggesting that cell blocks constitute relevant specimens for this analysis. Additionally, results using IHC and FISH, the latter performed in seven cases, correlated well [29]. HER2 status by IHC and FISH correlated less well in another study of 35 effusions (31 breast and 4 ovarian carcinomas), in part due to chromosome 17 polyploidy [30]. Arihiro et al. compared HER2 status by FISH in 100 pairs of primary breast carcinoma and locoregional recurrences or metastases, including 7 effusions, and found discrepancy in 9 cases, including both negative-to-positive and positive-to-negative conversions [31]. In a recent, smaller study, concordance in HER2 status was seen in eight pleural effusions compared to the primary breast carcinoma, whereas one ascites specimen showed positive-to-negative conversion [32].

Data for gastric carcinoma is more limited. However, analysis of 72 patient-matched primary and metastatic gastric carcinomas, including 15 effusions, showed high concordance rates for HER2 status by both FISH (98.5%) and IHC (94.9%) [33].

Fig. 6.3 HER2 amplification by silver in situ hybridization (SISH). (**a**) H&E-stained section from a breast carcinoma pleural effusion (×200 magnification); (**b**) HER2 immunostaining, score = 3 (×200 magnification); (**c**) HER2 SISH analysis. Tumor cells have aggregates of black dots, corresponding to HER2 amplification. Chromosome 17 copy number (red dots) does not exceed 2/cell (×400 magnification)

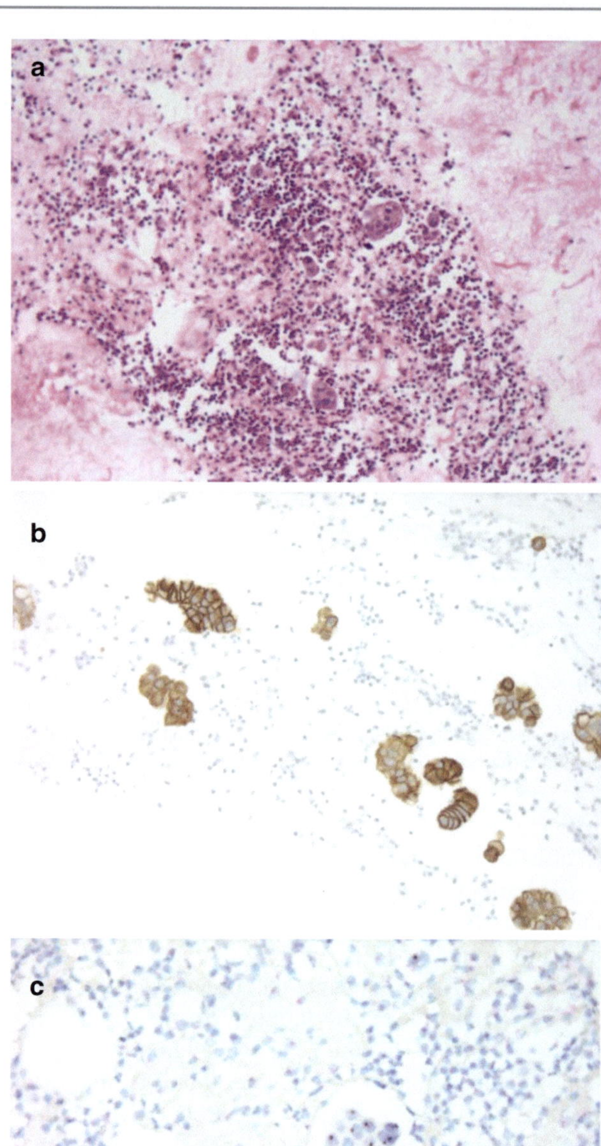

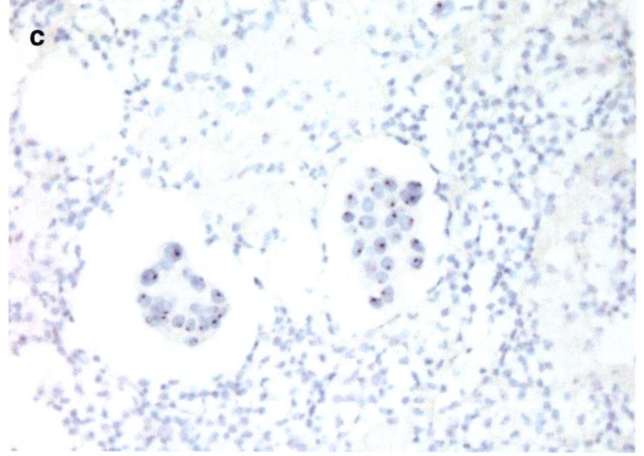

6.3.2   EGFR and Related Molecules

Analysis of *EGFR* mutation status is mandatory prior to TKI treatment and is currently performed in the presence of advanced disease in several cancers, of which the most relevant in the context of effusion cytology is non-small cell lung carcinoma (NSCLC) (Fig. 6.4). *EGFR* mutations are found in 15–20% of lung adenocarcinomas and are limited to exons 18–24, the majority located in exons 18–21. Exon 19 mutations, mainly in-frame deletions, and L858R substitution at exon 21 constitute 85–90% of *EGFR* mutations. The TKIs erlotinib (Tarceva®), gefitinib (Iressa®), and afatinib are approved to the treatment of patients with advanced or recurrent lung cancer which have sensitizing *EGFR* mutations [34].

Testing for *EGFR* mutations can be done using different methods, including direct sequencing, denaturing high-performance liquid chromatography (dHPLC),

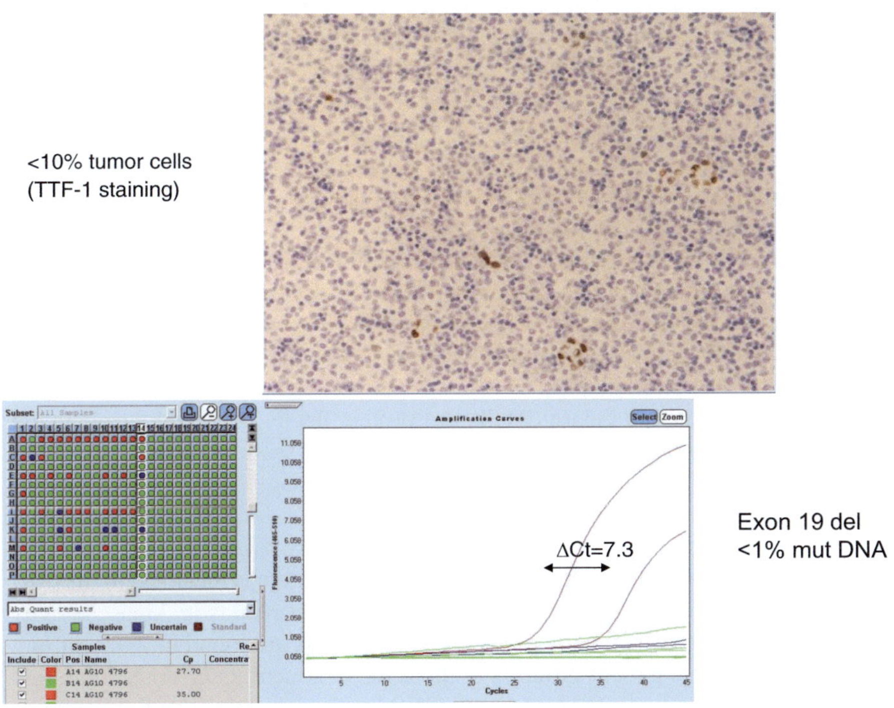

Fig. 6.4   EGFR mutation analysis. Pleural effusion from a NSCLC patient. TTF1 immunostaining shows nuclear expression in tumor cells, which constitute <10% of the cell population. EGFR exon 19 del mutation was nevertheless detected using the therascreen EGFR PCR kit (Qiagen, Manchester, UK) on LightCycler 480 (Roche, Basel, Switzerland). The sample was previously negative using dHPLC, which has lower sensitivity. Mutation was later confirmed in a needle biopsy containing more tumor material (Courtesy Dr. Lilach Kleinberg, Oslo University Hospital)

high-resolution melting analysis (HRMA), pyrosequencing, amplification-refractory mutation system (ARMS) PCR, and PCR-restriction fragment length polymorphisms (PCR-RFLP) [35]. The majority of laboratories use multiplex qPCR-based platforms, such as Cobas (Roche) and Therascreen (Qiagen). Next-generation sequencing (NGS) is likely to play an increasing role in this area in the future [34].

Cytological specimens, including effusions, are considered adequate material for testing *EGFR* mutation status [34, 35], and a growing number of studies have focused on this area in recent years. Success rate was 100% for 5 different methods applied to *EGFR* mutation status analysis in 20 pleural effusions [36]. A concordance rate of 91.7% for histology and cytology was shown in analysis of specimens from 60 patients, in which cytology specimens included 16 pleural effusions and one ascites specimen [37]. Tissue sections, cell blocks, pleural effusions, and sera were studied for *EGFR* mutation status in another study of 37 NSCLC with malignant pleural effusion, in which peptide nucleic acid (PNA)-mediated real-time PCR clamping and direct sequencing were compared. Analysis of the pleural fluid was associated with sensitivity and specificity of 89% and 100%, respectively, compared to tumor tissue and cell blocks using PNA clamping, and 67% and 90%, respectively, using direct sequencing [38].

Comparable values were seen for *KRAS* mutation analysis in another study by the same group, in which 57 malignant effusions, the majority of lung origin, were analyzed using these two methods [39].

In analysis of 48 cytological specimens, including 15 pleural effusions, from patients whose tumors had *EGFR* mutation in tissue specimens, NGS was superior to direct sequencing in detecting *EGFR* mutations (81% vs. 16%, respectively), and mutations were found also in some of the effusions diagnosed as negative for carcinoma based on morphology [40].

Anaplastic lymphoma kinase (ALK) is a protein involved in fetal development, which is lost in adult tissues with the exception of the brain. ALK is expressed in several tumors, including NSCLC, due to genetic rearrangements, most often thorough inversion of chromosome 2p, where the *ALK* gene is located, leading to fusion with the echinoderm microtubule-associated protein-like 4 gene *EML4*, located on the same chromosome arm. The EML4-ALK fusion protein is localized in the cytoplasm following loss of its transmembrane domain, but retains its kinase activity, resulting in pro-survival signaling. *ALK* rearrangements are found in 2–8% of lung carcinomas, and this patient group is eligible for treatment using ALK inhibitors, including crizotinib and newer ALK inhibitors such as ceritinib and alectinib, as well as other drugs currently in development [41].

Soda et al. analyzed 808 lung carcinoma specimens from 754 patients using multiplex PCR and found *EML4-ALK* transcripts in 36 specimens, including 5 pleural effusions, from 32 patients [42]. Wu and co-workers studied pleural effusions from 116 patients with wild-type *EGFR*. *EML4-ALK* fusion was detected in 39 tumors (34%) using RT-PCR. FISH analysis was positive in 10/12 PCR-positive cases in which a paraffin block from biopsy or surgical resection was available [43]. In another study, *EML4-ALK* fusion was detected in 5/46 pleural effusions with wild-type *EGFR* using multiplex PCR, whereas 67 specimens with *EGFR* mutation were negative [44].

Other genomic aberrations described in NSCLC affect the *RET, ROS1, NRG1, MET, BRAF, HER2, NF1*, and *MEK1* genes. *RET* rearrangements at chromosome 10 lead to fusion with the *KIF5B* gene, and patients with *RET* rearrangements are currently under consideration for TKI treatment [45]. Analysis of *RET* rearrangements in a series of 722 pleural effusions from patients with lung adenocarcinoma was positive in 17 (2.4), of which 11 and 6 had *KIF5B- RET* and *CCDC6-RET* fusion, respectively [46].

Akamatsu et al. analyzed 100 pleural effusion specimens from 84 patients for *EGFR, KRAS, BRAF, PIK3CA, NRAS, MEK1, AKT1, PTEN*, and *HER2* mutations; *EGFR, MET, FGFR1, FGFR2*, and *PIK3CA* amplifications; and *ALK, ROS1*, and *RET* fusion genes. *EGFR* mutation was found in specimens from 24 patients, *EML4-ALK* rearrangement in 4 patients, *KRAS* mutation and *EGFR* amplification in 3 patients, and *PIK3CA* mutation and *MET* amplification in 2 patients. *BRAF* mutation, *NRAS* mutation, *AKT* mutation, *ROS1* fusion, and *FGFR1* amplification, the latter reflecting *KIF5B-RET* fusion, were found in one patient each [47].

6.4 Future Directions

While the number of molecular assays that are currently performed on effusion specimens as part of the routine practice of pathology labs is still relatively limited, this is likely to change dramatically over the coming years, as already exemplified by the increasing complexity of lung carcinoma management. While it is fairly certain to assume that FISH and PCR will continue to be an integral part of molecular testing, NGS is expected to have an increasingly central role in this area. Analyzing tumors for genetic changes that are characteristic of each tumor with focus on few dozens of genes is the more relevant assay for assessing patient-tailored therapy, whereas more large-scale platforms are used as discovery tools.

Several recent publications on lung carcinoma are examples of the potential of NGS in this respect. Roscilli and co-workers recently performed mutation analysis of 22 genes in short-term cultures from 16 lung adenocarcinoma effusions and identified mutations in *EGFR, KRAS, BRAF, PIK3CA, MET, TP53*, and *STK11*, with high variation across tumors. Whole-exome sequencing was performed in five cases and detected multiple mutations affecting critical cellular pathways, particularly in chromosomes 1, 11, and 19 [48]. Analysis of 38 NSCLC pleural effusions using the TruSight™ tumor sequencing panel, which interrogates mutational hotspots in 174 amplicons of 26 genes, identified mutations in *EGFR, KRAS, BRAF, PIK3CA, MAPK21, PTEN*, and *SMAD4* [49]. DiBardino et al. analyzed 49 NSCLC specimens, including both biopsies and cytological specimens, of which 36 were found to be adequate for full sequencing of 255 genes, including 6/6 pleural effusion specimens, highlighting the value of the latter for such analysis. Using the Illumina HiSeq2500 platform, 179 alterations were found, of which 63 were clinically relevant, including *EGFR, KRAS, ERBB2*, and *PIK3CA* mutations [50]. The adequacy of cytological material for NGS was also shown in analysis of 17 specimens, including 4 effusions, tested for alterations in 47 genes, in which mutations in *EGFR*, *KRAS*, *BRAF*, *NRAS*, and *TP53* were found [51].

Studies of other cancers have to date focused on large-scale analyses aimed at mapping the genetic landscape of these tumors.

Lim and co-workers compared normal gastric mucosa, primary carcinoma, and malignant effusions from eight patients and identified mutations characteristic of tumor cells in effusions, which may promote the metastatic process in this cancer [52].

Three studies applied NGS to analysis of ovarian carcinoma effusions. Castellarin and co-workers applied whole-exome sequencing to analysis of serial effusions from three high-grade serous carcinoma (HGSC) patients, including the primary diagnosis specimen, first recurrence, and second recurrence. *TP53* mutations were found in all specimens, and the mutation spectrum of the primary specimen was generally conserved in the subsequent ones, suggesting that chemoresistant clones that are present in the tumor at diagnosis are the origin for recurrent disease [53]. Shah et al. compared the effusion specimen, frozen tumor, and formalin-fixed paraffin-embedded tumor from 5 patients using the IMPACT assay which targets 281 genes. Among 17 mutations found, 10 were detected in both biopsy specimens and effusions and were listed in the Cancer Genome Atlas (TCGA) study, whereas the remaining 7 were detected only in the IMPACT assay. Among the latter, two mutations (in *FGFR3* and *MYB*) were detected only in the effusion specimen from one of the patients [54]. Reinartz et al. analyzed separately tumor-associated macrophages and tumor cells from 28 HGSC and 1 serous borderline tumor effusions using the Illumina HiSeq1500 platform and characterized expression profiles and signaling pathways for each of these cell populations [55].

Effusions are specimens that are relatively easy to obtain, and often contain numerous viable cells, making them ideal for molecular analyses. The studies discussed in this chapter suggest a central role for effusions in cancer diagnosis, as well as tailoring of targeted therapy in the future.

References

1. Davidson B, Firat P, Michael CW, editors. Serous effusions. London: Springer; 2011.
2. Davidson B. Serous effusions. In: Bartlett JMS, Shabaan A, Schmitt F, editors. Molecular pathology: a practical guide for the surgical pathologist and cytopathologist. Cambridge: Cambridge University Press; 2015. p. 356–72.
3. Han J, Cao S, Zhang K, et al. Fluorescence in situ hybridization as adjunct to cytology improves the diagnosis and directs estimation of prognosis of malignant pleural effusions. J Cardiothorac Surg. 2012;7:121.
4. Rosolen DC, Kulikowski LD, Bottura G, et al. Efficacy of two fluorescence in situ hybridization (FISH) probes for diagnosing malignant pleural effusions. Lung Cancer. 2013;80:284–8.
5. Fiegl M, Massoner A, Haun M, et al. Sensitive detection of tumour cells in effusions by combining cytology and fluorescence in situ hybridisation (FISH). Br J Cancer. 2004;91:558–63.
6. Illei PB, Ladanyi M, Rusch VW, et al. The use of CDKN2A deletion as a diagnostic marker for malignant mesothelioma in body cavity effusions. Cancer. 2003;99:51–6.

7. Matsumoto S, Nabeshima K, Kamei T, et al. Morphology of 9p21 homozygous deletion-positive pleural mesothelioma cells analyzed using fluorescence in situ hybridization and virtual microscope system in effusion cytology. Cancer Cytopathol. 2013;121:415–22.

8. Onofre FB, Onofre AS, Pomjanski N, et al. 9 p21 deletion in the diagnosis of malignant mesothelioma in serous effusions additional to immunocytochemistry, DNA-ICM, and AgNOR analysis. Cancer. 2008;114:204–15.

9. Hida T, Matsumoto S, Hamasaki M, et al. Deletion status of p16 in effusion smear preparation correlates with that of underlying malignant pleural mesothelioma tissue. Cancer Sci. 2015;106:1635–41.

10. Hwang HC, Sheffield BS, Rodriguez S, et al. Utility of BAP1 immunohistochemistry and p16 (CDKN2A) FISH in the diagnosis of malignant mesothelioma in effusion cytology specimens. Am J Surg Pathol. 2016;40:120–6.

11. Walts AE, Hiroshima K, McGregor SM, et al. BAP1 immunostain and CDKN2A (p16) FISH analysis: clinical applicability for the diagnosis of malignant mesothelioma in effusions. Diagn Cytopathol. 2016;44:599–606.

12. Flores-Staino C, Darai-Ramqvist E, Dobra K, et al. Adaptation of a commercial fluorescent in situ hybridization test to the diagnosis of malignant cells in effusions. Lung Cancer. 2010;68:39–43.

13. Savic S, Franco N, Grilli B, et al. Fluorescence in situ hybridization in the definitive diagnosis of malignant mesothelioma in effusion cytology. Chest. 2010;138:137–44.

14. Shin HJ, Shin DM, Tarco E, et al. Detection of numerical aberrations of chromosomes 7 and 9 in cytologic specimens of pleural malignant mesothelioma. Cancer. 2003;99:233–9.

15. O'Connell JT, Hacker CM, Barsky SH. MUC2 is a molecular marker for pseudomyxoma peritonei. Mod Pathol. 2002;15:958–72.

16. Li X, Wan L, Shen H, et al. Thyroid transcription factor-1 amplification and expressions in lung adenocarcinoma tissues and pleural effusions predict patient survival and prognosis. J Thorac Oncol. 2012;7:76–84.

17. Yu CJ, Shew JY, Liaw YS, et al. Application of mucin quantitative competitive reverse transcription polymerase chain reaction in assisting the diagnosis of malignant pleural effusion. Am J Respir Crit Care Med. 2001;164:1312–8.

18. Sakaguchi M, Virmani AK, Ashfaq R, et al. Development of a sensitive, specific reverse transcriptase polymerase chain reaction-based assay for epithelial tumour cells in effusions. Br J Cancer. 1999;79:416–22.

19. Hofmann M, Ruschenburg I. mRNA detection of tumor-rejection genes BAGE, GAGE, and MAGE in peritoneal fluid from patients with ovarian carcinoma as a potential diagnostic tool. Cancer. 2002;96:187–93.

20. Saito T, Kobayashi M, Harada R, et al. Sensitive detection of small cell lung carcinoma cells by reverse transcriptase-polymerase chain reaction for prepro-gastrin-releasing peptide mRNA. Cancer. 2003;97:2504–11.

21. Fiegl M, Haun M, Massoner A, et al. Combination of cytology, fluorescence in situ hybridization for aneuploidy, and reverse-transcriptase polymerase chain reaction for human mammaglobin/mammaglobin B expression improves diagnosis of malignant effusions. J Clin Oncol. 2004;22:474–83.

22. Mohamed F, Vincent N, Cottier M, et al. Improvement of malignant serous effusions diagnosis by quantitative analysis of molecular claudin 4 expression. Biomarkers. 2010;15:315–24.

23. Salani R, Davidson B, Fiegl M, et al. Measurement of cyclin E genomic copy number and strand length in cell-free DNA distinguish malignant versus benign effusions. Clin Cancer Res. 2007;13:5805–9.

24. Wang T, Qian X, Wang Z, et al. Detection of cell-free BIRC5 mRNA in effusions and its potential diagnostic value for differentiating malignant and benign effusions. Int J Cancer. 2009;125:1921–5.

25. Tiwari SR, Mishra P, Abraham J. Neratinib, a novel HER2-targeted tyrosine kinase inhibitor. Clin Breast Cancer. 2016;16:344–8.

26. Lordick F, Janjigian YY. Clinical impact of tumour biology in the management of gastro-esophageal cancer. Nat Rev Clin Oncol. 2016;13:348–60.
27. Graham DM, Coyle VM, Kennedy RD, et al. Molecular subtypes and personalized therapy in metastatic colorectal cancer. Curr Colorectal Cancer Rep. 2016;12:141–50.
28. Yeung C, Hilton J, Clemons M, et al. Estrogen, progesterone, and HER2/neu receptor discordance between primary and metastatic breast tumours-a review. Cancer Metastasis Rev. 2016;35:427–37.
29. Shabaik A, Lin G, Peterson M, et al. Reliability of Her2/neu, estrogen receptor, and progesterone receptor testing by immunohistochemistry on cell block of FNA and serous effusions from patients with primary and metastatic breast carcinoma. Diagn Cytopathol. 2011;39:328–32.
30. Schlüter B, Gerhards R, Strumberg D, et al. Combined detection of Her2/neu gene amplification and protein overexpression in effusions from patients with breast and ovarian cancer. J Cancer Res Clin Oncol. 2010;136:1389–400.
31. Arihiro K, Oda M, Ogawa K, et al. Discordant HER2 status between primary breast carcinoma and recurrent/metastatic tumors using fluorescence in situ hybridization on cytological samples. Jpn J Clin Oncol. 2013;43:55–62.
32. Nakayama Y, Nakagomi H, Omori M, et al. Benefits of using the cell block method to determine the discordance of the HR/HER2 expression in patients with metastatic breast cancer. Breast Cancer. 2016;23:633–9.
33. Bozzetti C, Negri FV, Lagrasta CA, et al. Comparison of HER2 status in primary and paired metastatic sites of gastric carcinoma. Br J Cancer. 2011;104:1372–6.
34. Sheikine Y, Rangachari D, McDonald DC, et al. EGFR testing in advanced non-small-cell lung cancer, a mini-review. Clin Lung Cancer. 2016;17:483–92.
35. Ellison G, Zhu G, Moulis A, et al. EGFR mutation testing in lung cancer: a review of available methods and their use for analysis of tumour tissue and cytology samples. J Clin Pathol. 2013;66:79–89.
36. Goto K, Satouchi M, Ishii G, et al. An evaluation study of EGFR mutation tests utilized for non-small-cell lung cancer in the diagnostic setting. Ann Oncol. 2012;23:2914–9.
37. Sun PL, Jin Y, Kim H, et al. High concordance of EGFR mutation status between histologic and corresponding cytologic specimens of lung adenocarcinomas. Cancer Cytopathol. 2013;121:311–9.
38. Yeo CD, Kim JW, Kim KH, et al. Detection and comparison of EGFR mutations in matched tumor tissues, cell blocks, pleural effusions, and sera from patients with NSCLC with malignant pleural effusion, by PNA clamping and direct sequencing. Lung Cancer. 2013;81:207–12.
39. Kang JY, Park CK, Yeo CD, et al. Comparison of PNA clamping and direct sequencing for detecting KRAS mutations in matched tumour tissue, cell block, pleural effusion and serum from patients with malignant pleural effusion. Respirology. 2015;20:138–46.
40. Buttitta F, Felicioni L, Del Grammastro M, et al. Effective assessment of egfr mutation status in bronchoalveolar lavage and pleural fluids by next-generation sequencing. Clin Cancer Res. 2013;19:691–8.
41. Facchinetti F, Tiseo M, Di Maio M, et al. Tackling ALK in non-small cell lung cancer: the role of novel inhibitors. Transl Lung Cancer Res. 2016;5:301–21.
42. Soda M, Isobe K, Inoue A, North-East Japan Study Group, ALK Lung Cancer Study Group, et al. A prospective PCR-based screening for the EML4-ALK oncogene in non-small cell lung cancer. Clin Cancer Res. 2012;18:5682–9.
43. Wu SG, Kuo YW, Chang YL, et al. EML4-ALK translocation predicts better outcome in lung adenocarcinoma patients with wild-type EGFR. J Thorac Oncol. 2012;7:98–104.
44. Chen YL, Lee CT, Lu CC, et al. Epidermal growth factor receptor mutation and anaplastic lymphoma kinase gene fusion: detection in malignant pleural effusion by RNA or PNA analysis. PLoS One. 2016;11:e0158125.
45. Saito M, Shiraishi K, Kunitoh H, et al. Gene aberrations for precision medicine against lung adenocarcinoma. Cancer Sci. 2016;107:713–20.
46. Tsai TH, Wu SG, Hsieh MS. Clinical and prognostic implications of RET rearrangements in metastatic lung adenocarcinoma patients with malignant pleural effusion. Lung Cancer. 2015;88:208–14.

47. Akamatsu H, Koh Y, Kenmotsu H, et al. Multiplexed molecular profiling of lung cancer using pleural effusion. J Thorac Oncol. 2014;9:1048–52.
48. Roscilli G, De Vitis C, Ferrara FF, et al. Human lung adenocarcinoma cell cultures derived from malignant pleural effusions as model system to predict patients chemosensitivity. J Transl Med. 2016;14:61.
49. Puglisi M, Stewart A, Thavasu P, et al. Characterisation of the phosphatidylinositol 3-kinase pathway in non-small cell lung cancer cells isolated from pleural effusions. Oncology. 2016;90:280–8.
50. DiBardino DM, Saqi A, Elvin JA, et al. Yield and clinical utility of next-generation sequencing in selected patients with lung adenocarcinoma. Clin Lung Cancer. 2016;17:517–522.e3.
51. Wei S, Lieberman D, Morrissette JJ, et al. Using "residual" FNA rinse and body fluid specimens for next-generation sequencing: an institutional experience. Cancer Cytopathol. 2016;124:324–9.
52. Lim B, Kim C, Kim JH, et al. Genetic alterations and their clinical implications in gastric cancer peritoneal carcinomatosis revealed by whole-exome sequencing of malignant ascites. Oncotarget. 2016;7:8055–66.
53. Castellarin M, Milne K, Zeng T, et al. Clonal evolution of high-grade serous ovarian carcinoma from primary to recurrent disease. J Pathol. 2013;229:515–24.
54. Shah RH, Scott SN, Brannon AR, et al. Comprehensive mutation profiling by next-generation sequencing of effusion fluids from patients with high-grade serous ovarian carcinoma. Cancer Cytopathol. 2015;123:289–97.
55. Reinartz S, Finkernagel F, Adhikary T, et al. A transcriptome-based global map of signaling pathways in the ovarian cancer microenvironment associated with clinical outcome. Genome Biol. 2016;17:108.

Molecular Cytology Applications on Urine

7

Spasenija Savic

7.1   Introduction

Worldwide bladder cancer (BC) is the ninth most common cancer, and urothelial carcinoma (UC) is by far the most common morphological subtype [1, 2]. Symptoms leading to the diagnosis are nonspecific (e.g., hematuria), and unfortunately already 25% of patients present with muscle-invasive BC, harboring a poor prognosis and high mortality rate despite radical surgery. Seventy-five percent are non-muscle-invasive urothelial carcinomas (NMIBC), a heterogeneous group of superficial carcinomas including low-grade (LGUC, in 70%) and high-grade UC (HGUC). NMIBC are treated by bladder-sparing transurethral resection and receive, based on a clinico-pathological risk assessment, an adjuvant intravesical immuno- (e.g., Bacillus Calmette-Guérin, BCG) or chemotherapy (e.g., mitomycin) [3]. Despite this attempt of local control, both LG- and HGUC have a high recurrence rate (50–70%), and HGUC has a significant risk of progression to life-threatening muscle-invasive carcinomas—urothelial carcinoma in situ (CIS) in as many as 50% [2]. To detect recurrence and progression, patients therefore require frequent and long, with HGUC lifelong, surveillance with cystoscopy and cytology, the standard of care for both initial diagnosis and follow-up of patients with BC [3].

Cystoscopy is quite invasive and expensive and can show a false-negativity rate of >10% [4]. The strength of cytology as a noninvasive adjunct to cystoscopy is the high specificity of >95% for HGUC with a sensitivity of 44% for papillary noninvasive HGUC, 70% for CIS, and 81% for invasive carcinoma [5, 6]. Cytology can detect HGUC, especially CIS, which might be missed by cystoscopy and random biopsies. A positive voided urine cytology can indicate UC from anywhere in the urinary tract, including the urethra and upper urinary tract (UTT). However, a

S. Savic
Institute of Pathology, University Hospital Basel, Basel, Switzerland
e-mail: spasenija.savicprince@usb.ch

© Springer International Publishing AG, part of Springer Nature 2018   117
F. C. Schmitt (ed.), *Molecular Applications in Cytology*,
https://doi.org/10.1007/978-3-319-74942-6_7

negative cytology cannot exclude UC, and cytology has a low sensitivity for LGUC ranging from 10 to 44% [7, 8]. Furthermore, urinary tract cytology is regarded as one of the more difficult fields in cytopathology, which is mainly due to morphologically challenging cases with equivocal cytological atypia. Such an inconclusive cytology puts the urologist into uncertainty, especially if cystoscopy is negative or shows only equivocal findings, as there are no clinical management guidelines for this scenario: Observation of the patients bears a risk of missing a potential HGUC, whereas performing re-endoscopy with biopsies in a potentially benign condition is associated with discomfort and risk of bladder injury.

These limitations of cystoscopy and cytology have driven the discovery of molecular tumor markers in the urine with the goal to improve noninvasive diagnosis of UC.

7.2   General Overview on Molecular Urine Markers

Numerous DNA, RNA, protein- and epigene-based urine tumor markers have been identified for detection of UC, and few of them have been developed into US Food and Drug Administration (FDA)-approved commercially available diagnostic tests [9, 10]. The most widely studied molecular urine tests are the FDA-approved protein-based NMP22 (Alere), BTA (Polymedicol), and uCyt+ (Scimedx) and the DNA-based UroVysion fluorescence in situ hybridization (U-FISH, Abbott Molecular) tests. NMP22 and BTA measure tumor-associated proteins in the urine and are available as in-office assays used by the urologists. U-FISH and uCyt+ are performed on cells from cytology preparations, and U-FISH is by far the most commonly used test in cytology laboratories.

There is a plentitude of literature reporting data on performance of urine tumor markers in different clinical settings including screening, hematuria evaluation, surveillance of patients with a history of UC, and equivocal cytological atypia [4, 9, 11]. However, the lack of standardized study design makes comparison between different studies and data interpretation nearly impossible. Test performance critically depends on the pretest probability of a positive result and the prevalence of the disease in the studied population (screening population, high-risk population with symptoms of UC, surveillance population with history of UC), the studied tumors (proportion of LGUC and HGUC), the clinical endpoint and follow-up time, the specimen cellularity for cell-based tests (voided urines versus washings), technical procedures, and finally test evaluation and interpretation, including the definition of a positive result. Additionally, there is a lack of independent validation of some promising molecular markers by prospective clinical trials including marker-guided clinical management.

Though many studies did not even compare the performance of the molecular urine test to matched cytology, the markers generally seem to be less specific and more sensitive than cytology, which is mostly due to improved detection of LGUC. For example, U-FISH has a pooled sensitivity and specificity for detection of UC of 63% and 87% as compared to cytology with 44% and 96%, respectively [6, 10]. Despite the improved sensitivity U-FISH, like cytology, has a lower sensitivity for the detection of LGUC compared to HGUC [12]. The sensitivity and negative predictive values of U-FISH and other molecular markers are in general still insufficient to exclude UC and therefore cannot reduce the number of diagnostic (e.g., in patients with nonspecific symptoms like microhematuria or irritative bladder symptoms) and follow-up cystoscopies. The lower specificity and higher rate of false-positive results compared to cytology can even lead to unnecessary diagnostic procedures.

Therefore no molecular marker is recommended by current clinical guidelines for UC screening, hematuria evaluation, or surveillance of patients with a history of UC [3]. The most promising application so far has been shown for U-FISH as ancillary test in the setting of equivocal cytology, which is acknowledged by the recent AUA/SUO (American Urological Association/Society of Urologic Oncology) guidelines [13]. Though interpretation of the available scientific evidence on the added clinical benefit of ancillary U-FISH is very difficult due to the lack of comparable prospective studies, when performed in a specific clinico-morphological context, with standardized pre-analytic/analytic procedures and a standardized test evaluation, U-FISH can help clarify equivocal cytology and may provide clinically relevant results. A comprehensive review of all available molecular urine markers is beyond the scope of this chapter, which will focus on ancillary U-FISH testing in equivocal cytology, as it is the most promising indication of this widely used molecular test in cytology.

7.3 Ancillary UroVysion FISH Testing for Clarification of Equivocal Urothelial Cell Atypia

U-FISH is a multitarget, multicolor assay that detects numerical and structural chromosomal aberrations for chromosomes 3, 7, and 17 and the 9p21 locus on interphase nuclei of cytology preparations [14]. These are the most common chromosomal aberrations in UC, and a loss of 9p21 is one of the earliest events in the tumorigeneses of both LG- and HGUC. The indication to perform U-FISH should be based on cytology and endoscopy findings in order to provide a clinical benefit that justifies the added costs.

Cells of a HGUC are invariably U-FISH positive; however a cytological diagnosis of HGUC is highly accurate and will induce appropriate clinical workup and treatment. HGUC is therefore not an indication for ancillary U-FISH testing, as it does not add any clinical benefit.

Also in negative cytology, ancillary U-FISH has no added value [15, 16].

Though the low sensitivity for the detection of LGUC is often pointed as a weakness of cytology, this is hardly clinically relevant as they are usually well visible by cystoscopy, and a delay in diagnosis by a false-negative cytology will not impact patient's outcome. U-FISH can increase the sensitivity of cytology for LGUN from

25 to 60–75%, but as already mentioned, these tumors are usually well visible by endoscopy, and therefore the U-FISH result will, in most cases, not have an impact on clinical management. In selected cases, U-FISH might be useful to clarify a cytology showing a monotonous population of urothelial cells with mild nuclear atypia suggestive but not definite for LGUC and inconclusive findings by endoscopy. A positive FISH result will allow for a LGUC diagnosis. However, 30% of LGUC do not show chromosomal aberrations by U-FISH, and a negative result thus cannot exclude it.

Based on two prospective studies, U-FISH is most useful in patients with equivocal cytology that show a negative or equivocal cystoscopy, but it is unnecessary in patients with an obvious tumor on cystoscopy [17, 18]. Reflex-FISH testing of all equivocal cytologies is therefore not a cost-effective approach. More reasonable is testing upon request of the urologist, who decides based on cystoscopy findings and all available clinico-pathological factors that influence the risk of malignancy (age, smoking history, grade, stage, number and size of previous UC, previous recurrences, etc.) if an ancillary U-FISH test will influence clinical management.

Equivocal urothelial cell atypia are particularly challenging and common after intravesical treatment (e.g., BCG) for HGUC and in upper urinary tract cytology, where cytology has a lower sensitivity and up to 60% of UC are invasive at time of diagnosis (in contrast to only 15% in urinary bladder) [19, 20]. Even invasive urothelial carcinoma of the upper urinary tract can have only mild nuclear atypia and mimic reactive urothelial cell change. In a prospective study on washings of upper urinary tracts from 55 consecutive patients, the sensitivity of U-FISH for detecting urothelial neoplasms was significantly higher than for cytology (100% and 21%, respectively). The specificity was 90% for FISH and 97.4% for cytology [21]. On the other hand, reactive urothelial cell change, especially common after intravesical treatment for HGUC (e.g., BCG), can be worrisome and even lead to a SHGUC interpretation. A negative U-FISH test in urothelial cells with equivocal atypia and a negative or equivocal cystoscopy result makes their origin from a UC very unlikely suggesting that re-endoscopies with bladder biopsies can safely be avoided [17, 18]. A positive U-FISH result in cells classified as SHGUC supports a final diagnosis of HGUC. Equivocal cytology with a positive ancillary U-FISH result is associated with a higher rate of UC on follow-up than those with a negative U-FISH result [17, 18, 22].

Therefore, ancillary FISH can push the interpretation into an unequivocal diagnostic category and better stratify the risk for UC in patients with equivocal cytology and a negative or equivocal cystoscopy: These findings suggest that patients with a negative U-FISH result can safely avoid a biopsy and patients with a positive result are at higher risk for harboring HGUC and need additional diagnostic workup [18]. Such a U-FISH-guided approach needs to be validated in an appropriately designed prospective clinical trial.

Well-defined morphological criteria for equivocal urothelial cell atypia, corresponding to the diagnostic categories of atypical urothelial cells (AUC) and suspicious for high-grade urothelial carcinoma (SHGUC), have only recently been proposed by the Paris System for Reporting Urinary Cytology [23]. The lack of standardized criteria for equivocal cytology in previous studies resulted in a great variability of the reported prevalence and associated risk of malignancy. With the use of the strict criteria proposed by the Paris System, first studies show a decrease in prevalence of AUC with an increase in its risk of malignancy [24]. This might even better stratify patients for ancillary U-FISH and have an influence on the test performance, which depends on the pretest probability of a positive result.

7.4 Optimized Criteria Defining a FISH-Positive Result

Despite the mentioned promising results, in the three largest studies, the positive predictive value of U-FISH for UC in equivocal cytology ranged only from 47 to 57% [12, 18, 25]. A high rate of false-positive U-FISH was observed in 75% of patient with equivocal cytology and a negative cystoscopy [18]. Such a high false-positivity rate of >50% was also reported by a recent retrospective study evaluating atypical urothelial cells (AUC) by ancillary U-FISH [25].

All of these studies have performed FISH on residual urinary specimens without targeted evaluation of the atypical cells and have used the criteria for a positive U-FISH result as suggested by the manufacturer. These criteria include cells showing a tetraploid pattern in as few as four cells ($\geq$4 cells; see also below under FISH scoring). However, balanced polyploidy with a tetra- or even octaploid pattern (four or eight signals for each of the four FISH probes) can be observed in reactive benign urothelial cells, especially in umbrella cells, and are most likely responsible for the high rate of false-positive results [26–29]. Applying the manufacturer's criteria, a FISH-positive result was reported in 64% of 77 benign urinary tract conditions with clearly benign reactive cell change [29]. Modified criteria for a U-FISH-positive result have therefore been proposed defining balanced polyploidy as a negative FISH result, unless the cells are numerous ($\geq$10 cells) suggesting a clonal process and additionally including a heterozygous loss of 9p21 as a positive result [19, 30, 31]. These modified criteria with targeted evaluation of cells with equivocal atypia, avoiding clearly benign cells (e.g., umbrella cells), improve the performance of U-FISH and reduce significantly the rate of false-positive results. Unbalanced numerical chromosomal aberration are very rare in benign conditions and are mainly observed after pelvic irradiation that can cause permanent chromosomal aberrations (e.g., for cancer of the prostate or the uterus). Loss of 9p21 is specific for neoplasia and in our experience is never present in cells with reactive change or after irradiation [11, 27]. Therefore, in a patient with a history of pelvic irradiation, a positive FISH result is only associated with cancer in the presence of a 9p21 deletion.

7.5 Pre-analytic and Analytic Procedures

For optimal morphology and ancillary testing, urinary tract specimens (voided, catheterized, and ileal conduit urines, bladder, and UTT washings) are ideally processed in the cytology laboratory within 4 h after collection, though they can be refrigerated overnight. If the anticipated delay between collection and processing is greater than 24 h, the cells can be preserved for a few days by adding an equal volume of 50% alcohol to the freshly collected specimen [32, 33].

All kinds of cytology preparations (direct smears, cytocentrifugation and liquid-based preparations, alcohol-fixed or air-dried) are suited for U-FISH. As urinary tract specimens have typically a low cellularity, cytocentrifugation preparations (Shandon Cytospin®, Thermo Fisher Scientific) are particularly useful. They have the advantage of minimal cell loss and produce an evenly distributed cell monolayer of only 6 mm in diameter on the glass slide, which facilitates screening of the Papanicolaou (PAP)-stained slides and safes reagents of the U-FISH assay. Two PAP-stained cytocentrifugation preparations are representative of the whole specimen.

To be able to clarify equivocal urothelial cell atypia, which are typically sparse and can be strongly intermixed with normal cells, U-FISH is best performed on the diagnostic, PAP-stained slide with targeted evaluation of the atypical cells in question [32, 34]. In order to prevent cell loss after uncovering of the PAP-stained slide during pretreatment and DNA denaturation, the use of adhesive slides with electrostatic positive charge is recommended. Distaining of the PAP-stained slide is not necessary before FISH. The assay is often performed on unstained cellular material, which can be problematic because without visual control, one cannot be sure that the rare atypical cells in question are even present and, as mentioned above, reactive cell change with a balanced polysomy could lead to a false-positive result.

It can be difficult or even impossible to manually relocate the sparse target cells for U-FISH on the 4′,6-diamidino-2-phenylindole (DAPI) counterstain after hybridization, as morphological details are lost. Targeted FISH evaluation of these cells can easily be achieved using a standard fluorescence microscope equipped with a camera and an automated stage coupled with a relocation software. Recording the location of the photo-documented target cells on the PAP-stained slides before uncovering and hybridization enables not only to accurately identify the target cells but also to save a lot of time. The same can also be achieved with an automated imaging system by pre-scanning the PAP-stained slides. As mentioned above, this targeted FISH evaluation under visual control of the photo-documented cells avoiding benign cells (e.g., umbrella cells) improves the sensitivity and specificity of FISH analyses.

U-FISH is a multitarget, multicolor assay with four directly fluorescence-labeled single-stranded DNA probes: Three chromosome enumeration probes (CEP) targeting the centromeric region of chromosomes 3, 7, and 17 and one locus-specific probe (LSI) for 9p21, which harbors the tumor suppressor gene *p16*.

The basic steps for U-FISH, which can be done manually or automatically, are as follows [32]: First an appropriate area containing the target cells is selected for hybridization and marked on the PAP-stained slide. The coverslip is then removed from the slide in xylene. The cells on the slides are pretreated with protease to uncover target DNA. Heat is applied to the slide and the U-FISH probes in order to denaturate the target and probe DNA to its single strands, respectively. After applying the denaturated U-FISH probes to the marked area, the slides are coverslipped and sealed with rubber cement and incubated overnight at 37 °C, leading to hybridization of the probes to the target DNA sequence of chromosomes 3, 7, and 17 and 9p21. Following hybridization excess probes are removed by a series of washes. As a final step, the cell nuclei are counterstained with DAPI, a DNA stain with blue fluorescence, and coverslipped. The hybridized slide is stored at −20 °C in the dark before scoring in order to prevent fading of the fluorescence signals.

7.6 Targeted FISH Scoring

The fluorescent signals of the probes are visualized on interphase nuclei under a fluorescence microscope with appropriate excitation and emission filters after the fluorophore is excited with light at an appropriate wavelength. With the spectrally distinct fluorophore labels (CEP 3 SpectrumRed, CEP 7 SpectrumGreen, CEP 17 Spectrum Aqua and LSI 9p21 SpectrumGold) and matched filter sets, the multiple hybridization probes can be evaluated simultaneously. Z-stacked imaging throughout the cell nucleus greatly facilitates signal evaluation on a computer screen and allows for documentation of FISH findings.

FISH scoring is best supervised by an experienced cytotechnician or cytopathologist in order to correlate the FISH signal pattern with morphology. At least twenty-five, well-hybridized, non-overlapping target cells have to be scored, which is greatly facilitated by automated relocation as described above. In addition to manual scoring under the microscope, several automated imaging systems are on the market which allow scoring of the FISH signals on representative digitalized images of scanned FISH slides. These systems are more commonly used in institutions with a high volume of FISH tests [32].

Normal cell nuclei are diploid and contain a set of paired autosomal chromosomes (2N) with two signals for each U-FISH probe. Chromosomal aberrations are a characteristic feature of cancer cells. Aneuploidy refers to numerical chromosomal abnormalities with gains (polysomy) or losses of single (monosomy) or multiple chromosomes. A polysomy is commonly present in cancer cells. A 9p21 deletion is a structural chromosomal abnormality which results in inactivation of the tumor suppressor gene *p16*.

As mentioned above, the following optimized criteria for a U-FISH-positive result are suggested [19, 30, 31]: (1) the presence of ≥ 4 cells with gains in ≥ 2 centromeric probes, (2) the presence of a homozygous (one signal) or heterozygous (no signal) deletion of 9p21 in at least 12 cells, or (3) the presence of ≥ 10 cells with a balanced polyploidy (i.e., 4N or 8N). This definition of a positive FISH result differs from the manufacturer's recommendation, which does not consider balanced polyploidy and does not include heterozygous deletion of 9p21. A heterozygous deletion of 9p21 is a common finding in UC and can occur without additional gains in the chromosomes 3, 7, and 17 (isolated heterozygous 9p21 deletion). For scoring a cell as having an isolated 9p21 deletion, hybridization quality must be good with a visible disomic 9p21 pattern (2 signals) in adjacent clearly benign cells.

Representative FISH images should be performed in order to document the result.

FISH evaluation under morphological control avoiding clearly benign cells and using modified criteria for a U-FISH-positive result is crucial for an accurate interpretation.

Representative images of U-FISH findings are shown in Fig. 7.1.

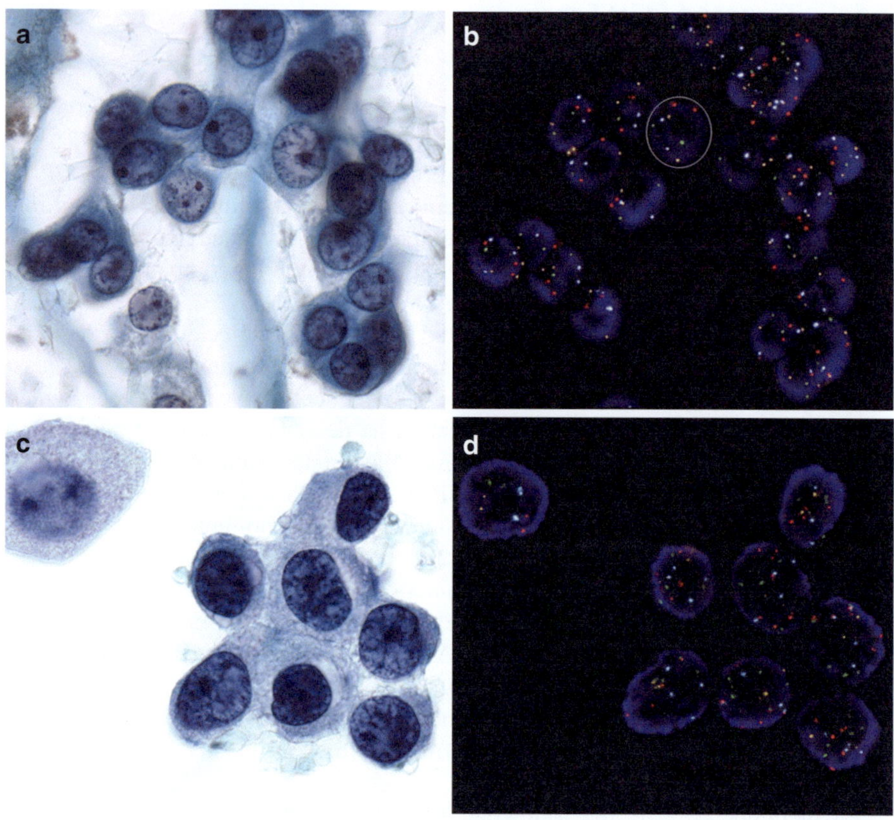

Fig. 7.1 UroVysion FISH (Abbott Molecular, Abbott Park, IL, USA) with four fluorescence-labeled DNA probes targeting the centromeric region of chromosomes 3 (SpectrumRed), 7 (SpectrumGreen), and 17 (Spectrum Aqua) and the chromosomal locus 9p21 (SpectrumGold). (**a, b**) Renal pelvic washing of a patient evaluated for microhematuria: (**a**) Papanicolaou-stained atypical urothelial cells (cytospin, original magnification 400×). (**b**) Targeted FISH shows a negative result: Encircled a non-overlapping cell nucleus with two signals for each probe (diploid pattern). (**c, d**) Bladder washing of a patient with a history of high-grade urothelial carcinoma: (**c**) Papanicolaou-stained atypical urothelial cells and an umbrella cell in the left upper corner (cytospin, original magnification 400×). (**d**) Targeted FISH shows a positive result in the atypical cells with gains of the centromeric signals (4–6 blue, red, and green signals) and a relative loss of 9p21 (2–3 yellow signals). The umbrella cell shows a regular diploid signal pattern (original magnification 600×). Following the FISH result the patient was reexamined and diagnosed with a recurrent pT1G3 high-grade urothelial carcinoma. *FISH* fluorescence in situ hybridization

Conclusions

Despite many available diagnostic molecular urine markers, there is currently only a very limited indication for ancillary testing. As illustrated for U-FISH, the most commonly used molecular test in urinary cytology, clinically meaningful results can only be achieved in the context of patient's history, cystoscopy, and cytology findings. Well-designed prospective clinical trials to show that U-FISH in equivocal cytology improves clinical management and earlier detection of HGUC are still lacking.

References

1. Ferlay J, Soerjomataram I, Dikshit R, et al. Cancer incidence and mortality worldwide: sources, methods and major patterns in GLOBOCAN 2012. Int J Cancer. 2015;136:E359–E86.
2. Moch HPP, Ulbright TM, Reuter VE. WHO classification of tumours of the urinary system and male genital organs. 4th ed. Lyon: IARC; 2016.
3. Babjuk M, Bohle A, Burger M, et al. EAU guidelines on non-muscle-invasive urothelial carcinoma of the bladder: update 2016. Eur Urol. 2017;71:447–61.
4. Clinton T, Lotan Y. Review of the clinical approaches to the use of urine-based tumor markers in bladder cancer. Rambam Maimonides Med J. 2017;8:4.
5. Garbar C, Mascaux C, Wespes E. Is urinary tract cytology still useful for diagnosis of bladder carcinomas? A large series of 592 bladder washings using a five-category classification of different cytological diagnoses. Cytopathology. 2007;18:79–83.
6. Mowatt G, Zhu S, Kilonzo M, et al. Systematic review of the clinical effectiveness and cost-effectiveness of photodynamic diagnosis and urine biomarkers (FISH, ImmunoCyt, NMP22) and cytology for the detection and follow-up of bladder cancer. Health Technol Assess. 2010;14:1–331. iii-iv
7. Li HX, Wang MR, Zhao H, Cao J, Li CL, Pan QJ. Comparison of fluorescence in situ hybridization, NMP22 bladderchek, and urinary liquid-based cytology in the detection of bladder urothelial carcinoma. Diagn Cytopathol. 2013;41:852–7.
8. Yafi FA, Brimo F, Auger M, Aprikian A, Tanguay S, Kassouf W. Is the performance of urinary cytology as high as reported historically? A contemporary analysis in the detection and surveillance of bladder cancer. Urol Oncol. 2014;32:e1–6.
9. Schmitz-Drager BJ, Droller M, Lokeshwar VB, et al. Molecular markers for bladder cancer screening, early diagnosis, and surveillance: the WHO/ICUD consensus. Urol Int. 2015;94:1–24.
10. Chou R, Gore JL, Buckley D, et al. Urinary biomarkers for diagnosis of bladder cancer: a systematic review and meta-analysis. Ann Intern Med. 2015;163:922–31.
11. Bubendorf L. Multiprobe fluorescence in situ hybridization (UroVysion) for the detection of urothelial carcinoma - FISHing for the right catch. Acta Cytol. 2011;55:113–9.
12. Dimashkieh H, Wolff DJ, Smith TM, Houser PM, Nietert PJ, Yang J. Evaluation of urovysion and cytology for bladder cancer detection: a study of 1835 paired urine samples with clinical and histologic correlation. Cancer Cytopathol. 2013;121:591–7.
13. Chang SS, Boorjian SA, Chou R, et al. Diagnosis and treatment of non-muscle invasive bladder cancer: AUA/SUO guideline. J Urol. 2016;196:1021–9.
14. Sokolova IA, Halling KC, Jenkins RB, et al. The development of a multitarget, multicolor fluorescence in situ hybridization assay for the detection of urothelial carcinoma in urine. J Mol Diagn. 2000;2:116–23.
15. Youssef RF, Schlomer BJ, Ho R, Sagalowsky AI, Ashfaq R, Lotan Y. Role of fluorescence in situ hybridization in bladder cancer surveillance of patients with negative cytology. Urol Oncol. 2012;30:273–7.

16. Todenhofer T, Hennenlotter J, Guttenberg P, et al. Prognostic relevance of positive urine markers in patients with negative cystoscopy during surveillance of bladder cancer. BMC Cancer. 2015;15:155.

17. Lotan Y, Bensalah K, Ruddell T, Shariat SF, Sagalowsky AI, Ashfaq R. Prospective evaluation of the clinical usefulness of reflex fluorescence in situ hybridization assay in patients with atypical cytology for the detection of urothelial carcinoma of the bladder. J Urol. 2008;179:2164–9.

18. Schlomer BJ, Ho R, Sagalowsky A, Ashfaq R, Lotan Y. Prospective validation of the clinical usefulness of reflex fluorescence in situ hybridization assay in patients with atypical cytology for the detection of urothelial carcinoma of the bladder. J Urol. 2010;183:62–7.

19. Savic S, Zlobec I, Thalmann GN, et al. The prognostic value of cytology and fluorescence in situ hybridization in the follow-up of nonmuscle-invasive bladder cancer after intravesical Bacillus Calmette-Guerin therapy. Int J Cancer. 2009;124:2899–904.

20. Roupret M, Babjuk M, Comperat E, et al. European association of urology guidelines on upper urinary tract urothelial cell carcinoma: 2015 update. Eur Urol. 2015;68:868–79.

21. Mian C, Mazzoleni G, Vikoler S, et al. Fluorescence in situ hybridisation in the diagnosis of upper urinary tract tumours. Eur Urol. 2010;58:288–92.

22. Skacel M, Fahmy M, Brainard JA, et al. Multitarget fluorescence in situ hybridization assay detects transitional cell carcinoma in the majority of patients with bladder cancer and atypical or negative urine cytology. J Urol. 2003;169:2101–5.

23. Rosenthal DL, Wojcik E, Kurtycz DFI. The Paris system for reporting urinary cytology. New York: Springer; 2016.

24. Wang Y, Auger M, Kanber Y, Caglar D, Brimo F. Implementing the Paris system for reporting urinary cytology results in a decrease in the rate of the "atypical" category and an increase in its prediction of subsequent high-grade urothelial carcinoma. Cancer Cytopathol. 2017;126(3):207–14.

25. Virk RK, Abro S, de Ubago JMM, et al. The value of the UroVysion(R) FISH assay in the risk-stratification of patients with "atypical urothelial cells" in urinary cytology specimens. Diagn Cytopathol. 2017;45:481–500.

26. Wojcik EM, Brownlie RJ, Bassler TJ, Miller MC. Superficial urothelial (umbrella) cells. A potential cause of abnormal DNA ploidy results in urine specimens. Anal Quant Cytol Histol. 2000;22:411–5.

27. Tapia C, Glatz K, Obermann EC, et al. Evaluation of chromosomal aberrations in patients with benign conditions and reactive changes in urinary cytology. Cancer Cytopathol. 2011;119:404–10.

28. Zhou AG, Liu Y, Cyr MS, et al. Role of Tetrasomy for the diagnosis of urothelial carcinoma using urovysion fluorescent in situ hybridization. Arch Pathol Lab Med. 2016;140:552–9.

29. Moatamed NA, Apple SK, Bennett CJ, et al. Exclusion of the uniform tetraploid cells significantly improves specificity of the urine FISH assay. Diagn Cytopathol. 2013;41:218–25.

30. Bubendorf L, Grilli B, Sauter G, Mihatsch MJ, Gasser TC, Dalquen P. Multiprobe FISH for enhanced detection of bladder cancer in voided urine specimens and bladder washings. Am J Clin Pathol. 2001;116:79–86.

31. Zellweger T, Benz G, Cathomas G, et al. Multi-target fluorescence in situ hybridization in bladder washings for prediction of recurrent bladder cancer. Int J Cancer. 2006;119:1660–5.

32. Bubendorf LCN, Fischer AH, Katz RL, Olson MT, Schmitt F, Stojan Flezar M, Van der Kwast TH, Vielh P. Ancillary studies in urinary cytology. The Paris system for reporting urinary cytology. New York: Springer; 2016.

33. Layfield LJ, Elsheikh TM, Fili A, Nayar R, Shidham V, Papanicolaou Society of C. Review of the state of the art and recommendations of the Papanicolaou Society of Cytopathology for urinary cytology procedures and reporting : the Papanicolaou Society of Cytopathology Practice Guidelines Task Force. Diagn Cytopathol. 2004;30:24–30.

34. Savic S, Bubendorf L. Common fluorescence in situ hybridization applications in cytology. Arch Pathol Lab Med. 2016;140:1323–30.

Molecular Cytology Applications on Gynecological Cytology

8

Francesca Carozzi, Giovanni Negri, and Cristina Sani

8.1 Introduction

Cervical cancer is still one of the most frequent cancers and one major cause of mortality worldwide. In the last decades, however, the introduction of the Pap test has led to a drastic reduction of the incidence of invasive cervical neoplasia. Regular Pap screening decreases cervix cancer incidence and mortality by at least 70%. Cervical cytology, nevertheless, has several limitations particularly concerning reproducibility and sensitivity, latter being about 60% [1, 2].

In more recent years, the better understanding of the role of human papillomaviruses (HPV) in the carcinogenesis of cervical neoplasia has led to the development of new molecular techniques, which are supposed to progressively replace the Pap test in several countries. At the same time, the development of liquid-based cytology (LBC) has filled the gap that progressively became evident in the last decades between histopathology and conventional cytology, the former allowing the use of a progressively increasing number of special stains and novel techniques, the latter being stuck to the bare morphological evaluation. In fact, LBC allows the use of biomarkers and molecular tests on the residual cellularity, adding valuable molecular informations to cell morphology.

In these days, screening for cervical cancer has several options, including the traditional Pap smear, which may still be a valuable choice in some settings, and primary HPV-based screening. Latter may be based on different techniques and mostly needs a triage for HPV-positive women, which may be purely cytological, or aided by different bimolecular techniques.

F. Carozzi (✉) · C. Sani
Institute for cancer research, prevention and clinical network, Cancer Prevention Laboratory,
HPV Laboratory and Molecular Oncology Unit, Florence, Italy
e-mail: f.carozzi@ispro.toscana.it; c.sani@ispro.toscana.it

G. Negri
Department of Pathology, Central Hospital Bolzano, Bolzano, Italy

© Springer International Publishing AG, part of Springer Nature 2018
F. C. Schmitt (ed.), *Molecular Applications in Cytology*,
https://doi.org/10.1007/978-3-319-74942-6_8

Most of these techniques are based on the detection of HPV or surrogate markers of the viral oncogenic activity.

HPV is a double-stranded, circular DNA virus approximately 8000 base pairs in size. The distribution of CpG sites is uneven throughout the viral genome. All oncogenic HPV types code for six early genes (E6, E7, E1, E2, E4, and E5) involved in viral gene expression and replication and two late genes [L2 and L1 gene of human papillomavirus (L1)] involved in capsid formation [3]. The L1 protein self-assembles into viral-like particles and is the active component in the currently licensed HPV vaccines. The upstream regulatory region (URR) located between the L1 and E6 genes contains the E6 promoter and an enhancer region with *cis*-responsive elements that regulate viral gene expression, replication, and packaging into viral particles [4, 5]. The primary HPV oncogenes, E6 and E7, interact with a large number of cellular targets, including the cellular tumor suppressor proteins p53 and pRb, which are central regulators of apoptosis and cell cycle, respectively [6–9]. During productive infection, E6 and E7 are expressed at relatively low levels, in part due to transcriptional repression by E2 gene of human papillomavirus (E2). During the carcinogenic process, transcription of E6 and E7 is deregulated, leading to their overexpression [10]. This deregulation may be mediated by the integration of HPV DNA into the host genome, often resulting in disruption of the E2 gene with increased E6 and E7 transcripts spliced into host sequences, causing increased HPV oncogene expression [11, 12]. However, HPV integration is not a necessary step in malignant transformation, and other mechanisms, such as alterations of the E2 binding sites in the URR or altered expression of E2, may be implicated [13, 14]. On the basis of these molecular mechanisms of HPV oncogenesis, a number of biomarkers have been developed including those associated with HPV oncogene activity (i.e., E6 and E7 mRNA expression) and with cell cycle deregulation [15, 16].

8.2   Classification of Cervical Lesions

The Bethesda system [17] is the worldwide most used classification for cervical cytology. TBS divides precancerous squamous lesions in two categories, merging HPV-induced changes and mild dysplasia in low-grade squamous intraepithelial lesions (LSIL), whereas moderate and severe dysplasia are included together in high-grade squamous intraepithelial lesions (HSIL). Adenocarcinoma in situ (AIS) is used for noninvasive glandular lesions of the endocervical epithelia, while smears with borderline changes with LSIL, HSIL, and AIS or adenocarcinoma may be classified as atypical squamous cells unknown significance (ASC-US), atypical squamous cells unknown significance, a high-grade lesion cannot be excluded (ASC-H), and atypical glandular cells (AGC), respectively. Invasive cancer is divided in squamous cell cancer and adenocarcinoma.

8.2.1 Squamous Lesions

LSILs include large squamous cells which may show nuclear enlargement, binucleation, hyperchromasia, pycnosis with typical "smudged" chromatin, and sometimes koilocytosis, which shows distinct perinuclear halos with sharp borders. LSILs are expression of the early phase of cervical carcinogenesis, which is characterized by the production of new viruses. In this productive phase, the main molecular event is the expression of the HPV-L1 capsidic protein, while the proliferative activity of the epithelium and the expression of markers of oncogenic activity are still negligible [18]. High-risk HPV is found in 82% of all LSILs [19].The main HPV types are 16, which is found in 26% of lesions, followed by 31, 51, and 53 which are found in 10–12% of LSILs [20].

The main differential diagnosis of LSIL is other conditions which may show large abnormal cells. Reactive changes may be observed in inflammatory smears and may show nuclear enlargement up to 2×, albeit lacking hyperchromasia and nucleoli. Borderline changes may be classified as ASC-US according to TBS. Tissue repair typically shows sheets of epithelia with evident nucleoli, while isolated atypical cell and tumor diathesis are absent. Both reactive and reparative changes are independent from HPV, although they may be associated with a transitory HPV infection. *Invasive squamous cancer* may also include large atypical cells, which however show high-grade nuclear atypia and sometimes nucleoli, while tumor diathesis is often evident on the background; most cancers express HPV and biomarkers that are typical for high-grade lesions.

HSILs typically include small squamous cells with definite hyperchromasia, variability of nuclear size and shape, abnormal n/c ratio, and indentations of the nuclear membrane. Conventional smears may show a typical "Indian filing," which is however lost in LBC. HSILs are expression of the second part of carcinogenesis, which is characterized by the abnormal proliferation of the cervical epithelium. In this phase, the main molecular event is the expression of markers of oncogenic activity, particularly E6 and E7, while in most cases, L1 is no more detectable [21]. High-risk HPV (HR HPV) is found in up to 98% of all HSILs. The main HPV types are 16, which are found in about 50% of lesions, followed by 18 and 31 [22]. Accordingly, most HSILs and squamous cancers strongly express biomarkers of oncogenic activity [23, 24].

The main differential diagnosis of HSIL is other conditions that may be associated with abnormal small cells, including particularly invasive cancer and immature metaplasia. When small cells show marked nuclear atypia and nucleoli or tumor diathesis is present, an invasive cancer should be ruled out. Reactive changes on metaplastic cells usually lack hyperchromasia and show a modest nuclear enlargement as well as a slight anisocariosis. Metaplastic cells may occasionally express oncogenic or proliferative markers, being a potential pitfall in the interpretation of these lesions [25]. Borderline changes, particularly in smears with immature metaplastic cells, may be classified as *ASC-H* according to TBS.

8.2.2 Glandular Lesions of the Cervix

Atypical glandular cells may be found in *adenocarcinoma in situ (AIS)*, endocervical adenocarcinoma, endometrial adenocarcinoma, and metastasis of extrauterine malignancy. Particularly in LBC specimens, AIS is often characterized by a high cellularity. Already at low magnification, several hyperchromatic sheets are mostly readily evident. At higher magnification, the sheets consist of abnormally pseudostratified columnar cells with crowded, enlarged, elongated, and often hyperchromatic nuclei. The cytoplasm is typically reduced due to the nuclear enlargement, and nucleoli are mostly inconspicuous or small. Feathering is often observed at the periphery of the strips, and pseudorosettes may be also present. Since in about 50% of endocervical lesions a SIL may coexist, atypical squamous cells are often found. Borderline findings that are suspicious but not definite for glandular neoplasia may be classified as *AGC* according to TBS. AGC is further divided in AGC NOS and AGC favor neoplastic, depending on the severity of the cytologic features. The origin of the atypical cells (endocervical, endometrial, or extrauterine) should be specified when possible.

AIS is typically of usual type and accordingly HPV associated. HR HPV is found in 94% of all AIS. The main HPV types are 16, which are found in up to 57% of lesions, followed by type 18 which is found in up to 38% of AIS [26]. Biomarkers of oncogenic activity are mostly strongly expressed in AIS [27, 28] and may be useful for the differential diagnosis with reactive changes on endocervical cells, which are potentially the main mimic of endocervical neoplasia.

Tumor diathesis is not a feature of AIS, and its presence, as well as the loss of cell cohesion and highly atypical, polymorphic cells, strongly indicates the possibility of an invasive *adenocarcinoma*. Differently from AIS and squamous cancers, invasive adenocarcinomas of the cervix may be HPV negative in up to 25% of cases [24, 26]. Accordingly, HPV-negative variants of adenocarcinomas of non-usual type do not express most of the biomarkers of oncogenic activity. Moreover, up to 18% of AGC with negative HPV testing after the menopause harbor a non-cervical cancer, mostly of endometrial type [29].

8.3 Biomarkers in Cervical Cytology

The use of biomarkers in cervical cytology has some potential advantages compared with histology. The cytological sampling can be easily obtained noninvasively during routine testing, while histological sampling requires colposcopy. Moreover, a good cytologic sample may include a more representative part of the lesion compared with a small punch biopsy, leading to a better sensitivity and predictive value [30]. In both cervical cytology and histology most biomarkers are surrogate markers of the oncogenic activity of HPV. Thus, while the expression of a biomarker may correlate with a specific phase of the HPV-induced carcinogenesis, the lack of expression does not negate the possibility of an HPV infection or even the future development of a lesion, as well as the overexpression of a marker does not always correlate with the gravity of a precancerosis. In fact, it is important to keep in mind that most biomarkers that were developed for cervical pathology are functional markers that not always correlate with definite morphological features.

Basically, biomarkers may be used as diagnostic tools, particularly in borderline cases (ASC-US, ASC-H, AGC) in which the differentiation between reactive changes and neoplasia is morphologically difficult, and/or as markers of progression risk in LSILs or negative specimens with positive HPV test. The usefulness of biomarkers in latter case may be due to the identification of cases that in spite of a normal or low-grade morphology will progress to high-grade, or high-grade cells that have not been identified or have been incorrectly interpreted by cytology alone. Particularly in the setting of an HPV-based primary screening biomarkers may have the potentiality to improve the accuracy of cytology triage, thus allowing a better management of HPV-positive women while reducing the burden of unnecessary colposcopies.

From a practical point of view, biomarkers may be divided in two categories according to the main phases of HPV-induced carcinogenesis: markers of the early productive phase and markers of the advanced proliferative phase.

8.3.1 Biomarkers of the Productive Phase of the HPV-Induced Carcinogenesis

The early phase of cervical carcinogenesis is the productive phase. The morphological correlate of this phase is the LSIL, which shows an abnormal enlargement of the basal epithelial layers and typical cytopathic changes of the superficial layers (koilocytes). The productive phase is characterized by expression of late viral genes (particularly the major capsidic protein L1) which are involved in the viral capsid assembly and are restricted to differentiated superficial squamous cells. [21].

HPV-L1 is a marker which may detect immunohistochemically in tissue sections and immunocytochemically in conventional smears (CS) and liquid-based cytology (LBC) the viral L1 capsidic protein. In tissue sections, HPV-L1 is typically detected in superficial cells of the epithelium of low-grade lesions. Immunocytochemically, HPV-L1 is expressed in up to 69% of HPV-positive LSILs, whereas the expressions in HSILs with moderate dysplasia are found in 44% of samples [31, 32]. Histologically, HPV-L1 was described in up to 40% LSIL (CIN1), 6% HSIL (CIN2), and no HSIL with severe dysplasia (CIN3) [33, 34]. Galgano et al. described, however, HPV-L1 positivity in 16.5% of CIN3 lesions [35].

In cytologic specimens from HPV-positive women, HPV-L1-positive LSILs and even HSILs with moderate dysplasia have a higher potential of spontaneous regression compared with HPV-L1-negative lesions. Melhorn et al. described that 20% of HPV-L1-positive LSIL and HSIL (with moderate dysplasia) may progress to histological CIN3, while HPV-L1-negative SILs of the same grade show a progression to CIN3 in 84% of cases. [31]. This data are confirmed by further studies, which describe a significant difference between the progression risk of HPV-L1 positive and negative LSILs [36–38]. Thus, HPV-L1 may be useful in the management of

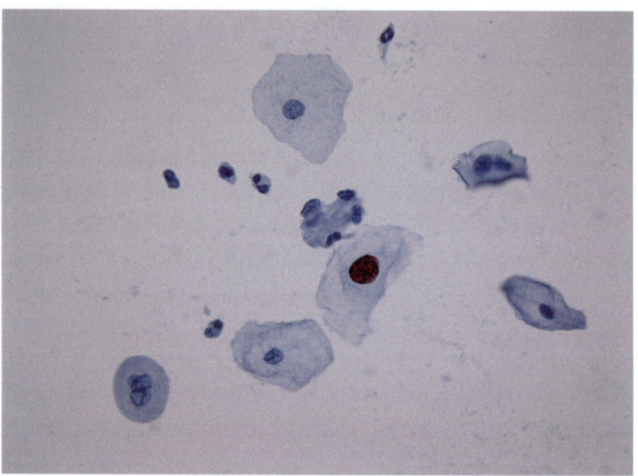

Fig. 8.1 L1-immunocytochemistry. LSIL with intense nuclear stain

HPV-positive women, allowing a less aggressive management in those who stain positive, even when cytology already shows features of HSIL with moderate dysplasia. The utility of HPV-L1 as a marker of regressive lesions may be limited, however, by the occasional expression in severe dysplasia (CIN3) [35]. A promising approach, using both HPV-L1 and a marker of the proliferative phase (e.g. p16), may allow a better differentiation of risk categories among LSILs [34, 37, 39] but still needs to be validated in large studies.

Positive HPV-L1 cells show an intense nuclear staining (Fig. 8.1). Some cytoplasmic staining was described in cervical samples [31], which however do not impair the evaluation of the immunoreaction.

8.3.2 Biomarkers of the Proliferative Phase of the HPV-Induced Carcinogenesis

The morphological correlate of the proliferative phase of the carcinogenesis of the squamous epithelia of the cervix is HSIL and squamous cancer. In this phase, a deregulation of the expression of the viral transforming proteins E6 and E7 leads to an abnormal cell proliferation and to the inability to repair mutations in the host cell DNA [8].

ProEx C (Becton Dikinson, USA) is a cocktail of MCM2 and TOP2a, two proteins that are involved in the control of DNA replication. MCM2 is a replicative helicase and is a member of the DNA licensing factor family that is required in an early stage of DNA replication as a key step during the G1 phase. TOP2a is a nucleic enzyme that affects the DNA structure and is involved in DNA replication, transcription, chromosome segregation, and cell cycle progression [40]. Both MCM2 and TOP2A are overexpressed when the S-phase cell cycle induction is aberrant [40, 41]. Several studies have evaluated ProEx C in cytologic specimens showing promising results. The marker is prevalently expressed in the nucleus of high-grade lesions, while the prevalence in LSILs is low particularly in women with negative follow-up (15%) and higher in those with LSIL persistence (30%) or progression to HSIL (43%) [43]. In a ASC-US population, Kelly et al. describe a sensitivity of 85% with a PPV of 44% and a NPV of 94% for CIN2+ [42]. As a triage test following primary HPV screening, ProEx C showed a sensitivity of 76%, a PPV of 41.7%, and a specificity of 98.3% compared with 85% sensitivity and 9.3% PPV of the HPV test alone [43]. Compared with other techniques, ProEx C showed results similar to molecular mRNA tests [44], making it an interesting option particularly in a setting of screening with primary HPV test. When compared with the classic proliferation marker Mib1, ProExC showed similar or more specific results [45].

Proex C was developed for the BD-SurePath LBC as well as for histology, but the possibility to use it with ThinPrep (Hologic, USA) LBC was described [46].

Immunostains with ProEx C in cytological specimens show a definite nuclear reaction (Fig. 8.2), although normal endocervical and metaplastic cells may also be stained [42, 46].

p16INK4a (p16) is a cyclin-dependent kinase inhibitor that physiologically counteracts the phosphorylation of pRB thus leading to a cycle arrest in normal somatic cells [47]. In cervical lesions, pRB may be inactivated by the HPV E7 viral oncoprotein, causing a loss of control of the cell cycle and, eventually, an overexpression of p16. Immunohistochemically, normal cervical epithelia mostly do not or only focally express p16. Conversely, a diffuse expression of p16 in at least the lower third of the squamous epithelium is considered characteristic for proliferative lesions in HPV-associated cervical carcinogenesis. In a meta-analysis of studies investigating p16 in histological specimens, p16 was diffusely expressed in 2% normal samples, 38% CIN1 (LSIL), 68% CIN2 (HSIL), and 83% CIN3 (HSIL) [48]. In LSILs, p16 expression is mostly restricted in the lower third of the epithelium, whereas in HSILs the protein may be detected also in the middle and upper third. In HPV-associated glandular neoplasia of usual type, p16 was detected in more than

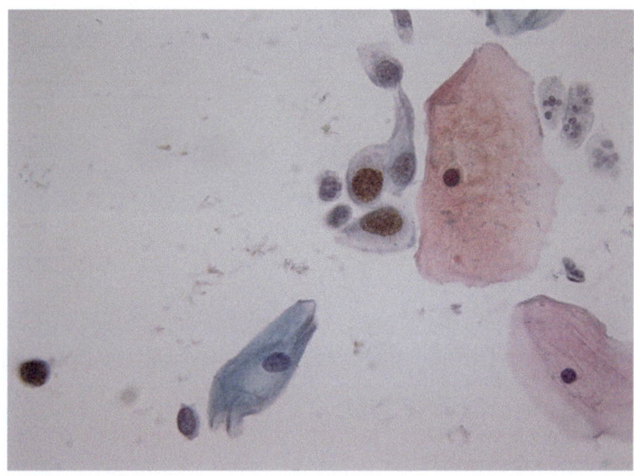

Fig. 8.2 ProEx C immuno-cytochemistry. HSIL with nuclear staining. Note the modified Papanicolaou counterstaining

90% of AIS and invasive adenocarcinomas [27, 49–51]. Conversely, p16 is often absent or only focally expressed in non-HPV-related variants of cervical adenocarcinoma [52, 53]. In both squamous and glandular lesions, p16 is usually detected in the cytoplasm and nucleus of dysplastic and cancer cells.

In histological specimens with low-grade dysplasia, several studies showed that p16-negativity is mostly associated with a regression of the lesion, while p16-positive CIN1 may progress to high-grade lesions [30, 54–56]. However, in spite of a significant difference in progression risk between p16-positive and p16-negative low-grade lesions, most p16-positive LSILs eventually regress, thus making a different management of these lesions still not feasible [57].

Cytologically, p16 immunocytochemistry was shown to be a sensitive marker of high-grade dysplasia and useful for the discrimination of borderline cases with a higher specificity than the HPV test [58]. In a setting of primary HPV screening, it was demonstrated that p16 triage cytology gives a significant increase in sensitivity compared with cytology alone [59, 60]. p16 alone may however be expressed also in occasional metaplastic, atrophic, and endocervical cells [25, 61]. While in histological specimens this may be readily differentiated from the typical diffuse staining of a true positivity, the occurrence of isolated p16-positive cells in a cytologic sample may be more challenging to evaluate. In more recent years, a combination of p16 and the proliferation marker ki67 was proposed as a marker of cervical lesions in cytologic specimens (CINtec PLUS, Roche, Switzerland). Simultaneous staining of p16 in nucleus and cytoplasm and Ki67 in the nucleus was described as specific for cell cycle deregulation in neoplasia. In both conventional smears and LBCs, positive cells show a brown (p16) cytoplasmic staining with a bright red (Ki67) nuclear stain (Fig. 8.3). Only cells with a definite dual staining are interpreted as positive, cells that stain only for p16 or ki67 are judged negative for the biomarker (Fig. 8.4). Dual staining with p16/ki67 demonstrated a better specificity compared with p16 alone [62]. Specificity and sensitivity were better than cytology alone in primary screening, while compared with HPV test immunocytochemistry was less

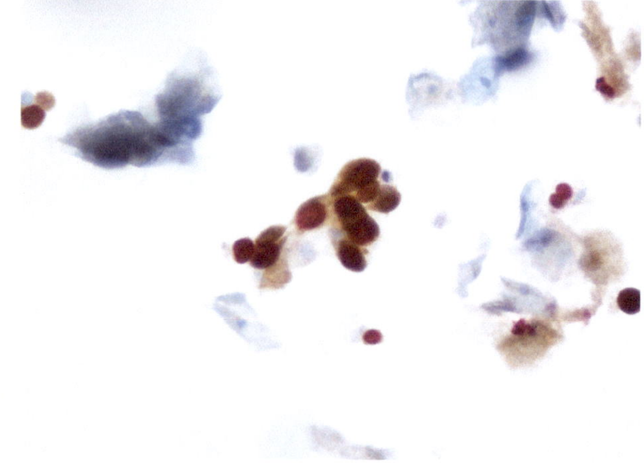

Fig. 8.3 CINtec PLUS p16/
Ki67 dual staining. HSIL
with brown cytoplasmic (p16)
and red nuclear (Ki67)
staining in the same cells

Fig. 8.4 CINtec PLUS p16/Ki67 dual staining. Atrophic epithelia with sole p16 staining. Unless both p16 and Ki67 are co-expressed in the same cell, the immunostaining is judged negative

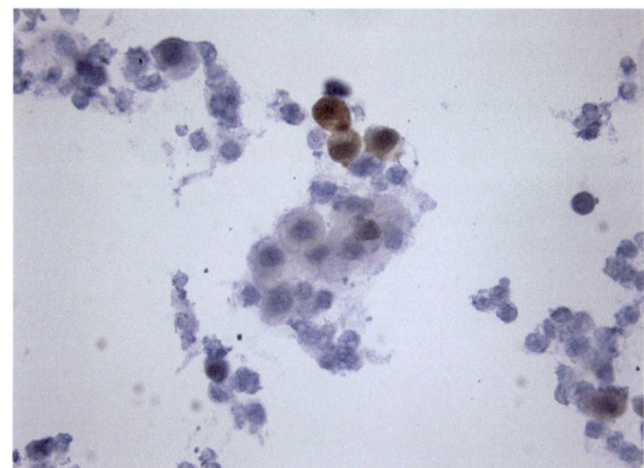

Fig. 8.5 CINtec PLUS p16/Ki67 dual staining. Adenocarcinoma in situ (AIS) of the cervix with intense, diffuse immunostaining

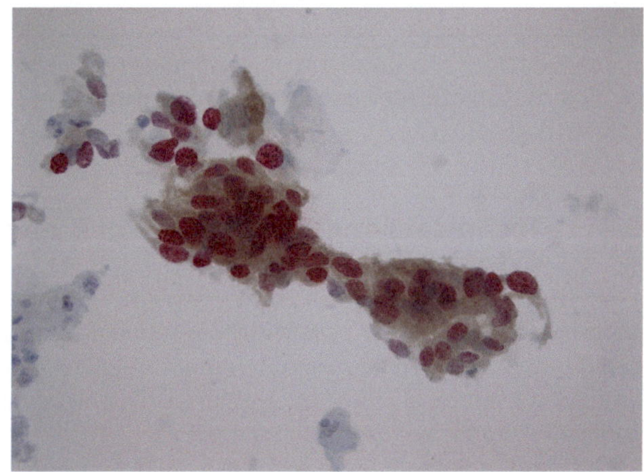

sensitive but more specific [63]. Furthermore, dual staining was shown to improve agreement between cytologists [64] with a better specificity (58.9% vs 49.6%), PPV (21.0 vs 16.6), and NPV (96.4 vs 94.2) compared with cytology alone in HPV-positive women [65]. Thus, particularly in a setting of primary HPV screening, p16/ki67 dual stain could allow a better risk stratification for HPV-positive women with normal cytology, allowing longer control intervals for those that do not express the biomarker while referring to colposcopy women with dual stain positivity [65]. In glandular lesions of the cervix, p16/ki67 was described in 92.5% of in situ and invasive adenocarcinomas of usual type, while only 6.2% of negative samples expressed the biomarker [28]. In glandular lesions, particularly in AIS, dual staining is mostly evident in sheets of adjacent neoplastic cells which show a diffuse and strong staining (Fig. 8.5), while the occurrence of occasional cell staining (Fig. 8.6) in large endocervical sheets should not be regarded as positive. Immunocytochemistry of samples in which a glandular lesion is suspected should always be associated with

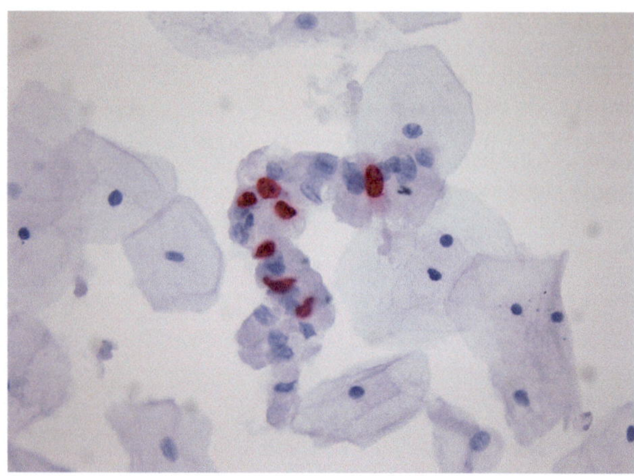

Fig. 8.6 CINtec PLUS p16/Ki67 dual staining. Normal endocervical epithelia with sole nuclear Ki67 staining (negative immunostaining). In neoplastic glandular sheets p16 and Ki67 are typically co-expressed in more adjacent cells

a careful morphological evaluation. Up to 25% of cervical adenocarcinomas, particularly the mucinous variants [24], are not associated with HPV and thus do not stain with p16/Ki67. Furthermore, particularly in menopausal women, most adenocarcinomas are of endometrial or extrauterine origin [29] and do not express surrogate markers of HPV.

8.4 Technical Aspects of the Use of Biomarkers in Cervical Cytology

Most biomarkers may be used with conventional smears, LBC, and cell blocks prepared from LBC residual material. Immunocytochemistry may be performed on the original conventional smear or original LBC or on a new LBC slide, which may be prepared from the residual sample material.

Performing immunocytochemistry on the original slide requires the careful unmounting of the cover glass and implicates a loss of the original cytologic staining. When immunocytochemistry is performed on conventional smears, the evaluation may be disturbed by cell overlapping, excess at blood or mucus. Several published studies, however, have successfully immunostained original conventional and LBC slides [31, 36] (Fig. 8.7). A possible solution to the loss of Papanicolaou staining is the use of a modified Pap counterstain after immunocytochemistry, which may also improve the diagnostic agreement of immunostained slides [25] (Fig. 8.2); the feasibility of this technique with dual immunostains as p16/ki67 has however still to be evaluated.

The main advantage of using a new LBC slide for immunostaining is the preservation of the original slide. In these cases, the immunocytochemical sample includes a cell population that is not the same of the original smear, and in some cases, particularly when only few abnormal cells were present in the original slide, there is the possibility that the new slide lacks diagnostic cells at all. Inadequate slides from the residual LBC material have been described in 4–9% of cases [62, 65]. On the other

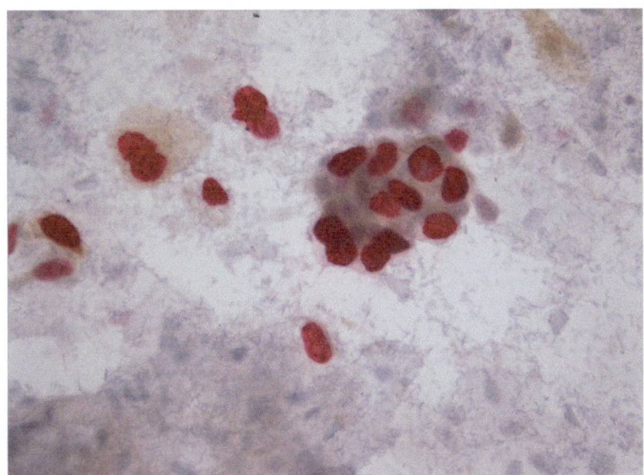

Fig. 8.7 CINtec PLUS p16/Ki67 dual staining in HSIL in a conventional smear

hand, the preparation of a further slide may also result in adding new valuable cells to the diagnostic evaluation.

The use of cell blocks of LBC residual material for immunohistochemistry of cervical lesions was described in few studies [66–68] with promising results. Cell blocks theoretically could allow multiple immunostains, but in about 25% of cases, a lack of diagnostic cells was reported [66, 69].

8.5 Molecular Application in Cervical Samples

Most of the guidelines on cervical cancer prevention consider reflex cytology (i.e., the evaluation of the cytological sample collected at the time of primary HPV DNA testing) a valuable triage tool for HR HPV DNA-positive women. Nevertheless, up to 8% of HR HPV-positive women with normal cytology have or will develop in the subsequent years a CIN2+ lesion. Therefore, there is a strong need for biomarkers that may allow risk stratification of HPV-positive women with normal cytology or, alternatively, potentially capable of replacing cytology as a triage tool (Fig. 8.8) [70–72].

Increasing evidence shows that several ancillary techniques are potentially useful in triaging HPV-positive women to increase the specificity of the test. These include (1) HPV molecular markers (HPV genotyping, mRNA), (2) molecular markers involved in cell cycling (hyperexpression of p16, HPV viral load, and integration), and (3) molecular markers related to epigenetic changes (methylation of human and viral genes, microRNAs (miRNAs)) [73] and cervical microbiome.

Molecular markers can be evaluated in purposely sampled cervical cells, on the residual cellularity of LBC, or on already stained Pap smears. In fact, a cervical cytology biobank could be established as an extension of current cytopathology laboratory practices implementing the systematic storage of Pap smears or LBC samples from women participating to the cervical cancer screening. This would also allow the standardization of cervical sample processing which is an important

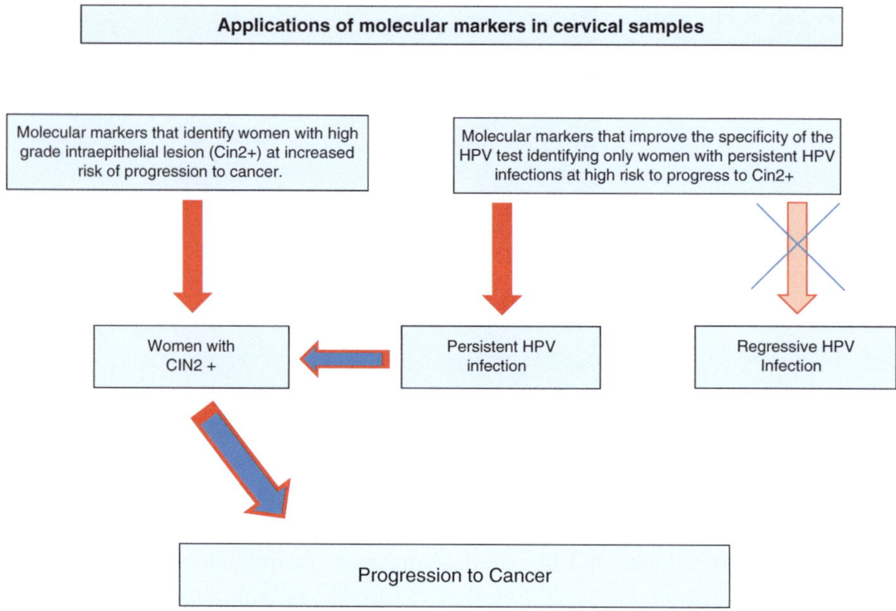

Fig. 8.8 Applications of molecular markers in cervical samples

step to preserve DNA, RNA, and proteins. The samples collected in LBC can be used for several months after collection for DNA analysis, while for RNA test, it is necessary to store the residual material as soon as possible at −80 °C [74]. In general, the storage of LBC specimens at room temperature decreases the stability of nucleic acids compared with frozen specimens. The recovery of DNA and RNA from specimens collected using ThinPrep (Hologic, Boxborough, Mass) was reported as reliable [75, 76]. Protocols for the efficient recovery of nucleic acids from specimens processed using SurePath (Becton Dickinson) have also been reported [77, 78]. Checking the length of the DNA fragments or the amount of ribosomal RNA to evaluate the quality of DNA and RNA in these samples is always recommended.

Archived, Pap-stained conventional smears may be used for the amplification of human or viral genomic sequences after scraping the cells from the slide. [79, 80]

8.6 HPV Molecular Markers

8.6.1 HPV Genotyping

HPV DNA typing is the technique that allows the detection of a specific HPV type in a biological sample.

Several methods have been described to identify different virus types in cytological samples: PCR with generic primers, RFLP (restriction fragment length polymorphism), hybridization with specific probes, reverse hybridization line probe assay, reverse line-blot hybridization, nucleotide sequencing, Luminex, and DNA Chip. Independently from the technique, it is important that a laboratory involved in genotyping participates at external quality control (EQA). The risk of precancer and cancer varies substantially for the different HPV types. The HPV genotypes 16 and 18 were shown to be cross-sectionally [81] and longitudinally [82] most often associated with high-grade CIN (hgCIN). Also HPV 31 and HPV 33 infections [83] have a higher risk to progression compared to the other carcinogenic types [84] detected by most commercial HPV assays [85]. However, while HPV genotyping can predict an increased risk of precancer, it cannot definitively differentiate between a transient infection and a prevalent precancer. Several commercial HPV assays offer partial genotyping and US guidelines recommend immediate referral of HPV16/18 positive women with normal cytology to colposcopy in a HPV-cytology cotesting strategy. Thus genotyping, combined with cytology, can be a suitable technique for identifying women with clinically relevant lesions already at the first test, or to select HPV infections at increased risk of developing precancer in the future. Moreover a complete HPV genotyping on cytological samples is already applied in epidemiological studies , in the follow-up and sometimes prior to HPV vaccination in adult women.

8.6.2   mRNA

Transcription of the circular HPV genoma lead to increasing level of messanger RNA (mRNA) that cause genetic instability and imply a risk of cellular changes, resulting in a selective growth advantage.

Expression of viral oncogenes E6 and E7 is higher in cervical precancer compared to transient HPV infection. In fact the progression to cervical malignancy requires the overexpression of the E6 and E7 genes of the integrated HR HPV genome [86, 87]. Thus, in cervical samples, HR HPV E6/E7 transcripts might be more specific than HR HPV DNA testing alone for the detection of CIN2+ lesions. Transcript analysis is feasible on LBC, which preserves RNA sufficiently to allow in vitro amplification and detection. Several studies have investigated mRNA on cervical biopsy and cytology samples, showing that the ratio of hrHPV E6/E7 mRNA positivity to HR HPV DNA positivity increases along with the severity of dysplasia. This suggests a higher specificity of the mRNA assay for high-grade cervical lesions compared to HPV DNA assays [88–92]. These studies stressed the possible relevance of mRNA detection in the clinical management of women screened for cervical cancer precursors. mRNA might be of value for the prediction of the risk of progression of cervical precancer thus allowing to select hrHPVDNA-positive women with normal cytology requiring immediate referral to colposcopy [93], but at this time, is used mainly in research studies. Long-term longitudinal studies (> = 6 years) are required to demonstrate that HPV DNA positive but HPV mRNA negative women have no risk to develop clinically relevant disease.

8.7   Molecular Markers Involved in Cell Cycling

8.7.1   Viral Load and Integration

HPV viral load and physical state of the viral genome are important determinants of HPV infection which influence the tumorigenic transformation of normal cervical epithelium and progression of the disease. Several studies suggested that viral copy number and physical state of viral genome (episomal vs integrated or mix) may have important clinical implications in the viral persistence and progression of cervical neoplasia [94, 95]. The amount of HPV DNA in cervical samples can be determined by real-time PCR and is feasible in LBC.

Integration is considered a key event in cervical carcinogenesis, which results in loss of episomal viral DNA. It is well-documented that E2 gene product derived from episomal DNA has an inhibitory effect on viral oncogene expression [96] and integrants are spontaneously selected during cancer progression due to selective growth advantage and endogenous antiviral response [97]. Integration of HPV16 viral DNA into the host genome and a high viral copy number within infected epithelial cells have been associated with an increased persistence of HPV infection and an increased risk of developing cervical intraepithelial neoplasia 2/3 (CIN2/3) or cancer [94, 95, 98, 99].

The clinical usefulness of these results has however still to be evaluated in large prospective studies.

8.8   Molecular Markers Related to Epigenetic Changes

8.8.1   DNA Methylation

Host DNA methylation involving CpG islands within gene promoters leads to silencing of gene expression, and its association with carcinogenesis has been widely described in many cancer sites. In human cells, DNA methylation is facilitated by a family of DNA methyltransferases that catalyze the addition of a methyl group to cytosines at the $5'$ position of a CpG dinucleotide pair and is typically detected by bisulfite modification of DNA [100, 101]. The methyl group can alter chromatin conformation and DNA topology resulting in displacement of transcription factors and alterations in expression [102, 103]. Methylation of CpG-rich stretches of human DNA located in promoter regions of genes, termed "CpG Islands," is essential for normal biologic processes [104]. Disruption of CpG island methylation has been documented in malignant cellular transformation [105]. Although there are no classical CpG islands within the HPV genome, regions of high density and conservation of CpG sites [106] suggest the potential for a functional role. The molecular basis and covalent alterations of methylation at individual CpG sites are poorly understood.

The human papillomavirus (HPV) DNA includes a total of 113 CpGs that could be potentially methylated. Several studies, mostly based on small convenience samples, showed different patterns of HPV DNA methylation in cervix cancer and precancerous cervical lesions compared to cervical cells with transient HPV infection. In the uterine cervix, DNA methylation in the host cell genes and in the virus genome could be an indicator of transforming HPV infection as well as a potential biomarker of aggressiveness. Targeted methylation of CpG sites may represent a mechanism by which HPV switches from a productive infection to one leading to transformation [107]. Alternatively, methylation of HPV DNA may serve as a host defense mechanism for silencing viral replication and transcription. Recent studies have shown that methylation status of HPV viral DNA could help to identify the presence of CIN2+ lesion in HPV infected women. [108–111]. Similar associations between HPV methylation and other HPV-associated anogenital and head and neck cancers have also been reported [112–115]. Among the several cell genes (>70) investigated for methylation status, some showed consistently elevated methylation in cervical cancers across the studies [116]. Different frequencies of methylation at specific sites were found in association with high-grade lesions, and the results were somehow not conclusive. [108, 109, 117] Although the results are already highly promising, a valuation of the methylation of the viral genome of other oncogenic HPV types is still needed before clinical application.

8.9   MiRNA

MiRNAs are endogenous, small noncoding single-stranded RNAs (~22 nt) that regulate gene expression by interacting with multiple of RNAs and inducing either translation suppression or degradation of RNA. Evidence suggests that alteration of miRNAs might be involved in the pathogenesis of a variety of human cancers, including cervical carcinoma. These differences frequently occur in tumor-specific microRNA signatures which may be helpful for the determination of the origin of the neoplasia and, sometimes, also specific tumor subtypes. Those specific microRNAs are frequently located in cancer-related genomic regions, which include fragile sites at or near HPV integration sites as well as common breakpoint regions [118].

Several miRNAs have been shown to be dysregulated in cervical carcinoma and could have a clinical use in the management of HPV-positive women as markers of the risk of developing hgCIN as well as predictors of persistent infection, playing a prognostic role in cancer survival [119, 120]. Different levels of some specific miR-NAs have been observed in women with high-risk HPV, low-risk HPV, or HPV-free, suggesting an interaction between HPV and miRNA expression [121].

miRNAs expression could be determined by quantitative real-time PCR (RT qPCR), by microarray able to measure the expression of tens of thousands of mRNAs in a single assay depending on the microarray design or by NGS (next-generation sequencing). Total RNAs are extracted from cervical samples, converted into cDNA, analyzed. Results are then evaluated for miRNAs expression profiles using bioinformatics analysis. At the present time, *actually* miRNA analysis is used only in research studies.

8.10 Cervical Microbiota

The vaginal microenvironment plays an important role in reproductive health. Commensal vaginal *Lactobacillus* spp. are thought to defend against pathogens and sexually transmitted infections [122] through maintenance of a hostile pH [123]; production of species-specific metabolites, bacteriocins; and adherence to mucous and disruption of biofilms [124–127]. Bacterial community structure is dynamic and hormonally influenced with a propensity to become less stable during menstruation [128] and conversely more stable and less diverse during normal pregnancy [129, 130]. The stability and composition of the vaginal microbiome may play an important role in determining host innate immune response and susceptibility to infection.

It has been recently proposed that abnormal vaginal microbiota could play an important role in the development of cervical neoplasm [131], but there are still several gaps in knowledge regarding the association between vaginal and cervical microbiomes and *CC* cancer development [132]. Microbiome could play a role in mechanisms associated with clearance or persistence of HPV infection and with CIN developing. Bacterial culture-based evidence indicates that some potential pro-oncogenic pathogens, which may be members of commensal microbiota, contribute to tumor initiation and development [133, 134]. The vaginal microbiome, amplified from DNA isolated from exfoliated cervical cells, could be characterized by 16S rRNA gene sequencing using different platforms (Sanger, Roche 454, Illumina MiSeq). At the present time, vaginal microbiota analysis in cervical samples is applied only in research studies.

References

1. Cuzick J, Clavel C, Petry KU, et al. Overview of the European and North American studies on HPV testing in primary cervical cancer screening. Int J Cancer. 2006;119(5):1095–101.
2. Nanda K, McCrory DC, Myers ER, et al. Accuracy of the Papanicolaou test in screening for and follow-up of cervical cytologic abnormalities: a systematic review. Ann Intern Med. 2000;132(10):810–9.
3. Schiffman M, Castle PE, Jeronimo J, et al. Human papillomavirus and cervical cancer. Lancet. 2007;370:890–907.
4. Bernard HU. Gene expression of genital human papillomaviruses and considerations on potential antiviral approaches. Antivir Ther. 2002;7:219–37.
5. zur Hausen H. Papillomaviruses and cancer: from basic studies to clinical application. Nat Rev Cancer. 2002;2:342.
6. McLaughlin-Drubin ME, Meyers J, Munger K. Cancer associated human papillomaviruses. Curr Opin Virol. 2012;2:459–66.
7. Ghittoni R, Accardi R, Hasan U, et al. The biological properties of E6 and E7 oncoproteins from human papillo-maviruses. Virus Genes. 2010;40:1–13.
8. Doorbar J. Molecular biology of human papillomavirus infection and cervical cancer. Clin Sci. 2006;110:525–41.
9. Moody CA, Laimins LA. Human papillomavirus oncoproteins: path-ways to transformation. Nat Rev Cancer. 2010;10:550–60.
10. Doorbar J, Quint W, Banks L, et al. The biology and life-cycle of human papillomaviruses. Vaccine. 2012;30S:55–70.

11. el Awady MK, Kaplan JB, O'Brien SJ, Burk RD. Molecular analysis of integrated human papillomavirus 16 sequences in the cervical cancer cell line SiHa. Virology. 1987;159:389–98.

12. Wentzensen N, Vinokurova S, Von Knebel Doeberitz M. Systematic review of genomic integration sites of human papillomavirus genomes in epithelial dysplasia and invasive cancer of the female lower genital tract. Cancer Res. 2004;64:3878–84.

13. Snellenberg S, Schutze DM, Claassen-Kramer D, et al. Methylation status of the E2 binding sites of HPV16 in cervical lesions determined with the Luminex(R) xMAP system. Virology. 2012;422:357.

14. Wentzensen N, von Knebel Doeberitz M. Biomarkers in cervical cancer screening. Dis Markers. 2007;23:315–30.

15. Reuschenbach M, Clad A, von Knebel Doeberitz C, et al. Performance of p16INK4a-cytology, HPV mRNA, and HPV DNA testing to identify high grade cervical dysplasia in women with abnormal screening results. Gynecol Oncol. 2010;119:98–105.

16. Sahasrabuddhe VV, Luhn P, Wentzensen N. Human papillomavirus and cervical cancer: biomarkers for improved prevention efforts. Future Microbiol. 2011;6:1083–98.

17. Nayar R, Wilbur DC. The bethesda system for reporting cervical cytology. 3rd ed. New York: Springer; 2014.

18. Izadi-Mood N, Sarmadi S, Eftekhar Z, et al. Immunohistochemical expression of p16 and HPV L1 capsid proteins as predictive markers in cervical lesions. Arch Gynecol Obstet. 2014;289(6):1287–92. https://doi.org/10.1007/s00404-013-3124-1.

19. ALTS Group. Human papillomavirus testing for triage of women with cytologic evidence of low-grade squamous intraepithelial lesions: baseline data from a randomized trial. The Atypical Squamous Cells of Undetermined Significance/Low-Grade Squamous Intraepithelial Lesions Triage Study (ALTS) Group. J Natl Cancer Inst. 2000;92(5):397–402.

20. Clifford GM, Rana RK, Franceschi S, et al. Human papillomavirus genotype distribution in low-grade cervical lesions: comparison by geographic region and with cervical cancer. Cancer Epidemiol Biomark Prev. 2005;14(5):1157–64.

21. Doorbar J. The papillomavirus life cycle. J Clin Virol. 2005;32(Suppl 1):S7–15.

22. Guan P, Howell-Jones R, Li N, et al. Human papillomavirus types in 115,789 HPV-positive women: a meta-analysis from cervical infection to cancer. Int J Cancer. 2012;131(10):2349–59. https://doi.org/10.1002/ijc.27485.

23. Doorbar J. Papillomavirus life cycle organization and biomarker selection. Dis Markers. 2007;23(4):297–313.

24. Stoler M, Bergeron C, Colgan TJ, et al. Squamous cell tumours and precursors. In: Kurman RJ, Carcangiu ML, Herrington CS, Young RH, editors. WHO classification of tumours of female reproductive organs. Lyon: IARC; 2014.

25. Negri G, Moretto G, Menia E, Vittadello F, et al. Immunocytochemistry of p16INK4a in liquid-based cervicovaginal specimens with modified papanicolaou counterstaining. J Clin Pathol. 2006;59(8):827–30.

26. Holl K, Nowakowski AM, Powell N, et al. Human papillomavirus prevalence and type-distribution in cervical glandular neoplasias: results from a European multinational epidemiological study. Int J Cancer. 2015;137(12):2858–68.

27. Negri G, Egarter-Vigl E, Kasal A, et al. p16INK4a is a useful marker for the diagnosis of adenocarcinoma of the cervix uteri and its precursors: an immunohistochemical study with immunocytochemical correlations. Am J Surg Pathol. 2003;27(2):187–93.

28. Ravarino A, Nemolato S, Macciocu E, et al. CINtec PLUS immunocytochemistry as a tool for the cytologic diagnosis of glandular lesions of the cervix uteri. Am J Clin Pathol. 2012;138(5):652–6.

29. Verdoodt F, Jiang X, Williams M, et al. High-risk HPV testing in the management of atypical glandular cells: a systematic review and meta-analysis. Int J Cancer. 2016;138(2):303–10.

30. Pacchiarotti A, Ferrari F, Bellardini P, et al. Prognostic value of p16-INK4A protein in women with negative or CIN1 histology result: a follow-up study. Int J Cancer. 2014;134(4):897–904.

31. Mehlhorn G, Obermann E, Negri G, et al. HPV L1 detection discriminates cervical precancer from transient HPV infection: a prospective international multicenter study. Mod Pathol. 2013;26(7):967–74.

32. Grapsa D, Frangou-Plemenou M, Kondi-Pafiti A, et al. Immunocytochemical expression of P53, PTEN, FAS (CD95), P16INK4A and HPV L1 major capsid proteins in ThinPrep cervical samples with squamous intraepithelial lesions. Diagn Cytopathol. 2014;42(6):465–75.

33. Yemelyanova A, Gravitt PE, Ronnett BM, et al. Immunohistochemical detection of human papillomavirus capsid proteins L1 and L2 in squamous intraepithelial lesions: potential utility in diagnosis and management. Mod Pathol. 2013;26(2):268–74.

34. Gatta LB, Berenzi A, Balzarini P, et al. Diagnostic implications of L1, p16, and Ki-67 proteins and HPV DNA in low-grade cervical intraepithelial neoplasia. Int J Gynecol Pathol. 2011;30(6):597–604.

35. Galgano MT, Castle PE, Atkins KA, et al. Using biomarkers as objective standards in the diagnosis of cervical biopsies. Am J Surg Pathol. 2010;34(8):1077–87.

36. Griesser H, Sander H, Walczak C, Hilfrich RA. HPV vaccine protein L1 predicts disease outcome of high-risk HPV+ early squamous dysplastic lesions. Am J Clin Pathol. 2009;132(6):840–5.

37. Yoshida T, Sano T, Kanuma T, et al. Immunochemical analysis of HPV L1 capsid protein and p16 protein in liquid-based cytology samples from uterine cervical lesions. Cancer. 2008;114(2):83–8.

38. Xiao W, Bian M, Ma L, et al. Immunochemical analysis of human papillomavirus L1 capsid protein in liquid-based cytology samples from cervical lesions. Acta Cytol. 2010;54(5):661–7.

39. Huang MZ, Li HB, Nie XM, et al. An analysis on the combination expression of HPV L1 capsid protein and p16INK4a in cervical lesions. Diagn Cytopathol. 2010;38(8):573–8.

40. Shroyer KR, Homer P, Heinz D, Singh M. Validation of a novel immunocytochemical assay for topoisomerase II-alpha and minichromosome maintenance protein 2 expression in cervical cytology. Cancer. 2006;108(5):324–30.

41. Pinto AP, Degen M, Villa LL, Cibas ES. Immunomarkers in gynecologic cytology: the search for the ideal biomolecular papanicolaou test. Acta Cytol. 2012;56(2):109–21.

42. Kelly D, Kincaid E, Fansler Z, et al. Detection of cervical high-grade squamous intraepithelial lesions from cytologic samples using a novel immunocytochemical assay (ProEx C). Cancer. 2006;108(6):494–500.

43. Depuydt CE, Makar AP, Ruymbeke MJ. Benoy et al. BD-ProExC as adjunct molecular marker for improved detection of CIN2+ after HPV primary screening. Cancer Epidemiol Biomark Prev. 2011;20(4):628–37.

44. Alaghehbandan R, Fontaine D, Bentley J, et al. Performance of ProEx C and PreTect HPV-Proofer E6/E7 mRNA tests in comparison with the hybrid capture 2 HPV DNA test for triaging ASCUS and LSIL cytology. Diagn Cytopathol. 2013;41(9):767–75.

45. Beccati MD, Buriani C, Pedriali M, et al. Quantitative detection of molecular markers ProEx C (minichromosome maintenance protein 2 and topoisomerase IIa) and MIB-1 in liquid-based cervical squamous cell cytology. Cancer. 2008;114(3):196–203.

46. Oberg TN, Kipp BR, Vrana JA, et al. Comparison of p16INK4a and ProEx C immunostaining on cervical ThinPrep cytology and biopsy specimens. Diagn Cytopathol. 2010;38(8):564–72.

47. Klaes R, Friedrich T, Spitkovsky D, et al. Overexpression of p16(INK4A) as a specific marker for dysplastic and neoplastic epithelial cells of the cervix uteri. Int J Cancer. 2001;92(2):276–84.

48. Tsoumpou I, Arbyn M, Kyrgiou M, et al. p16(INK4a) immunostaining in cytological and histological specimens from the uterine cervix: a systematic review and meta-analysis. Cancer Treat Rev. 2009;35(3):210–20.

49. Negri G, Bellisano G, Carico E, et al. Usefulness of p16ink4a, ProEX C, and Ki-67 for the diagnosis of glandular dysplasia and adenocarcinoma of the cervix uteri. Int J Gynecol Pathol. 2011;30(4):407–13.

50. Riethdorf L, Riethdorf S, Lee KR, et al. Human papillomaviruses, expression of p16, and early endocervical glandular neoplasia. Hum Pathol. 2002;33(9):899–904.

51. Tringler B, Gup CJ, Singh M, et al. Evaluation of p16INK4a and pRb expression in cervical squamous and glandular neoplasia. Hum Pathol. 2004;35(6):689–96.

52. Carleton C, Hoang L, Sah S, et al. A Detailed immunohistochemical analysis of a large series of cervical and vaginal gastric-type adenocarcinomas. Am J Surg Pathol. 2016;40(5):636–44.
53. Park KJ, Kiyokawa T, Soslow RA, et al. Unusual endocervical adenocarcinomas: an immunohistochemical analysis with molecular detection of human papillomavirus. Am J Surg Pathol. 2011;35(5):633–46.
54. Negri G, Vittadello F, Romano F, et al. p16INK4a expression and progression risk of low-grade intraepithelial neoplasia of the cervix uteri. Virchows Arch. 2004;445(6):616–20.
55. Cortecchia S, Galanti G, Sgadari C, et al. Follow-up study of patients with cervical intraepithelial neoplasia grade 1 overexpressing p16Ink4a. Int J Gynecol Cancer. 2013;23(9):1663–9.
56. Liao GD, Sellors JW, Sun HK, et al. p16INK4A immunohistochemical staining and predictive value for progression of cervical intraepithelial neoplasia grade 1: a prospective study in China. Int J Cancer. 2014;134(7):1715–24.
57. Darragh TM, Colgan TJ, Cox JT, Members of LAST Project Work Groups, et al. The Lower anogenital squamous terminology standardization project for HPV-associated lesions: background and consensus recommendations from the college of American pathologists and the American society for colposcopy and cervical pathology. Arch Pathol Lab Med. 2012;136(10):1266–97.
58. Roelens J, Reuschenbach M, von Knebel Doeberitz M, et al. p16INK4a immunocytochemistry versus human papillomavirus testing for triage of women with minor cytologic abnormalities: a systematic review and meta-analysis. Cancer Cytopathol. 2012;120(5):294–307.
59. Carozzi F, Confortini M, Dalla Palma P, New Technologies for Cervival Cancer Screening (NTCC) Working Group, et al. Use of p16-INK4A overexpression to increase the specificity of human papillomavirus testing: a nested substudy of the NTCC randomised controlled trial. Lancet Oncol. 2008;9(10):937–45.
60. Carozzi F, Gillio-Tos A, Confortini M, et al. NTCC working group. Risk of high-grade cervical intraepithelial neoplasia during follow-up in HPV-positive women according to baseline p16-INK4A results: a prospective analysis of a nested substudy of the NTCC randomised controlled trial. Lancet Oncol. 2013;14(2):168–76.
61. Murphy N, Heffron CC, King B, et al. p16INK4A positivity in benign, premalignant and malignant cervical glandular lesions: a potential diagnostic problem. Virchows Arch. 2004;445(6):610–5.
62. Schmidt D, Bergeron C, Denton KJ, Ridder R, European CINtec Cytology Study Group. p16/ki-67 dual-stain cytology in the triage of ASCUS and LSIL papanicolaou cytology: results from the European equivocal or mildly abnormal Papanicolaou cytology study. Cancer Cytopathol. 2011;119(3):158–66.
63. Ikenberg H, Bergeron C, Schmidt D, PALMS Study Group, et al. Screening for cervical cancer precursors with p16/Ki-67 dual-stained cytology: results of the PALMS study. J Natl Cancer Inst. 2013;105(20):1550–7.
64. Wentzensen N, Fetterman B, Tokugawa D, et al. Interobserver reproducibility and accuracy of p16/Ki-67 dual-stain cytology in cervical cancer screening. Cancer Cytopathol. 2014;122(12):914–20.
65. Wentzensen N, Fetterman B, Castle PE, et al. p16/Ki-67 dual stain cytology for detection of cervical precancer in HPV-positive women. J Natl Cancer Inst. 2015;107(12):djv257.
66. Akpolat I, Smith DA, Ramzy I, et al. The utility of p16INK4a and Ki-67 staining on cell blocks prepared from residual thin-layer cervicovaginal material. Cancer. 2004;102(3):142–9.
67. Shidham VB, Mehrotra R, Varsegi G, et al. p16 immunocytochemistry on cell blocks as an adjunct to cervical cytology: potential reflex testing on specially prepared cell blocks from residual liquid-based cytology specimens. Cytojournal. 2011;8:1.
68. Tawfik O, Davis M, Diaz FJ, Fan F. Cell block preparation versus liquid-based thin-layer cervical cytology: a comparative study evaluating human papillomavirus testing by hybrid capture-2/cervista, in situ hybridization and p16 immunohistochemistry. Acta Cytol. 2016;60(2):145–53.
69. Keyhani-Rofagha S, Vesey-Shecket M. Diagnostic value, feasibility, and validity of preparing cell blocks from fluid-based gynecologic cytology specimens. Cancer. 2002;96(4):204–9.

70. Clarke MA, Wentzensen N, Mirabello L, et al. Human papillomavirus DNA methylation as a potential biomarker for cervical cancer. Cancer Epidemiol Biomark Prev. 2012;21(12):2125–37. https://doi.org/10.1158/1055-9965.EPI-12-0905.

71. Ronco G, Giorgi-Rossi P, Carozzi F, New Technologies for Cervical Cancer screening (NTCC) Working Group, et al. Efficacy of human papillomavirus testing for the detection of invasive cervical cancers and cervical intraepithelial neoplasia: a randomised controlled trial. Lancet Oncol. 2010;11:249–25.

72. Rodríguez AC, Schiffman M, Herrero R, et al. Longitudinal study of human papillomavirus persistence and cervical intraepithelial neoplasia grade 2/3: critical role of duration of infection. J Natl Cancer Inst. 2010;102:315–24.

73. McCredie MR, Sharples KJ, Paul C, et al. Natural history of cervical neoplasia and risk of invasive cancer in women with cervical intraepithelial neoplasia 3: a retrospective cohort study. Lancet Oncol. 2008;9:425–34.

74. Carozzi F, De Marco L, Gillio-Tos A, NTCC Working Group, et al. Age and geographic variability of human papillomavirus high-risk genotype distribution in a large unvaccinated population and of vaccination impact on HPV prevalence. J Clin Virol. 2014;60(3):257–63.

75. Tarkowski TA, Rajeevan MS, Lee DR, Unger ER. Improved detection of viral RNA isolated from liquid-based cytology samples. Mol Diagn. 2001;6:125–30.

76. Cuschieri KS, Beattie G, Hassan S, et al. Assessment of human papillomavirus mRNA detection over time in cervical specimens collected in liquid d based cytology medium. J Virol Methods. 2005;124:211–5.

77. Murphy PG, Henderson DT, Adams MD, et al. Isolation of RNA from cell lines and cervical cytology specimens stored in BD SurePath preservative fluid and downstream detection of housekeeping gene and HPV E6 expression using real time RT-PCR. J Virol Methods. 2009;156:138–44.

78. Dixon EP, Lenz KL, Doobay H, et al. Recovery of DNA from BD SurePath cytology specimens and compatibility with the Roche AMPLICOR human papillomavirus (HPV) test. J Clin Virol. 2010;48:31–5.

79. Carozzi F, Ronco G, Confortini M, et al. Prediction of high-grade cervical intraepithelial neoplasia in cytologically normal women by human papillomavirus testing. Br J Cancer. 2000;83(11):1462–7.

80. Canfell K, Gray W, Snijders P, et al. Factors predicting successful DNA recovery from archival cervical smear samples. Cytopathology. 2004;15:276–82.

81. Castle PE, Stoler MH, Wright TC Jr, et al. Performance of carcinogenic human papillomavirus (HPV) testing and HPV16 or HPV18 genotyping for cervical cancer screening of women aged 25 years and older: a subanalysis of the ATHENA study. Lancet Oncol. 2011;12:880–90.

82. Kjaer S, Høgdall E, Frederiksen K, et al. The absolute risk of cervical abnormalities in high-risk human papillomavirus-positive, cytologically normal women over a 10-year period. Cancer Res. 2006;66:10630–6.

83. Kjaer SK, Frederiksen K, Munk C, Iftner T. Long-term absolute risk of cervical intraepithelial neoplasia grade 3 or worse following human papillomavirus infection: role of persistence. J Natl Cancer Inst. 2010;102(19):1478–88. https://doi.org/10.1093/jnci/djq356.

84. Bouvard V, Baan R, Straif K, et al. WHO International Agency for Research on Cancer Monograph Working Group A review of human carcinogens--Part B: biological agents. Lancet Oncol. 2009;10(4):321–2.

85. Wentzensen N, Schiffman M, Palmer T, Arbyn M. Triage of HPV positive women in cervical cancer screening. J Clin Virol. 2016;76(Suppl 1):S49–55. https://doi.org/10.1016/j.jcv.2015.11.015.

86. Johansson H, Bjelkenkrantz K, Darlin L, et al. Presence of high-risk HPV mRNA in relation to future high-grade lesions among high-risk HPV DNA positive women with minor cytological abnormalities. PLoS One. 2015;10(4):e0124460. https://doi.org/10.1371/journal.pone.0124460.

87. Cattani P, et al. Clinical performance of human papillomavirus E6 and E7 mRNA testing for high-grade lesions of the cervix. J Clin Microbiol. 2009;47(12):3895–901. https://doi.org/10.1128/JCM.01275-09.

88. Monsonego J, et al. Risk assessment and clinical impact of liquid-based cytology, oncogenic human papillomavirus (HPV) DNA and mRNA testing in primary cervical cancer screening (The FASE Study). Gynecol Oncol. 2012;125(1):175–80. https://doi.org/10.1016/j.ygyno.2012.01.002.

89. Ratnam S, et al. Clinical performance of the PreTect HPV-Proofer E6/E7 mRNA assay in comparison with that of the Hybrid Capture 2 test for identification of women at risk of cervical cancer. J Clin Microbiol. 2010;48(8):2779–85. https://doi.org/10.1128/JCM.00382-10.

90. Rijkaart DC, et al. High-risk human papillomavirus (hrHPV) E6/E7 mRNA testing by PreTect HPV-proofer for detection of cervical high-grade intraepithelial neoplasia and cancer among hrHPV DNA-positive women with normal cytology. J Clin Microbiol. 2012;50:2390–6. https://doi.org/10.1128/JCM.06587-11.

91. Munkhdelger J, et al. Performance of HPV E6/E7 mRNA RT-qPCR for screening and diagnosis of cervical cancer with ThinPrep® Pap test samples. Exp Mol Pathol. 2014;97(2):279–84. https://doi.org/10.1016/j.yexmp.2014.08.004.

92. Verdoodt F, et al. Triage of women with minor abnormal cervical cytology: meta-analysis of the accuracy of an assay targeting messenger ribonucleic acid of 5 high-risk human papillomavirus types. Cancer Cytopathol. 2013;121(12):675–87. https://doi.org/10.1002/cncy.21325.

93. Arbyn M, et al. The APTIMA HPV assay versus the Hybrid Capture 2 test in triage of women with ASC-US or LSIL cervical cytology: a meta-analysis of the diagnostic accuracy. Int J Cancer. 2013;132(1):101–8. https://doi.org/10.1002/ijc.27636.

94. Dalstein V, Riethmuller D, Pretet JL, et al. Persistence and load of high-risk HPV are predictors for development of high-grade cervical lesions: a longitudinal French cohort study. Int J Cancer. 2003;106:396–403.

95. Josefsson AM, Magnusson PK, Ylitalo N, et al. Viral load of human papilloma virus 16 as a determinant for development of cervical carcinoma in situ: a nested case-control study. Lancet. 2000;355:2189–93.

96. Pett M, Coleman N. Integration of high-risk human papillomavirus: a key event in cervical carcinogenesis? J Pathol. 2007;212:356–67.

97. Pett MR, Herdman MT, Palmer RD, et al. Selection of cervical keratinocytes containing integrated HPV16 associates with episome loss and an endogenous antiviral response. Proc Natl Acad Sci U S A. 2006;103:3822–7.

98. Lorincz AT, Castle PE, Sherman ME, et al. Viral load of human papillomavirus and risk of CIN3 or cervical cancer. Lancet. 2002;360:228–9.

99. Woodman CB, Collins SI, Young LS. The natural history of cervical HPV infection: unresolved issues. Nat Rev Cancer. 2007;7:11–22.

100. Herman JG, Baylin SB. Gene silencing in cancer in association with promoter hypermethylation. N Engl J Med. 2003;2042(54):349.

101. Jurkowska RZ, Jurkowski TP, Jeltsch A. Structure and function of mammalian DNA methyltransferases. Chembiochem. 2011;12:206.

102. Stein RA. DNA methylation pro filing: a promising tool and a long road ahead for clinical applications. Int J Clin Pract. 2011;65:1212–3.

103. Deaton AM, Bird A. CpG islands and the regulation of transcription. Genes Dev. 2011;25:1010–22.

104. Illingworth RS, Bird AP. CpG islands—a rough guide. FEBS Lett. 2009;583:1713–20.

105. Rodriguez-Paredes M, Esteller M. Cancer epigenetics reaches main- stream oncology. Nat Med. 2011;17:330–9.

106. Galvan SC, Martinez-Salazar M, Galvan VM, et al. Analysis of CpG methylation sites and CGI among human papillomavirus DNA genomes. BMC Genomics. 2011;12:580.

107. Vinokurova S, von Knebel Doeberitz M. Differential methylation of the HPV 16 upstream regulatory region during epithelial differentiation and neoplastic transformation. PLoS ONE. 2011;6:e24451.

108. Mirabello L, Sun C, Ghosh A, et al. Methylation of human papillomavirus type 16 genome and risk of cervical precancer in a costa rican population. J Natl Cancer Inst. 2012;104:556.

109. Wentzensen N, Sun C, Ghosh A, et al. Methylation of HPV18, HPV31, and HPV45 genomes and cervical intraepithelial neoplasia grade 3. J Natl Cancer Inst. 2012;104(22):1738–49.
110. Xi LF, Jiang M, Shen Z, et al. Inverse association between methylation of human papillomavirus type 16 DNA and risk of cervical intraepithelial neoplasia grades 2 or 3. PLoS ONE. 2011;6:e23897–65.
111. Hong D, Ye F, Lu W, et al. Methylation status of the long control region of HPV 16 in clinical cervical specimens. Mol Med Rep. 2008;1:555–60.
112. Wiley DJ, Huh J, Rao JY, et al. Methylation of human papillomavirus genomes in cells of anal epithelia of HIV-infected men. J Acquir Immune Defic Syndr. 2005;39:143.
113. Kalantari M, Villa LL, Calleja-Macias IE, Bernard HU. Human papillomavirus-16 and -18 in penile carcinomas: DNA methylation, chromo-somal recombination and genomic variation. Int J Cancer. 2008;123:1832–40.
114. Balderas-Loaeza A, Anaya-Saavedra G, Ramirez-Amador VA, et al. Human papillomavirus-16 DNA methylation patterns support a causal association of the virus with oral squamous cell carcinomas. Int J Cancer. 2007;120:2165–9.
115. Park IS, Chang X, Loyo M, et al. Characterization of the methylation patterns in human papillomavirus type 16 viral DNA in head and neck cancers. Cancer Prev Res (Phila). 2011;4:207–17.
116. Wentzensen N, et al. Utility of methylation markers in cervical cancer early detection. Gynecol Oncol. 2009;112:293.
117. Mirabello L, Schiffman M, Ghosh A, et al. Elevated methylation of HPV16 DNA is associated with the development of high grade cervical intraepithelial neoplasia. Int J Cancer. 2013;132:1412.
118. Mo W, Tong C, Zhang Y, Lu H. microRNAs' differential regulations mediate the progress of Human Papillomavirus (HPV)-induced Cervical Intraepithelial Neoplasia (CIN). BMC Syst Biol. 2015;9:4. https://doi.org/10.1186/s12918-015-0145-3.
119. Gadducci A, Guerrieri ME, Greco C. Tissue biomarkers as prognostic variables of cervical cancer. Crit Rev Oncol Hematol. 2012;86(2):104–29.
120. Cheung TH, Man KN, Yu MY, et al. Dysregulated microRNAs in the pathogenesis and progression of cervical neoplasm. Cell Cycle. 2012;11(15):2876–84.
121. Li Y, Liu J, Yuan C, et al. High-risk human papillomavirus reduces the expression of microRNA-218 in women with cervical intraepithelial neoplasia. J Int Med Res. 2010;38:1730–6.
122. Martin DH. The microbiota of the vagina and its influence on women's health and disease. Am J Med Sci. 2012;343:2. https://doi.org/10.1097/MAJ.0b013e31823ea228.
123. Boskey ER, Cone RA, Whaley KJ, Moench TR. Origins of vaginal acidity: high D/L lactate ratio is consistent with bacteria being the primary source. Hum Reprod. 2001;16:1809–13.
124. McMillan A, et al. Disruption of urogenital biofilms by lactobacilli. Colloids Surf B Biointerfaces. 2011;86(1):58–64. https://doi.org/10.1016/j.colsurfb.2011.03.016.
125. Boris S, Barbes C. Role played by lactobacilli in controlling the population of vaginal pathogens. Microbes Infect. 2000;2:543–6.
126. Aroutcheva A, et al. Defense factors of vaginal lactobacilli. Am J Obstet Gynecol. 2001;185(2):375–9. https://doi.org/10.1067/mob.2001.115867.
127. Ocana VS, Pesce De Ruiz Holgado AA, Nader-Macias ME. Characterization of a bacteriocin-like substance produced by a vaginal Lactobacillus salivarius strain. Appl Environ Microbiol. 1999;65:5631–5.
128. Gajer P, et al. Temporal dynamics of the human vaginal microbiota. Sci Transl Med. 2012;4(132):132ra52. https://doi.org/10.1126/scitranslmed.3003605.
129. MacIntyre DA, et al. The vaginal microbiome during pregnancy and the postpartum period in a European population. Sci Rep. 2015;5:8988. https://doi.org/10.1038/srep08988.
130. Romero R, et al. The composition and stability of the vaginal microbiota of normal pregnant women is different from that of non-pregnant women. Microbiome. 2014;2:4. https://doi.org/10.1186/2049-2618-2-4.

131. Dejea CM, Wick EC, Hechenbleikner EM, et al. Microbiota organization is a distinct feature of proximal colorectal cancers. Proc Natl Acad Sci U S A. 2014;111(51):18321–6. https://doi.org/10.1073/pnas.1406199111.
132. Chase D, Goulder A, Zenhausern F, et al. The vaginal and gastrointestinal microbiomes in gynecologic cancers: a review of applications in etiology, symptoms and treatment. Gynecol Oncol. 2015;138(1):190–200. https://doi.org/10.1016/j.ygyno.2015.04.036PMID:25957158.
133. Ito Y, Kishishita M, Yanase S. Induction of Epstein-Barr virus antigens in human lymphoblastoid P3HR1 cells with culture fluid of Fusobacterium nucleatum. Cancer Res. 1980;40(11):4329–30.
134. Han YW. Fusobacterium nucleatum: a commensal-turned pathogen. Curr Opin Microbiol. 2015;23:141.

Molecular Applications in Hematolymphoid Cytology

9

Joerg Schwock, Graeme R. Quest, and William R. Geddie

9.1 Introduction

Results from the College of American Pathologists Interlaboratory Comparison Program in Nongynecologic Cytopathology suggest that cytology laboratories perform surprisingly well in the diagnosis of lymphoma and are often able to identify the correct general diagnostic category even without immunophenotypic information [1]. A recent review focused on the extant literature on endoscopic/endobronchial ultrasound-guided fine needle sampling (FNS) of deep-seated lymphomas shows a favorable assessment in most studies [2]. Regardless, publications and guidelines have cast doubt on the use of cytology for the diagnosis of lymphoproliferative diseases [3, 4], an area where cytology has traditionally been restricted (or relegated) to special specimen types such as those which are quantitatively minimal or nonsolid (e.g., cerebrospinal fluid (CSF) or effusion samples). Even the casual observer will find, however, that cytologic samples, if obtained and processed correctly, provide an excellent substrate for morphologic assessment which today still remains the foundation of an accurate diagnosis in the vast majority of cases. On occasion alternative sampling methods such as core needle biopsy and surgical biopsy are indeed required. That may be the case in a number of situations in which a final diagnosis more crucially depends on architectural features (somewhat

J. Schwock (✉)
University of Toronto, University Health Network, Toronto General Hospital,
Toronto, ON, Canada
e-mail: joerg.schwock@uhn.ca

G. R. Quest
Queen's University, Kingston Health Science Centre,
Kingston, ON, Canada
e-mail: Graeme.Quest@kingstonhsc.ca

W. R. Geddie
Toronto, ON, Canada

© Springer International Publishing AG, part of Springer Nature 2018
F. C. Schmitt (ed.), *Molecular Applications in Cytology*,
https://doi.org/10.1007/978-3-319-74942-6_9

analogous to "follicular neoplasms" in thyroid cytology) or whenever extensive fibrosis or low tumor cell density preclude the acquisition of an adequate sample. However, cytology reports for inadequate samples are usually released within short time, and rapid on-site assessment provided in many centers often permits immediate addition of a core needle biopsy while the patient is still in the procedure room [5]. Another argument put forward is the risk of sampling error. However, multiple needle passes executed with proper technique may sample a lymph node more extensively than a limited number of core needle biopsies. A final point made by critics is often a lack of tissue for research purposes.

Although it is true that many cytologic samples are quantitatively more limited, numerous studies (some of which are included in the following text) provide evidence that modern pathology research can be performed successfully using cytology samples as substrate. In the appropriate context, which includes training, expertise, and access to ancillary techniques (in particular flow cytometry (FC)—after all nobody would suggest that histopathology is any more accurate without the use of immunohistochemistry), fine needle cytology with or without core needle biopsy should be considered the primary modality of assessment of nodal and extranodal masses *including* lymphoproliferative disease, while surgical excision should be reserved for those patients who have not had the benefit of a specific diagnosis or appropriate classification of their disease or whose clinical/radiologic presentation is not fully explained by the findings of the needle sample. After all, when the same result can be achieved with less invasive methods, is not the avoidance of costly and potentially harmful sampling procedures also a quality feature of the health care we should provide?

9.2 Handling and Triage of Lymphoid Specimens

Successful assessment of lymphoid tissue in cytologic specimens requires a dedicated approach to handling and laboratory processing [6]. Clinicians obtaining fine needle samples may not have the skills or insight required for this task which benefits greatly from rapid on-site evaluation (ROSE). ROSE has the dual goal of ensuring specimen adequacy and appropriate handling for requisite ancillary studies. Similarly, rapid assessment and laboratory-based triage (RALT) can be instituted for a predetermined set of specimens repeatedly received by a certain cytology laboratory. Both, ROSE and RALT are invaluable tools, which together guarantee the highest chance of successfully arriving at an accurate and clinically relevant diagnosis, and constitute a most fundamental approach to the widely emphasized theme of personalized medicine.

ROSE is a process during which a cytopathologist or cytotechnologist performs an initial evaluation of a portion of the specimen in the course of the sampling procedure and provides immediate feedback to the clinician or radiologist. Beyond the immediate effect on adequacy, ROSE is used to triage material for FC which usually requires one or more dedicated needle passes which are rinsed into tissue culture medium such as RPMI-1640 or other suitable carrier solutions. Time to delivery for FC analysis should be minimized as much as possible, and refrigerated storage may be necessary if an extended time is required for delivery to the laboratory. A portion of the cell suspension may be retained either by removing a liquid aliquot, generating cytocentrifuge slides, or by storage of DNA on FTA™ cards. Cytocentrifuge slides further facilitate assessment for cellularity and morphology.

RALT permits evaluation of minimal specimens (e.g., CSF, vitreous fluid) or those suspected to be involved by lymphoma (e.g., body cavity effusions) in a similar fashion. Removal of an aliquot immediately after laboratory accessioning and processing as cytocentrifuge preparation permits assessment of specimen quality (e.g., cell preservation, admixture of blood, and other benign components), cellularity, and morphology. Potential outcomes of RALT are (1) morphologic assessment alone (e.g., paucicellular CSF specimen with non-specific clinical presentation and history), (2) morphology plus ancillary studies (e.g., FC for CSF with numerous morphologically abnormal lymphoid cells), and (3) selection of an alternative/more appropriate ancillary test (e.g., clonality analysis for paucicellular CSF with abnormal cells in a patient with history of lymphoproliferative disease and new neurologic symptoms).

9.3 Historical Perspective: Cytology and Ancillary Tests

Cozzolino et al. examined the history of FNS of lymph nodes and lymphoid organs [7]. One of the earliest scientific accounts stems from the hematologist Hirschfeld who studied lymphoproliferative lesions of the skin [8]. Because of the limitations of morphology alone, ancillary methods were sought for the diagnosis and classification of lymphoid lesions. Southern blotting for immunoglobulin gene rearrangement studies was proposed in the 1980s in order to enhance the diagnostic efficacy of FNS which was viewed as "safe, simple and economical" in most circumstances compared to excisional biopsy [9]. Southern blotting was embraced by some cytopathologists who found gene rearrangement studies useful in a subset of samples not conclusively classifiable due to absent or equivocal surface immunophenotype, T-cell derivation, or presence of a small or poorly differentiated neoplastic population [10, 11]. Karyotyping was initially used with cytology specimens for the detection of t(8;14) and variant translocations [12–14] as well as other, less common situations to enhance the accuracy of lymphoma subtyping [15]. The morphologic diversity of hematolymphoid neoplasms and continuously evolving classification systems made it apparent that no single diagnostic method (except for morphologic assessment) would be universally suitable, leading to the "birth" of the multiparameter approach in the cytologic diagnosis of incident or recurrent lymphadenopathies which in modernized form remains valid today [16–21]. Southern blotting, which is cumbersome and time-consuming and requires high-quality DNA, was eventually replaced by polymerase chain reaction (PCR) for the assessment of gene rearrangements. Similarly, traditional cytogenetics, which requires time-consuming and laborious cell culture for metaphase preparations, has been replaced for most mature lymphoid neoplasms by fluorescence in situ hybridization (FISH) on interphase nuclei which permits greater versatility and a turnaround time of hours if required. These technological advances were paralleled by significant progress in the classification of hematolymphoid neoplasms with much greater emphasis on surface immunophenotype, cytogenetic, and molecular parameters for classification [22]. Even more sophisticated methods have made inroads which now permit insight into changes at the genomic level (i.e., array comparative genomic hybridization, next-generation sequencing) [23]. Thus, the cooperation between hematopathologists and cytopathologists invoked in an early, eloquently written editorial [24] has become now more important than ever in order to exploit the full potential of the methods and technologies at the disposal of both specialties. Interestingly, although an article weighing the prós and cons of cytologic diagnosis of lymphoma finds that the sensitivity ranges widely (0–100%), 21 of the 30 articles (70%) included at the time of writing reported a sensitivity greater than 80% in their ability to definitively recognize non-Hodgkin lymphoma by FNA [25]. Others have reported an exceptionally high diagnostic efficacy in their practice setting with considerable sensitivity (96.9%), specificity (86.7%), positive predictive value (PPV) (96.9%), and negative predictive value (NPV) (86.7%) despite the potential for sampling error in a subset of fairly well-characterized scenarios such as Hodgkin lymphoma [26]. Thus, the experience of several groups contradicts the negative view voiced by some [3, 27] and supports FNA combined with FC as a suitable initial approach in the diagnosis of both primary and recurrent lymphoma which obviates the need for a surgical biopsy in a substantial number of patients either in isolation or through combination with core needle biopsy [28–32].

Although the use of FNS requires a minimum of technological infrastructure, which makes it attractive not only in resource-limited settings [33], the multiplicity of preparatory techniques at the disposal of the cytopathologist (as opposed to the relative uniformity of tissue preparation, processing, staining in surgical pathology) requires careful consideration of the pre-analytical factors such as the most appropriate sample storage medium [34, 35]. Assessment of the morphologic features (which includes microarchitectural clues such as the presence of numerous germinal center fragments in follicular lymphoma in conjunction with a lack of the distinct polymorphism normally encountered in reactive lymphoid hyperplasia) is the next step [36]. Diagnosis and subclassification especially of low-grade lymphomas relies substantially on data derived from appropriately chosen ancillary studies with immunophenotyping (either by FC or less commonly immunocytochemistry) as the cornerstone [37]. FISH and PCR are utilized in specific circumstances including those with limited or equivocal immunophenotype and, increasingly, to obtain additional data of prognostic or predictive value [6, 38].

Common situations in which the presence of lymphoma in a sample may be missed are those in which (1) ancillary tests are not performed (e.g., due to limited cellularity or erroneously omitted due to prevailing polymorphous morphology such as in marginal zone lymphoma or partial lymph node involvement by lymphoma), (2) neoplastic cells are rare (e.g., in Hodgkin lymphoma), or (3) reactive changes or admixed benign tissue (e.g., granulomatous inflammation) disguise the lymphoproliferative process both morphologically and immunophenotypically. Critical assessment of ancillary testing results in the context of morphologic, radiologic, and clinical findings is essential to avoid these pitfalls, and an algorithmic rather than a "shotgun" use of ancillary tests is more likely to be successful. For instance, PCR is most useful in the occasional B-cell neoplasm which lacks surface immunoglobulin light chain expression (the usual surrogate for a clonal population if monotypic) and in T-cell neoplasms. It must be kept in mind that the value of a negative result is limited due to the potential for a false-negative test arising from admixture of polyclonal cells (especially if lymphoid), lack of primer binding (due to somatic hypermutation), or other reasons [19]. Additionally, detection of a clonal population is not, on its own, diagnostic of neoplasia as small clonal populations may occur under physiologic conditions. An early study applying the multiparameter approach showed high sensitivity (91%), specificity (95%), and accuracy (97%) but found PCR analysis to be the least helpful ancillary test and occasionally misleading [39]. Similarly positive assessments are also seen in more recent reports which utilize the full spectrum of modern ancillary methods [20].

In conclusion, the value of ancillary studies to establish the immunophenotypic, cytogenetic, and molecular features of a hematolymphoid neoplasm cannot be overstated, but morphologic evaluation crucially guides their selection and clinical judgment (including patient history, disease presentation, sample adequacy, test characteristics, result communication, management decisions) is essential. Thorough training, familiarity with the pitfalls and dedication to proper specimen handling are at the heart of success in the cytopathological diagnosis and classification of lymphoma. Even when taking into account a recent critical assessment [27], cytopathology has the potential to avoid unnecessary surgery in well over half of the patients with lymphoma and certainly a much larger proportion of patients presenting for the initial workup of lymphadenopathy of unknown cause [32]. Keeping the pitfalls in mind, cytopathologists should have the courage to use the skills acquired in more traditional settings, such as effusion cytology [40], and apply them more extensively.

9.4   In Situ Hybridization (ISH) in Hematolymphoid Cytopathology

One of the earliest studies using the generation of DNA-RNA hybrids in cytological preparations of *Xenopus* oocytes was published by Gall and Purdue in 1969 [41]. Since then the method of in situ hybridization (ISH) for the detection of specific chromosomal sequences, in particular translocations and other structural chromosome rearrangements, has entered the standard repertoire of cytogenetics laboratories around the world with a wide array of applications using commercially available reagents. In the diagnosis of lymphoid neoplasms, ISH has largely replaced conventional cytogenetics which requires fresh tissue, time-consuming cell culture and meticulous specimen preparation now reserved for special circumstances or research applications [42–44]. The most common variation essentially utilizes fluorescently labelled DNA sequences (probes) for the detection of a sequence of interest in cells during interphase (I-FISH) observed with a fluorescence microscope (Fig. 9.1a, b). Replacement of the fluorescent label by a chromogen suitable for light microscopy is termed chromogenic in situ hybridization (CISH). Use of cells after culture and cell cycle arrest (metaphase FISH) permits the exact visualization of a sequence or rearrangement in the chromosomal

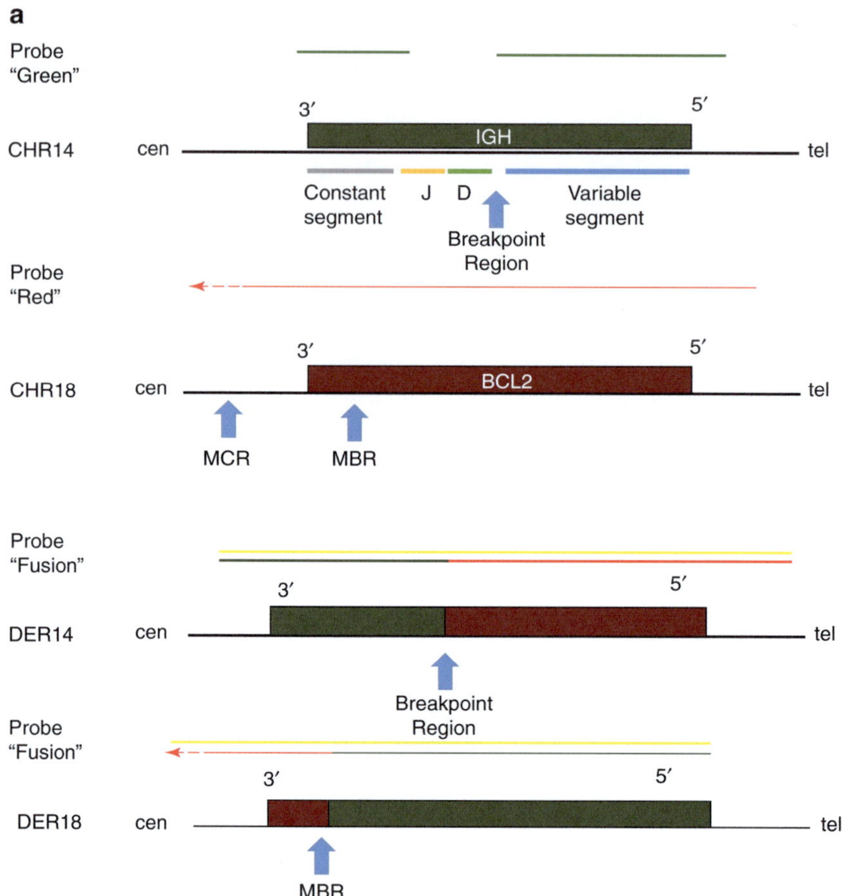

Fig. 9.1 FISH in hematolymphoid cytopathology. (**a**) Schematic of the t(14;18)(q32;q21) translocation (not to scale) involving IGH on chromosome 14 and BCL2 on chromosome 18. Probe location and color shown above each gene is to illustrate the dual-color dual-fusion design. BCL2 is shown with the major breakpoint region and the minor cluster region (arrows). BCL2 "Red" FISH probe with dashed line and arrow indicates extension of the probe to the left (not represented). (**b**) Two derivative chromosomes result from t(14;18)(q32;q21) rearrangement. Arrangement of the 5′ region of BCL2 next to D, J, and constant segments of IGH on derivative chromosome 14 causes illegitimate BCL2 expression driven by IGH downstream enhancers. Juxtaposition of red and green FISH probes results in a yellow fusion signal. Abbreviations: *CHR* chromosome, *DER* derivative, *cen* centromere, *tel* telomere. (**c**) I-FISH study using a dual-color dual-fusion design to detect t(11;14) (q13;q32) in mantle cell lymphoma. Fusion signals (horizontal yellow arrows) appear as adjacent red and green signals or overlapping yellow to orange dots. Each cell also shows the single red and green signal of the germline alleles. (**d**) I-FISH study of a Burkitt lymphoma illustrating the use of a break-apart probe spanning 8q24 to confirm a MYC translocation. Two interphase tumor cells and an adjacent metaphase have been photographed using a triple band pass filter (blue/green/red). Germline configuration is indicated by juxtaposed green and red fluorophores (vertical yellow arrows). Separation of the red (horizontal red arrows) and green signals (horizontal green arrows) indicates rearrangement. Inset shows a benign small lymphocyte (two yellow signals) and a lymphoma cell with one red, one green and one germline (arrow) signal. Size bar, 20 μm

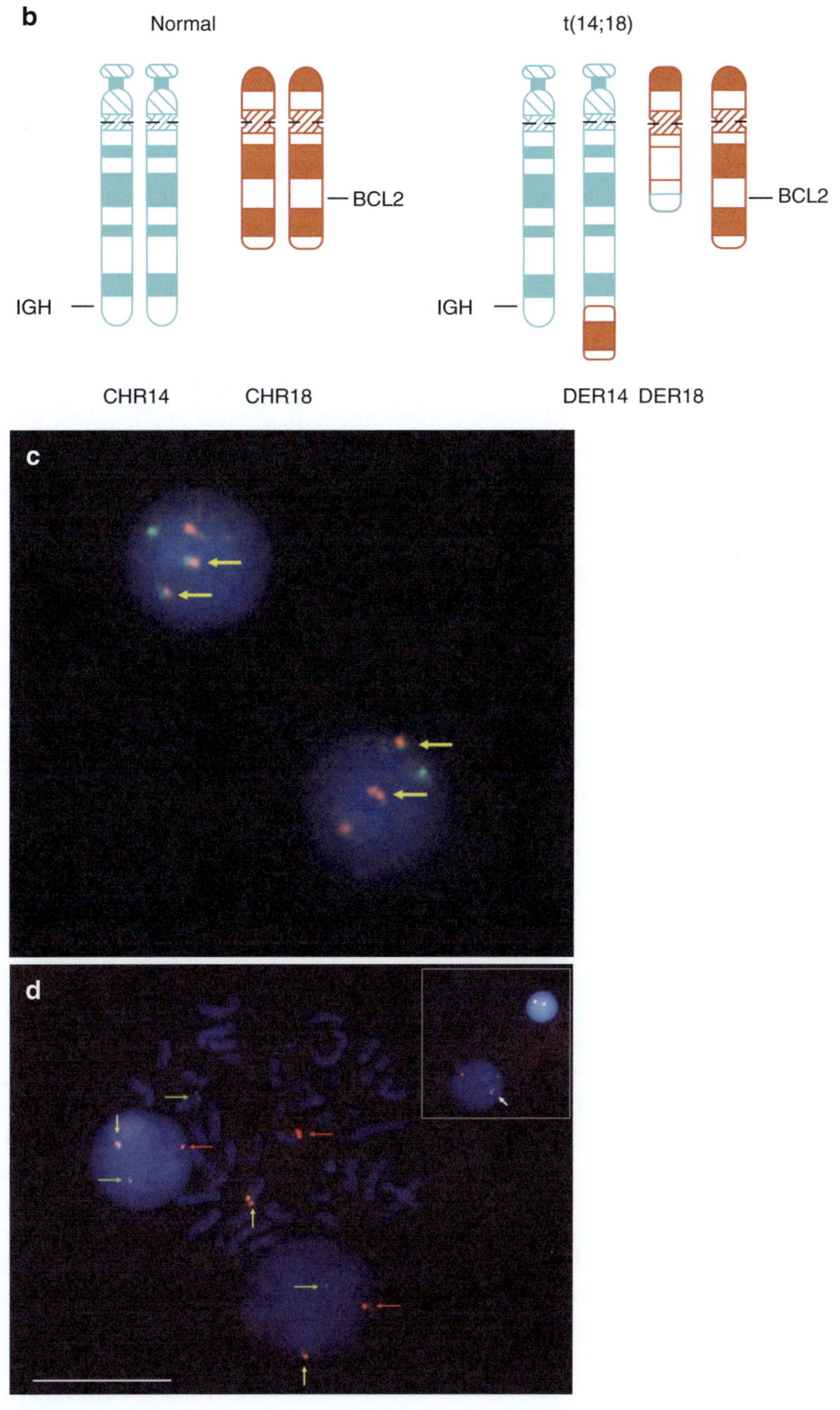

Fig. 9.1 (continued)

context. RNA (riboprobes) and peptide nucleic acids (PNAs) which consist of bases joined by a peptide-like backbone are alternatives to DNA probes.

I-FISH is a rapid and powerful technique for the clinical detection of numeric and structural abnormalities even in small subpopulations [45]. Unique sequence or locus-specific probes are used to detect the loss, gain, or structural rearrangement of genes or chromosomal regions of interest. The probes, which are labelled with different fluorophores, are designed to hybridize with two sequences on different loci in order to detect either their juxtaposition or separation. Single fusion probes designed to overlap either the 5′ or 3′ end of the two chromosomal areas would be expected to show two red and two green signals in a normal cell and one red, one green, and one yellow fusion signal in case of a translocation. A disadvantage of their simple design, especially for detection of gene fusions, is the possibility for random close proximity of the signals with resulting false-positive results. This has largely eliminated the use of single fusion probes in clinical applications. Much higher specificity and sensitivity is achieved with the use of two locus-specific probes which span the regions or genes involved in a balanced rearrangement (e.g., reciprocal translocation of IGH on chromosome 14 and CCND1 on chromosome 11 in mantle cell lymphoma) [46, 47] (Fig. 9.1c). This dual-color dual-fusion design produces two fusion signals (yellow ×2) with colocalization of the regions involved in the rearrangement and two signals (red ×1, green ×1) for the germline, unaffected allele [48, 49]. Dual-color break-apart probes are essentially the reverse design [49]. In this case the germline cell would show two yellow signals resulting from red and green fluorophores in close proximity, and a translocation would produce one red, one green, and one yellow signal. Break-apart probes are particularly useful in situations in which a translocation can involve multiple different partners. Centromeric probes targeted at repetitive alpha and beta satellite sequences of chromosomes can be, if unique, used for chromosome enumeration to detect aneuploidies. Telomeric probes are suitable for the detection of changes at the tandemly repeated chromosome ends. Complex rearrangements can be studied with whole-chromosome painting probes, multiplex-FISH using 24 colors, or spectral karyotyping, but the use of these methods in the routine clinical context is limited [49].

Direct smears, cytospin preparations, or formalin-fixed paraffin-embedded (FFPE) cell block material can be used as long as a monolayer is produced with limited overlap between neighboring nuclei. The basic steps consist of denaturation of probe and target, hybridization, washing to remove excess probe, and signal detection. Evaluation of FISH preparations and result reporting follows specific criteria which depend on the test substrate (intact cells or sections), the hybridization quality, probe design, and predetermined cutoff values (e.g., mean with three standard deviations or binominal distribution with 95% confidence interval). Cytologic preparations (i.e., direct smears, cytospin slides, tissue imprints, liquid-based preparations) have advantages over FFPE tissues such as lack of truncation artifact that arises from partial representation of nuclei in 4 μm thickness sections [50]. Some authors have proposed the extraction of nuclei from FFPE material [51], but upfront preparation of a cytologic sample easily circumvents this problem. Fine needle samples often contain less stromal tissue (compared to core needle or surgical biopsies) which facilitates scoring. The feasibility of sequential re-hybridization of single cytology slides has also been demonstrated [50]. Clinical use of FISH requires training to obtain the requisite analytical and post-analytical skills, probe and analytical validation, knowledge about interpretation and reporting of typical and atypical results, and administration of a quality program in accordance with the extant guidelines relevant to the individual laboratory [52].

The purpose of genetic studies including FISH in cytologic specimens with suspected hematolymphoid disorders is most commonly the detection of abnormalities that either serve as (1) proof of the clonal nature of the disease and/or provide (2) clues to the specific classification of a neoplasm or (3) are of prognostic and/or predictive value. In a study using both conventional cytogenetics and FISH, structural chromosomal abnormalities were more common than numerical abnormalities in mature B- and T-cell neoplasms, and FISH revealed rearrangements unsuspected by conventional cytogenetics in 48% of the cases [53]. The vast majority of the neoplasms encountered in the adult patient are mature B- or, less commonly, T-cell neoplasms. Some, such as the already mentioned mantle cell lymphoma, have more or less specific, recurrent abnormalities, most frequently translocation with the immunoglobulin heavy chain (IGH, 14q32) or one of the two (IGL, 22q11or IGK, 2p12) light chain loci. I-FISH is an invaluable tool due to the poor in vitro growth of these neoplasms which limits studies reliant on metaphase preparations.

Although no translocation is pathognomonic for a specific lymphoma type, detection of a recurrent abnormality is strong evidence in favor of a clonal process, especially in cases with equivocal or missing immunophenotypic data [54]. For instance, detection of a rearrangement involving IGH (14q32) can be used to distinguish a neoplastic from a reactive lymphoid process [48]. Using a break-apart IGH FISH-CISH approach (which takes advantage of antibodies specific to the FISH fluorochromes for chromogen labelling), high sensitivity (83%), specificity (100%), PPV (100%), and NPV (60%) for the diagnosis (although not classification) of lymphoma were reported [55]. FISH for t(14;18)(q32;q21) detects the IGH-BCL2 translocation and is one of the most commonly used studies in cytologic specimens where it is often performed for the purpose of classification in suspected follicular lymphomas [54, 56]. FISH is better suited than PCR for the detection of t(14;18) due to the wide variation in chromosomal break points which would require technically demanding long-distance PCR to ensure detection [57–59]. Approximately 80% of the follicular lymphomas harbor this translocation [60], but it is also found in 20–30% of diffuse large B-cell lymphomas (DLBCL) in which case it is characteristic of the germinal center B-like subtype, associated with better prognosis and raises the possibility of transformation from an occult follicular lymphoma. Similarly, a FISH-detectable rearrangement such as t(14;18) can support a clonal relationship between synchronous or metachronous neoplasms [61]. Notably, FISH detection of t(14;18) has been reported to be slightly more sensitive (85%) for the detection of follicular lymphoma in cytologic specimens than FC (75%) based on CD19+/CD10+ co-expression [62]. Another commonly encountered situation is suspected marginal zone lymphoma (MZL) where FISH studies can clinch the diagnosis in cases that would otherwise be equivocal due to the non-specific immunophenotype encountered in this lymphoma and/or the limitations posed by the material available for analysis (e.g., bronchoalveolar lavage fluid (BAL)) [63, 64].

FISH adds crucial prognostic information. In chronic lymphocytic leukemia/ small lymphocytic lymphoma (CLL/SLL), the detection of abnormalities associated with poor prognosis and poor treatment response (e.g., del17p, TP53) or Richter's transformation [65–69] is clinically important. Identification of aggressive, so-called "double-hit" or "triple-hit" large B-cell lymphomas with concurrent rearrangements of MYC (8q24) [70–72] with BCL2 (18q21) and/or BCL6 (3q27) [73] relies on FISH studies. Similarly, Burkitt lymphoma, which requires an accurate and expedited diagnosis due to its highly aggressive behavior, almost always shows rearrangement of MYC (8q24), mostly as t(8;14), which is readily detectable by FISH [74, 75] (Fig. 9.1d). Less common but often diagnostically challenging are lymphomas of T- and NK-cell differentiation which, with some geographic variation, constitute approximately 10% or less of the mature lymphoid neoplasms [22]. Among them anaplastic large cell lymphoma (ALCL) is a subtype which presents with several morphologic variants (including "common" anaplastic, small cell, Hodgkin-like, and lymphohistiocytic) and can mimic both carcinoma and sarcoma. Detection of rearrangements of ALK (2p23), mostly with NPM as partner resulting in t(2;5)(p23;q35), not only facilitates the diagnosis but also provides prognostic information due to a more favorable clinical course of the translocation-positive subgroup [76]. In addition, patients whose tumor harbors the t(2;5) translocation may benefit from newly developed targeted therapies [77].

Epstein-Barr virus (EBV) is a double-stranded DNA virus with tropism to lymphocytes and other human cells that has been linked to benign and malignant conditions including a spectrum of lymphoproliferative disorders such as Burkitt lymphoma, Hodgkin lymphoma, subtypes of large B-cell lymphoma, post-transplant lymphoproliferative disorder, lymphomatoid granulomatosis, and T-/NK-cell lymphomas [78]. EBV-encoded RNA (EBER) is detectable during acute infection as well as viral latency, which has three distinct types (I–III), and is associated with EBV-related malignancies [78]. EBER-ISH, as surrogate for latent EBV infection, aids in the classification of these neoplasms and often carries prognostic value. The test is commonly performed on FFPE tissue or similarly prepared cell block sections of cytologic specimens [79–81]. Cell block preparations using a proprietary system and methanol-based cytology fixative were found compatible [35]. Garady et al. examined the success rate in cytology preparations from FNAs and effusion specimen and found 4/10 failed assays performed on cytospin slides (mostly due to loss of material) as opposed to 2/50 failed assays for FFPE cell block sections with an otherwise high concordance between cytology and follow-up surgical samples [82].

In summary, ISH is a robust, versatile, and fast method to obtain information about cytogenetic alterations which may prove of diagnostic, prognostic, and/or predictive value. It may detect a broad variety of genetic rearrangements without requirement for knowledge about the exact sequence alteration, can give clinically useful results even in situations where breakpoints are widely dispersed or fusion partners vary, and is readily applicable to cytologic samples. In the context of a multiparameter approach to lymphoma diagnosis in cytologic samples, FISH is most often used as first- or second-line ancillary study after or in conjunction with immunophenotyping (mostly FC analysis) or in the context of lacking/equivocal immunophenotypic data. Due to the increasing use of cytogenetic information for appropriate treatment, the use of FISH in lymphoma diagnosis is expected to increase further, and cytologic preparations may gain in importance since they can circumvent some problems encountered with FFPE tissue sections. Cytologic preparations may be particularly worthwhile if automated FISH analysis for increased throughput is considered [83, 84], an area which requires further research.

9.5 Polymerase Chain Reaction (PCR) in Hematolymphoid Cytopathology

The next most important ancillary test in the evaluation of suspected lymphoid neoplasms, after immunophenotyping and ISH, is PCR which is currently utilized mostly if preceding studies yield insufficient or equivocal information [6] or up front in specimens in which paucicellularity precludes the use of other techniques. In some situations, depending on the individual laboratory setup, additional considerations such as turnaround time may come into play for the selection of the most appropriate ancillary test [85]. PCR for gene rearrangement studies was propelled to the forefront in the early 1990s by its technical simplicity and high sensitivity in comparison with Southern blotting [10, 16, 86–89]. PCR can be performed on DNA which is minimal in quantity (and therefore ideal in cytology specimens), obtained from fresh and archived—even FFPE—specimens [90–94], has a high sensitivity [94], permits fast turnaround especially if coupled with automated analysis [95], and avoids radioactivity in the detection of its reaction product(s) [88]. Stained slides, either Romanowsky or Papanicolaou, are convenient sources of DNA; however, immunocytochemistry stained slides have been found unsuitable in one study [96]. In situations where prior staining provides an obstacle, simple pretreatment steps may be beneficial [97].

The main role of PCR in hematolymphoid cytopathology is to detect clonal immunoglobulin (IG) heavy chain gene rearrangements and a subset of structural rearrangements with sufficiently repetitive breakpoints (Fig. 9.2). Some significant limitations and analytical requirements were recognized early and include the possibility of false-negative results which can arise from inadvertent sampling of residual nonneoplastic portions of an enlarged lymph node [98] or substantial admixture of polyclonal lymphoid cells which mask the detection of a small monoclonal component [99]. False-negative results may also occur due to mutational events that cause alteration or removal of primer binding sites, such as extensive and ongoing somatic hypermutation (e.g., follicular lymphoma, marginal zone lymphoma, DLBCL), atypical rearrangements, and translocation events that involve the IGH gene or germline configuration of the target sequence which effectively prevents the generation of a PCR product. A false-negative rate of approximately 10% even with modern PCR methods has been reported [100, 101]. High load of somatic hypermutation and abundant polyclonal lymphoid background hamper the detection of IGH rearrangements in Hodgkin lymphomas even with modern assays [102]. Sources of false-positive results include contamination with DNA from other samples,

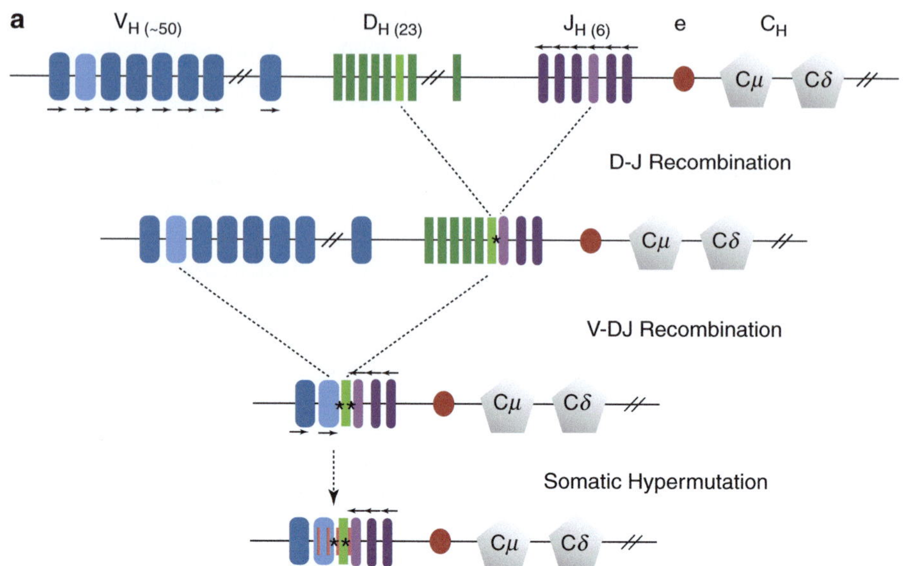

Fig. 9.2 PCR in hematolymphoid cytopathology. (**a**) Immunoglobulin heavy chain (IGH) diversity is generated through somatic recombination during pro-B cell development. Recombination is initiated first between diversity (D) and junction (J) regions which include an insertion of random nucleotides (asterisk) intervening the regions. After successful D-J recombination, the process is repeated with fusion of the variable (V) region to the DJ region in the same manner. Further maturation of the IGH region occurs in the germinal center through somatic hypermutation (illustrated by red banding) leading to further diversification of the IGH repertoire. The mu enhancer region (e) regulates transcription of the IGH locus in the functionally rearranged VDJ region. The enhancer may be coopted to drive abnormal expression of genes subsequent to translocation events (e.g., BCL2 in follicular lymphoma, CCND1 in mantle cell lymphomas, or MYC in Burkitt lymphoma). IGH clonality testing utilizes primer sequence homology within framework regions for each V region family and within the J regions (directional arrowheads). (**b**) Genomic spacing of IGH elements effectively prevents amplification of germline or partially rearranged sequences. Random insertion of nucleotides ensures that each "clone" is represented by a unique amplified fragment length polymorphism (AFLP)—even in instances of separate B-cell populations utilizing the same VDJ regions. IGH clonality testing relies on recombined B-cell IGH loci represented by unique AFLP peaks. Peak height/intensity is proportional to clone size: a single or markedly dominant peak is indicative of a clonal population. Codominant or multiple peaks may indicate bi-/oligoclonal populations. Sampling of a normal IGH repertoire results in a Gaussian distribution. (**c**) May-Grünwald-Giemsa stained direct smear of a fine needle sample obtained from a 23-year-old man with inguinal lymphadenopathy and chronic eosinophilia. A mixture of small lymphocytes, eosinophils, and blasts with immature chromatin and nucleoli is present. Flow cytometry confirmed T-cell acute lymphoblastic leukemia (ALL). (**d**) Real-time quantitative PCR performed on the sample shown in (**c**) demonstrated a FIP1L1-PDGFRA fusion which is susceptible to tyrosine kinase inhibition (TaqMan assay®, ABI 7900 sequence detector)

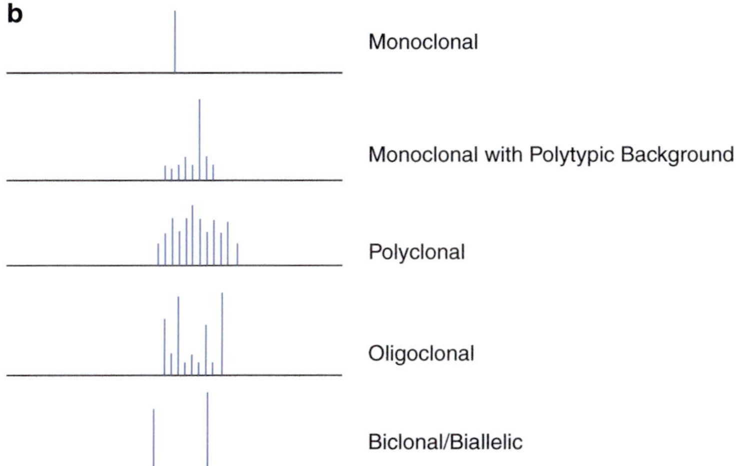

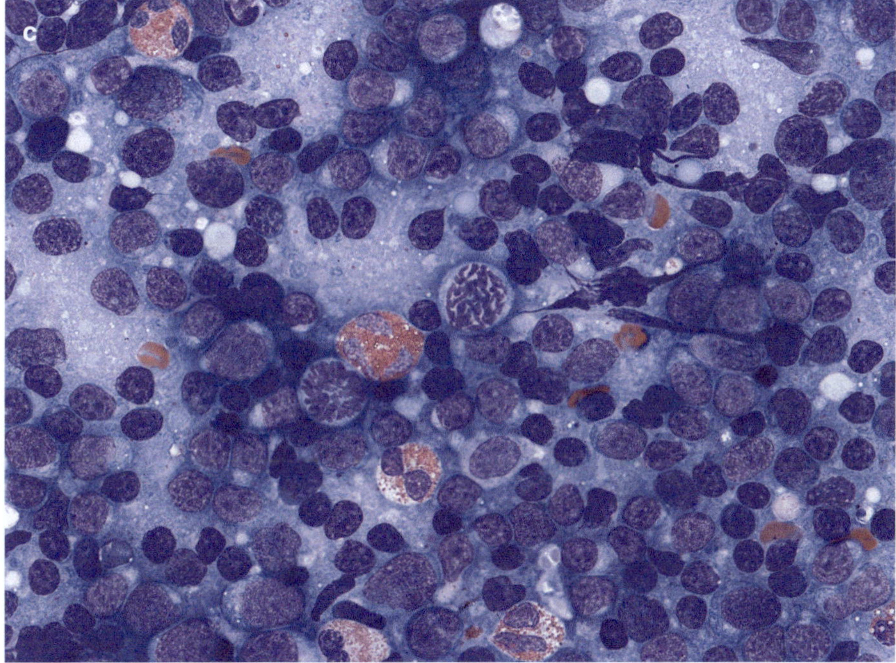

Fig. 9.2 (continued)

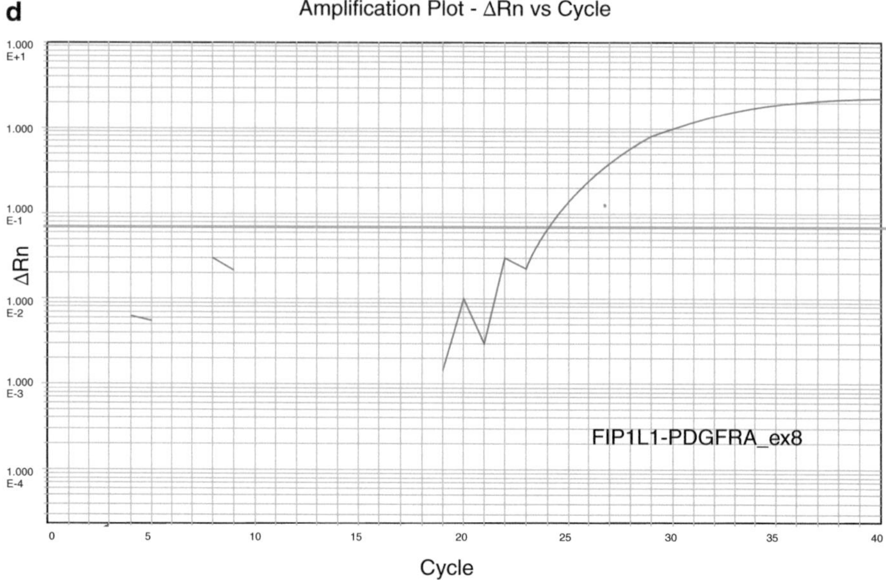

Fig. 9.2 (continued)

so-called pseudoclonality (especially with nested/semi-nested PCR designs), and/or preferential amplification of small lymphocyte populations in the context of a stimulated immune system or immunodeficiency/immunosenescence (e.g., HIV infection, autoimmune conditions, posttransplantation status, advanced age) [102, 103]. Recognition of these limitations resulted in emphasis on the need for proper laboratory procedures to prevent contamination, inclusion of controls, duplicate reactions, sequence-specific methods for result confirmation, and, most significantly, clinicopathologic correlation [104, 105].

Many different primer sets and PCR designs were explored initially by individual laboratories resulting in differences in sensitivity and applicability. While semi-nested PCR was commonly employed, an early study with single primer pair design, although less sensitive than FC, successfully detected an additional 14% of monoclonal cytology specimens [106]. Subsequent studies with single primer pair PCR showed sensitivities that rivaled or exceeded those of FC, and combination of both ancillary techniques showed high sensitivity (96%) with a relatively low number of false-positive results [96, 107, 108]. In 2003 the results of the BIOMED-2 Concerted Action Project, a collaboration of 47 institutes from seven European countries, were published which outlined in detail the experimental conditions for a series of multiplex PCR assays [109]. The adoption of standardized methodologies with commercially available reagents helped to decrease inaccurate, often false-negative results and facilitated comparison between laboratories. The subsequent publication of the EuroClonality/BIOMED-2 guidelines was aimed at standardization of the pre-analytical and post-analytical phase and included (a) technical description of possible multiplex PCR results and (b) guidance with respect to the interpretation of GeneScan and electrophoresis gel-based analysis applicable to at least 95% of routine cases [110]. This standard has been embraced worldwide and is applicable to a wide variety of specimens including material recovered from stained cytologic smear preparations [102]. A PPV of 100% has been reported for unequivocally monoclonal results [102]. However, sensitivity and specificity issues for certain targets remain and require a thoughtful selection of the most suitable test for a given clinical scenario [59, 102].

Body cavity fluids require accurate diagnosis due to the poor prognosis associated with malignant effusions, and PCR is readily applicable [111]. Frontline tests in most cases include FC or immunocytochemistry and ISH including EBER-ISH [112]. Pre-analytical variables, such as the submission of unfixed sample of sufficient quantity and refrigerated storage if assessment or triage for required tests is delayed, require attention. Studies targeting IGH, TCRG, and t(14;18) by PCR and Southern blotting have been found to support the diagnosis of lymphoma in effusions morphologically classified as suspicious and are especially valuable in cases with missing or inconclusive immunophenotype [113]. Clinical correlation is paramount and over-interpretation of isolated PCR results should be avoided [114]. However, if data from multiple sources are taken together, clonality assessment may assist greatly in the distinction between nonneoplastic conditions and neoplastic proliferations (e.g., plasmablastic lymphoma, primary effusion lymphoma) involving serous cavities [112, 115].

Another typical cytology specimen which often raises the differential diagnosis of inflammation versus lymphoid neoplasia is BAL fluid. Marginal zone lymphoma and other lymphoproliferative disorders may primarily or secondarily involve the pulmonary parenchyma where they can mimic inflammatory processes clinically as well as morphologically. PCR on BAL fluid may be a viable strategy if the cellularity is too low for FC or if reactive T-cells predominate [116]. A prospective study demonstrated good PPV and NPV (82% and 95%, respectively) of PCR coupled with sequencing and heteroduplex analysis; although the authors emphasize in their report that a detectable B-cell clone does not equal pulmonary lymphoma since several cases of autoimmune inflammation also showed monoclonal B-cell expansion [117]. Another organ site with frequent morphologic overlap between autoimmune inflammation and lymphoma is the thyroid gland. Judicious use of PCR and interpretation in the context of clinical, radiologic, morphologic, and immunophenotypic findings is warranted. Encouraging results have been reported with PCR supporting the diagnosis of MALT lymphoma [118, 119] or ruling out lymphoma in Hashimoto thyroiditis with skewed light chain ratio by FC [120, 121]. A somewhat analogous situation may be encountered in the context of lymphoid proliferations involving the skin, mucosal sites, and tributary lymph nodes. This may involve the assessment of nodules or tumors presenting with the clinical differential diagnosis of cutaneous lymphoma or, in cases of a previously established cutaneous lymphoma, the prognostically important assessment of potentially involved lymph nodes. The concept was examined in a study focused on cutaneous T-cell lymphomas with lymphadenopathy thought to represent either nodal lymphoma involvement or dermatopathic lymphadenopathy which found a poor correlation between PCR results and morphologic evaluation [122]. Correlation with FC was hampered by the limited number of cases. However, the authors felt that cytomorphologic assessment was still useful due to the strong correlation with histopathologic findings [122]. Authors of a more recent study provided results in favor of FNS of enlarged lymph nodes in mycosis fungoides and Sezary syndrome using cytomorphology and FC, while PCR was only applied in cases with missing or equivocal immunophenotype [123]. A similar strategy was employed successfully by Vigliar et al. [124]. Although few studies have examined FNS of mucosal sites in the context of lymphoproliferative disease and ancillary testing, Cozzolino et al. demonstrated its feasibility and usefulness even though final lymphoma classification may require deferral to tissue evaluation in a proportion of the cases [125]. PCR, again, was most useful if immunophenotypic data were equivocal or lacking [125].

Several studies examined the contribution of PCR to the assessment of cerebrospinal and vitreous fluid samples. Accurate and early detection of primary or secondary involvement by lymphoma in the central nervous system or eye is of great clinical importance but often fraught with difficulty due to quantitative and/or qualitative limitations of the specimen. Ancillary tests applicable to these limited specimens are needed, and PCR may fill this gap by improving the sensitivity of lymphoma detection beyond the level achieved by cytomorphology [126, 127]. PCR can facilitate detection of secondary lymphoma involvement in cases with equivocal morphology if a known molecular alteration of the neoplastic cells can be demonstrated [128] and can distinguish neoplastic disease from inflammation [129, 130] potentially avoiding more invasive tests including biopsy. Again, caution is warranted due to the potential for false-positive results [131]. Real-time PCR has been explored in pediatric patients with acute lymphoblastic leukemia and may be valuable if cytology and FC fail to detect the neoplastic cells, but central nervous system manifestations are present, or in cases with quantitatively insufficient samples [132]. Additional studies such as sequence analysis and comparison of the detected PCR product with previous samples may be necessary for clinically meaningful interpretation [133]. Modifications such as single-cell PCR [134] and PCR after direct cell lysis which may detect as little as 20 tumor cells [135] have been explored to improve the detection sensitivity. However, despite all technological advances, the pre-analytical steps with dedicated, cautious, and rapid processing followed by careful selection of the most suitable ancillary technique [136] remain among the most important factors and can be influenced by incorporation of early assessment steps such as RALT.

## 9.6	From Discovery Tools to Clinical Use: Next-Generation Sequencing and Other Technologies

Major scientific discoveries and technological progress have resulted from the competitive endeavor to sequence the human genome which shaped our understanding of neoplastic disease including the cancers of the hematolymphoid system [137]. Gene expression profiling, using cDNA after RNA reverse transcription, led to important inroads in the classification of DLBCL, a biologically heterogeneous disease which constitutes 25–30% of adult non-Hodgkin lymphomas in Western countries and an even higher percentage in the developing world [22]. This work revealed distinct gene expression patterns of activated (reminiscent of, but not identical to, activated peripheral blood B cells) B-like (ABC) and germinal center B-like (GCB) DLBCL which are not obviously related to histological subtypes but associated with statistically significant differences in overall survival and event-free survival [138]. Although considerable heterogeneity remains within each subgroup, the authors concluded that the use of molecular methods redefines our concept of what constitutes a disease entity [138]. Recent advancement has made interrogation of these so-called "cell-of-origin" (COO) categories applicable to FFPE (rather than frozen) tissue with a misassignment rate of only 2% which compares favorably to immunohistochemistry-based algorithms and combined with a rapid turnaround may enable prospective selection of patients for more appropriate management and potential clinical trials [139]. Data suggest that the COO classification remains prognostically relevant even in the context of BCL2 and MYC protein status [140], an immunohistochemical feature recently termed "double-expressor lymphoma" [141]. A 2006 study using Affymetrix technology demonstrated the feasibility of gene expression profiling for the identification of ABC and GCB signatures in fine needle samples as well as separation of DLBCL from follicular lymphoma [142]. In addition, a proof-of-principle study established that archival cytospin preparation is an adequate source of DNA for high-throughput multiplex mutation profiling using Sequenom's MassARRAY platform to detect mutations in EZH2, CD79B, and MYD88 which are related to the COO classification [143]. The same group previously demonstrated that other DNA sources such as direct smears and FTA cards are adequate, similar to frozen tissue, and suitable for the detection of tumor progression- or heterogeneity-related molecular events [144]. Post-transcriptional modification of histones appears to be of key importance in the pathogenesis of lymphomas of GCB phenotype with altered gene regulation due to deregulated histone modification as a core driver event in NHL [145].

A revised version of the monograph associated with the 2008 World Health Organization (WHO) classification of hematopoietic and lymphoid tumors continues the current development of a detailed molecular characterization and reclassification of traditionally defined entities [141]. This is exemplified in several areas such as the discovery of BRAF V600E mutations by genome-wide massively parallel sequencing in almost all cases of hairy cell leukemia (HCL), but not HCL-variant or other B-cell lymphomas, consistent with an alteration that constitutes a major driver (as opposed to a passenger mutation) of oncogenesis in this disease [146]. The same research group recently introduced a simple and sensitive allele-specific PCR assay which was used to confirm their initial results [147]. Although disease-defining in this particular context, BRAF V600E has been detected in numerous other neoplasms including Langerhans cell (LCH) and non-Langerhans cell histiocytosis (non-LCH) [148]. Indeed, the spectrum of molecular changes shows surprising similarities across different cell types such that activating MAP2K1 mutations seen with high prevalence in atypical/IGHV4-34 expressing HCL and HCL-variant

[149, 150] are also identified in BRAF V600E-negative LCH and non-LCH [151, 152]. The clinical relevance of a comprehensive genomic analysis is underlined by the fact that neoplastic proliferations driven by MAP2K1 are unlikely to respond to inhibitors targeting the upstream BRAF protein while more appropriately selected inhibitors may result in a treatment effect similar to that observed in their BRAF-mutant cousins [151, 152].

In several entities molecular characterization has led to refined models of pathogenesis. One example is mantle cell lymphoma for which two molecularly distinct subtypes (minimally mutated/unmutated immunoglobulin IGHV, SOX11+ versus hypermutated IGHV, SOX11-) of potential clinical significance are proposed [153]. A recent study using whole-genome sequencing (including paired tumor/germline samples) led to the discovery of MYD88 L265P mutations in 90% of Waldenström macroglobulinemia (WM) patients as well as, in a much small proportion of cases, CXCR4 and ARID1A mutations [154]. The authors of this study hypothesized that the multitude of molecular changes are a reflection of a multistep process for WM evolution from IgM MGUS [154]. The exact details of this process remain to be elucidated. The same MYD88 mutation, however, which is involved in NFκB signaling, has previously been identified in ABC-DLBCL [155]. Another example among the B-cell NHLs is splenic marginal zone lymphoma (SMZL) which shows recurrent somatic NOTCH2 mutations associated with an adverse clinical outcome in 25% of cases [156]. NOTCH2 mutations were not found in other B-cell lymphomas and leukemias [156]. More recent work with whole-exome sequencing succeeded in identifying KLF2 mutations in 42% of SMZL as most common genetic change and describes an association with IGHV1-2 rearrangement and 7q deletion, while MYD88 and TP53 mutations were found in SMZL without KLF2 mutation leading to the proposal of a dichotomous model of origin from T-cell-independent marginal zone B cells versus T-cell-dependent marginal zone B cells [157]. Making the information gleaned from time-consuming and complex research efforts accessible for clinical use is a priority. Methodologies are emerging such as a recently described high-throughput RNA expression profiling system which potentially permits a complete diagnostic and prognostic workup of chronic lymphocytic leukemia in a single assay based on a 61 gene panel [158].

Despite increasingly sophisticated molecular characterization, (cyto-)morphology and immunophenotype remain the pillars of lymphoma classification even though sample sizes will predictably decrease—a trend already seen in daily practice. A case in point is the newly discovered TBL1XR1/TP63 rearrangement involving two genes flanking the BCL6 locus on chromosome 3 which is detectable in 5% of GCB-DLBCL (and rarely in follicular lymphoma) and may be related to treatment-refractory disease [159]. Indeed, TP63 rearrangements are also found in 5.8% of peripheral T-cell lymphomas (PTCL) (including peripheral T-cell lymphoma - not otherwise specified, ALK-negative ALCL, and primary cutaneous ALCL), mostly with TBL1XR1 as partner gene and, again, associated with poorer prognosis [160]. Interestingly, p63 abnormalities were only one of five p53-related rearrangements detected in 67% of PTCLs in this study pointing toward a potential constellation of abnormalities with common endpoint in lymphoma pathogenesis [160].

Changes in the revised WHO monograph with advanced molecular characterization as underpinning also affect the classification of T-/NK-cell neoplasms. For instance, a combination of whole-exome and RNA sequencing led to the identification of activating STAT5B mutations in gamma-delta PTCL including monomorphic epitheliotropic intestinal T-cell lymphoma (previously EATL, type II) which may be pivotal in pathogenesis and as potential therapeutic target [161]. This abnormality was not detected in enteropathy-associated T-cell lymphoma (previously EATL, type I) which may be encountered in cytologic samples obtained by endoscopic ultrasound-guided or CT-guided procedures [162]. The translocation t(6;7) identified by next-generation sequencing using a mate-pair strategy for examination of the genome structure is the first recurrent translocation identified in ALK-negative ALCL (both primary cutaneous and systemic) and involves DUSP22 on chromosome 6, a dual-specific phosphatase and putative tumor suppressor which is down-regulated [163]. The experimental strategy used in this particular study, as opposed to transcriptome sequencing, permits the identification of rearrangements which do not result in the expression of a fusion gene [163]. Finally, the identification of frequent somatic mutation in RHOA, a GTPase protein belonging to the RAS family, by exome and transcriptome sequencing in 53–68% of angioimmunoblastic T-cell lymphomas is another example of a recently reported driver mutation in a T-cell malignancy [164–166].

Conclusion

Molecular testing is an integral part of the diagnostic workup and classification of hematolymphoid neoplasms as it adds not only essential information in the context of minimal sampling both by fine needle and needle core biopsies but also increasingly provides prognostic and predictive data of direct relevance to therapy selection. The use of sampling technique, ideally in combination with ROSE or RALT, has the potential to minimize procedure-related morbidity, patient discomfort, health-care cost, and wait time to diagnosis and treatment. Although areas of uncertainty remain which require a diagnostic problem to be resolved by surgical biopsy, as seen in nodular sclerosis classical Hodgkin lymphoma where insufficient core and fine needle samples are not infrequently encountered, this decision should be made on an individualized basis and after review of the often complimentary information obtained from less invasive samples. Interestingly, out of 42 studies included in a recent meta-analysis [27], only 2 used the full complement of ancillary techniques (i.e., immunohisto-/immunocytochemistry, FC, FISH) in combination with FNS, and only one of these two also included molecular diagnostics [167, 168]. This matches the experience of our institution which is that of a high accuracy with consequent use of the available diagnostic armamentarium and multiparameter approach. Indeterminate results which require additional or alternate sampling modalities are not uncommon in other areas of cytopathology. Considering this, the finding of a median rate of subtype-specific diagnosis of 74% by fine needle and core needle sampling is actually a hopeful sign and should encourage cytopathologists to renew their efforts in providing front-line care to patients with hematolymphoid disorders as they already do in many other areas.

Sample sizes will inevitably decrease as molecular techniques take center stage. However, microscopic characterization will remain as the entry point to diagnostic, prognostic, and predictive evaluation of hematolymphoid neoplasms. At a minimum an assessment of the presence of lesional tissue will be required prior to molecular testing due to the multitude of molecular abnormalities and occurrence of completely unrelated disease entities with similar or identical molecular alterations. Cytopathologists will have to demonstrate that they are up to the challenge to identify the most appropriate testing algorithm which leads to the best line of treatment for the exact disease subtype and clinical stage associated with a minimum of therapy-related morbidity, in short, to act as navigators of personalized medicine on behalf of the patient.

References

1. Young NA, et al. Fine-needle aspiration biopsy of lymphoproliferative disorders--interpretations based on morphologic criteria alone: results from the College of American Pathologists Interlaboratory Comparison Program in Nongynecologic Cytopathology. Arch Pathol Lab Med. 2006;130(12):1766–71.
2. Jin M, Wakely PE Jr. Endoscopic/endobronchial ultrasound-guided fine needle aspiration and ancillary techniques, particularly flow cytometry, in diagnosing deep-seated lymphomas. Acta Cytol. 2016;60(4):326–35.
3. Hehn ST, Grogan TM, Miller TP. Utility of fine-needle aspiration as a diagnostic technique in lymphoma. J Clin Oncol. 2004;22(15):3046–52.
4. Fine-needle aspirate for the evaluation of suspected lymphoma: clinical effectiveness and guidelines. 2015 March 31. http://www.choosingwiselycanada.org/wp-content/uploads/2015/12/CADTH-Rapid-Response-Report-Fine-Needle-Aspiration-in-Suspected-Lymphoma.pdf.
5. Joudeh AA, Shareef SQ, Al-Abbadi MA. Fine-needle aspiration followed by core-needle biopsy in the same setting: modifying our approach. Acta Cytol. 2016;60(1):1–13.
6. Safley AM, et al. The value of fluorescence in situ hybridization and polymerase chain reaction in the diagnosis of B-cell non-Hodgkin lymphoma by fine-needle aspiration. Arch Pathol Lab Med. 2004;128(12):1395–403.
7. Cozzolino I, et al. Lymph node and lymphoid organs fine needle aspiration cytology: historical background. Infez Med. 2012;20(Suppl 3):8–11.
8. Hirschfeld H. Über isolierte aleukämische Lymphadenose der Haut. Z Krebsforsch. 1912;11:397–407.
9. Hu E, et al. Diagnosis of B cell lymphoma by analysis of immunoglobulin gene rearrangements in biopsy specimens obtained by fine needle aspiration. J Clin Oncol. 1986;4(3):278–83.
10. Katz RL, et al. The role of gene rearrangements for antigen receptors in the diagnosis of lymphoma obtained by fine-needle aspiration. A study of 63 cases with concomitant immunophenotyping. Am J Clin Pathol. 1991;96(4):479–90.
11. Miyahara M, et al. Immunoglobulin gene rearrangement in T-cell-rich reactive pleural effusion of a patient with B-cell chronic lymphocytic leukemia. Acta Haematol. 1996;96(1):41–4.
12. Biggar RJ, et al. Direct cytogenetic studies by needle aspiration of Burkitt's lymphoma in Ghana, West Africa. J Natl Cancer Inst. 1981;67(4):769–76.

13. Kristoffersson U, et al. Cytogenetic studies in non-Hodgkin lymphomas--results from fine-needle aspiration samples. Hereditas. 1985;103(1):63–76.
14. Schmitz L, Beneke J, Kubic V. Diagnosis of small non-cleaved cell lymphoma by fine needle aspiration utilizing cytomorphologic features combined with cytogenetic analysis. Acta Cytol. 1997;41(3):759–64.
15. Hughes JH, Caraway NP, Katz RL. Blastic variant of mantle-cell lymphoma: cytomorphologic, immunocytochemical, and molecular genetic features of tissue obtained by fine-needle aspiration biopsy. Diagn Cytopathol. 1998;19(1):59–62.
16. Cartagena N Jr, et al. Accuracy of diagnosis of malignant lymphoma by combining fine-needle aspiration cytomorphology with immunocytochemistry and in selected cases, Southern blotting of aspirated cells: a tissue-controlled study of 86 patients. Diagn Cytopathol. 1992;8(5):456–64.
17. Caraway NP. Strategies to diagnose lymphoproliferative disorders by fine-needle aspiration by using ancillary studies. Cancer. 2005;105(6):432–42.
18. Dey P. Role of ancillary techniques in diagnosing and subclassifying non-Hodgkin's lymphomas on fine needle aspiration cytology. Cytopathology. 2006;17(5):275–87.
19. Krishnamurthy S. Applications of molecular techniques to fine-needle aspiration biopsy. Cancer. 2007;111(2):106–22.
20. Zhang S, et al. The role of fluorescence in situ hybridization and polymerase chain reaction in the diagnosis and classification of lymphoproliferative disorders on fine-needle aspiration. Cancer Cytopathol. 2010;118(2):105–12.
21. Bode B, Tinguely M. Role of cytology in hematopathological diagnostics. Pathologe. 2012;33(4):316–23.
22. Swerdlow SH, et al. WHO classifcation of tumours of haematopoietic and lymphoid tissues. World Health Organization classification of tumours. 4th ed. Lyon: IARC; 2008.
23. Kocjan G. Best practice No. 185. Cytological and molecular diagnosis of lymphoma. J Clin Pathol. 2005;58(6):561–7.
24. Young NA, Al-Saleem T. Hematopathologists and cytopathologists: enemies or allies? Diagn Cytopathol. 1999;21(5):305–6.
25. Wakely PE Jr. Fine-needle aspiration cytopathology in diagnosis and classification of malignant lymphoma: accurate and reliable? Diagn Cytopathol. 2000;22(2):120–5.
26. Swart GJ, et al. Fine needle aspiration biopsy and flow cytometry in the diagnosis of lymphoma. Transfus Apher Sci. 2007;37(1):71–9.
27. Frederiksen JK, et al. Systematic review of the effectiveness of fine-needle aspiration and/or core needle biopsy for subclassifying lymphoma. Arch Pathol Lab Med. 2015;139(2):245–51.
28. Young NA, et al. Utilization of fine-needle aspiration cytology and flow cytometry in the diagnosis and subclassification of primary and recurrent lymphoma. Cancer. 1998;84(4):252–61.
29. Allen EA, Ali SZ, Mathew S. Lymphoid lesions of the parotid. Diagn Cytopathol. 1999;21(3):170–3.
30. Meda BA, et al. Diagnosis and subclassification of primary and recurrent lymphoma. The usefulness and limitations of combined fine-needle aspiration cytomorphology and flow cytometry. Am J Clin Pathol. 2000;113(5):688–99.
31. Levine PH, Zamuco R, Yee HT. Role of fine-needle aspiration cytology in breast lymphoma. Diagn Cytopathol. 2004;30(5):332–40.
32. Katz RL. Modern approach to lymphoma diagnosis by fine-needle aspiration: restoring respect to a valuable procedure. Cancer. 2005;105(6):429–31.
33. Field AS, et al. Assisting cytopathology training in medically under-resourced countries: defining the problems and establishing solutions. Diagn Cytopathol. 2012;40(3):273–81.
34. Shetuni B, Lakey M, Kulesza P. Optimal specimen processing of fine needle aspirates of non-Hodgkin lymphoma. Diagn Cytopathol. 2012;40(11):984–6.
35. van Hemel BM, Suurmeijer AJ. Effective application of the methanol-based PreservCyt() fixative and the Cellient() automated cell block processor to diagnostic cytopathology, immunocytochemistry, and molecular biology. Diagn Cytopathol. 2013;41(8):734–41.

36. Schwock J, Geddie WR. Diagnosis of B-cell non-hodgkin lymphomas with small-/intermediate-sized cells in cytopathology. Pathol Res Int. 2012;2012:164934.
37. Mathiot C, et al. Fine-needle aspiration cytology combined with flow cytometry immunophenotyping is a rapid and accurate approach for the evaluation of suspicious superficial lymphoid lesions. Diagn Cytopathol. 2006;34(7):472–8.
38. Ochs RC, Bagg A. Molecular genetic characterization of lymphoma: application to cytology diagnosis. Diagn Cytopathol. 2012;40(6):542–55.
39. Stewart CJ, et al. Fine needle aspiration cytology diagnosis of malignant lymphoma and reactive lymphoid hyperplasia. J Clin Pathol. 1998;51(3):197–203.
40. Das DK. Serous effusions in malignant lymphomas: a review. Diagn Cytopathol. 2006;34(5):335–47.
41. Gall JG, Pardue ML. Formation and detection of RNA-DNA hybrid molecules in cytological preparations. Proc Natl Acad Sci U S A. 1969;63(2):378–83.
42. Al Omran S, Mourad WA, Ali MA. Gamma/delta peripheral T-cell lymphoma of the breast diagnosed by fine-needle aspiration biopsy. Diagn Cytopathol. 2002;26(3):170–3.
43. Yasuda I, et al. Endoscopic ultrasound-guided fine needle aspiration biopsy for diagnosis of lymphoproliferative disorders: feasibility of immunohistological, flow cytometric, and cytogenetic assessments. Am J Gastroenterol. 2012;107(3):397–404.
44. Perak RB, et al. Soft tissue B-cell lymphoma, unclassifiable, with features intermediate between diffuse large B-cell lymphoma and Burkitt's lymphoma diagnosed by fine needle aspiration cytology. Acta Cytol. 2015;59:355–7.
45. Jiang F, Katz RL. Use of interphase fluorescence in situ hybridization as a powerful diagnostic tool in cytology. Diagn Mol Pathol. 2002;11(1):47–57.
46. Bentz JS, et al. Rapid detection of the t(11;14) translocation in mantle cell lymphoma by interphase fluorescence in situ hybridization on archival cytopathologic material. Cancer. 2004;102(2):124–31.
47. Caraway NP, et al. The utility of interphase fluorescence in situ hybridization for the detection of the translocation t(11;14)(q13;q32) in the diagnosis of mantle cell lymphoma on fine-needle aspiration specimens. Cancer. 2005;105(2):110–8.
48. Cook JR. Paraffin section interphase fluorescence in situ hybridization in the diagnosis and classification of non-Hodgkin lymphomas. Diagn Mol Pathol. 2004;13(4):197–206.
49. Bishop R. Applications of fluorescence in situ hybridization (FISH) in detecting genetic aberrations of medical signficiance. Biosci Horiz. 2010;3(1):85–95.
50. Buno I, et al. Lymphoma associated chromosomal abnormalities can easily be detected by FISH on tissue imprints. An underused diagnostic alternative. J Clin Pathol. 2005;58(6):629–33.
51. Rowe LR, et al. Tumor cell nuclei extraction from paraffin-embedded lymphoid tissue for fluorescence in situ hybridization. Appl Immunohistochem Mol Morphol. 2006;14(2):220–4.
52. Wolff DJ, et al. Guidance for fluorescence in situ hybridization testing in hematologic disorders. J Mol Diagn. 2007;9(2):134–43.
53. Trcic RL, et al. Recurrent chromosomal abnormalities in lymphomas in fine needle aspirates of lymph node. Coll Antropol. 2010;34(2):387–93.
54. Monaco SE, et al. Fluorescence in situ hybridization studies on direct smears: an approach to enhance the fine-needle aspiration biopsy diagnosis of B-cell non-Hodgkin lymphomas. Cancer. 2009;117(5):338–48.
55. Zeppa P, et al. Immunoglobulin heavy-chain fluorescence in situ hybridization-chromogenic in situ hybridization DNA probe split signal in the clonality assessment of lymphoproliferative processes on cytological samples. Cancer Cytopathol. 2012;120(6):390–400.
56. Kishimoto K, et al. Cytologic differential diagnosis of follicular lymphoma grades 1 and 2 from reactive follicular hyperplasia: cytologic features of fine-needle aspiration smears with Pap stain and fluorescence in situ hybridization analysis to detect t(14;18)(q32;q21) chromosomal translocation. Diagn Cytopathol. 2006;34(1):11–7.
57. Jiang F, et al. Rapid detection of IgH/BCL2 rearrangement in follicular lymphoma by interphase fluorescence in situ hybridization with bacterial artificial chromosome probes. J Mol Diagn. 2002;4(3):144–9.

58. Albinger-Hegyi A, et al. High frequency of t(14;18)-translocation breakpoints outside of major breakpoint and minor cluster regions in follicular lymphomas: improved polymerase chain reaction protocols for their detection. Am J Pathol. 2002;160(3):823–32.

59. Stoos-Veic T, et al. Detection of t(14;18) by PCR of IgH/BCL2 fusion gene in follicular lymphoma from archived cytological smears. Coll Antropol. 2010;34(2):425–9.

60. Richmond J, et al. FISH detection of t(14;18) in follicular lymphoma on Papanicolaou-stained archival cytology slides. Cancer. 2006;108(3):198–204.

61. Mehrotra S, Pan Z. Fine needle aspiration cytology of histiocytic sarcoma with dendritic cell differentiation: a case of transdifferentiation from low-grade follicular lymphoma. Diagn Cytopathol. 2015;43(8):659–63.

62. Gong Y, et al. Evaluation of interphase fluorescence in situ hybridization for the t(14;18)(q32;q21) translocation in the diagnosis of follicular lymphoma on fine-needle aspirates: a comparison with flow cytometry immunophenotyping. Cancer. 2003;99(6):385–93.

63. Kido T, et al. Detection of MALT1 gene rearrangements in BAL fluid cells for the diagnosis of pulmonary mucosa-associated lymphoid tissue lymphoma. Chest. 2012;141(1):176–82.

64. Ko HM, et al. Cytomorphological and clinicopathological spectrum of pulmonary marginal zone lymphoma: the utility of immunophenotyping, PCR and FISH studies. Cytopathology. 2014;25(4):250–8.

65. Caraway NP, et al. Numeric chromosomal abnormalities in small lymphocytic and transformed large cell lymphomas detected by fluorescence in situ hybridization of fine-needle aspiration biopsies. Cancer. 2000;90(2):126–32.

66. Caraway NP, et al. Chromosomal abnormalities detected by multicolor fluorescence in situ hybridization in fine-needle aspirates from patients with small lymphocytic lymphoma are useful for predicting survival. Cancer. 2008;114(5):315–22.

67. Andrysiak-Mamos E, et al. Case report: rare case of infiltration of small lymphocytic B-cell lymphoma in the thyroid gland of female patient with B-cell chronic lymphocytic leukemia (CLL-B/SLL-B). Thyroid Res. 2013;6(1):1.

68. Woroniecka R, et al. Cytogenetic and flow cytometry evaluation of Richter syndrome reveals MYC, CDKN2A, IGH alterations with loss of CD52, CD62L and increase of CD71 antigen expression as the most frequent recurrent abnormalities. Am J Clin Pathol. 2015;143(1):25–35.

69. Wang L, et al. Richter transformation with c-MYC overexpression: report of three cases. Int J Clin Exp Pathol. 2015;8(6):7540–6.

70. da Cunha Santos G, et al. Targeted use of fluorescence in situ hybridization (FISH) in cytospin preparations: results of 298 fine needle aspirates of B-cell non-Hodgkin lymphoma. Cancer Cytopathol. 2010;118(5):250–8.

71. Elkins CT, Wakely PE Jr. Cytopathology of "double-hit" non-Hodgkin lymphoma. Cancer Cytopathol. 2011;119(4):263–71.

72. Kaplan A, et al. Follicular lymphoma transformed to "double-hit" B lymphoblastic lymphoma presenting in the peritoneal fluid. Diagn Cytopathol. 2013;41(11):986–90.

73. Wang W, et al. Triple-hit B-cell Lymphoma With MYC, BCL2, and BCL6 Translocations/Rearrangements: Clinicopathologic Features of 11 Cases. Am J Surg Pathol. 2015;39(8):1132–9.

74. Troxell ML, et al. Cytologic diagnosis of Burkitt lymphoma. Cancer. 2005;105(5):310–8.

75. McLean TW, et al. Diagnosis of Burkitt lymphoma in pediatric patients by thoracentesis. Pediatr Blood Cancer. 2007;49(1):90–2.

76. Shin HJ, et al. Detection of a subset of CD30+ anaplastic large cell lymphoma by interphase fluorescence in situ hybridization. Diagn Cytopathol. 2003;29(2):61–6.

77. Cleary JM, et al. Crizotinib as salvage and maintenance with allogeneic stem cell transplantation for refractory anaplastic large cell lymphoma. J Natl Compr Cancer Netw. 2014;12(3):323–6. quiz 326

78. Michelow P, Wright C, Pantanowitz L. A review of the cytomorphology of Epstein-Barr virus-associated malignancies. Acta Cytol. 2012;56(1):1–14.

79. Ohori NP, et al. Primary pleural effusion posttransplant lymphoproliferative disorder: distinction from secondary involvement and effusion lymphoma. Diagn Cytopathol. 2001;25(1):50–3.
80. Hecht JL, Cibas ES, Kutok JL. Fine-needle aspiration cytology of lymphoproliferative disorders in the immunosuppressed patient: the diagnostic utility of in situ hybridization for Epstein-Barr virus. Diagn Cytopathol. 2002;26(6):360–5.
81. Su XY, et al. Serous effusion cytology of extranodal natural killer/T-cell lymphoma. Cytopathology. 2012;23(2):96–102.
82. Garady C, et al. Epstein-Barr virus encoded RNA detected by in situ hybridization using cytological preparations. Cytopathology. 2014;25(2):101–7.
83. Reichard KK, et al. Automated analysis of fluorescence in situ hybridization on fixed, paraffin-embedded whole tissue sections in B-cell lymphoma. Mod Pathol. 2006;19(8):1027–33.
84. Liew M, et al. Validation of break-apart and fusion MYC probes using a digital fluorescence in situ hybridization capture and imaging system. J Pathol Inform. 2016;7:20.
85. Mayall F, Johnson S. Immunoflow cytometry compared with PCR for the identification of clonality in FNAs of T-cell-rich B-cell lymphomas. Cytopathology. 2007;18(2):117–9.
86. Price CG, et al. Polymerase chain reaction to confirm extranodal progression of follicular lymphoma. Lancet. 1989;1(8647):1132.
87. Wan JH, et al. Rapid method for detecting monoclonality in B cell lymphoma in lymph node aspirates using the polymerase chain reaction. J Clin Pathol. 1992;45(5):420–3.
88. Chen YT, Mercer GO, Chen Y. Polymerase chain reaction-based detection of B-cell monoclonality in cytologic specimens. Arch Pathol Lab Med. 1993;117(11):1099–103.
89. Kube MJ, et al. Use of archival and fresh cytologic material for the polymerase chain reaction. Detection of the bcl-2 oncogene in lymphoid tissue obtained by fine needle biopsy. Anal Quant Cytol Histol. 1994;16(3):174–82.
90. Greenberg ML, Cartwright L, McDonald DA. Histiocytic necrotizing lymphadenitis (Kikuchi's disease): cytologic diagnosis by fine-needle biopsy. Diagn Cytopathol. 1993;9(4):444–7.
91. Shivnarain D, Ladanyi M, Zakowski MF. Detection of BCL2 rearrangement in archival cytological smears of B-cell lymphomas. Mod Pathol. 1994;7(9):915–9.
92. Alkan S, et al. Polymerase chain reaction detection of immunoglobulin gene rearrangement and bcl-2 translocation in archival glass slides of cytologic material. Diagn Mol Pathol. 1995;4(1):25–31.
93. Grosso LE, Collins BT. DNA polymerase chain reaction using fine needle aspiration biopsy smears to evaluate non-Hodgkin's lymphoma. Acta Cytol. 1999;43(5):837–41.
94. Kikuchi M, et al. Diagnosis of B-cell lymphoma. Utility of the polymerase chain reaction for detecting clonality from archival cytologic smears. Acta Cytol. 2002;46(2):349–56.
95. Ruschenburg I, et al. Automated molecular genetic DNA analysis for detecting B-cell non-Hodgkin's lymphoma in cytologic specimens. Anal Quant Cytol Histol. 1997;19(3):255–63.
96. Torlakovic E, Berner A, Risberg B. Detection of immunoglobulin heavy chain gene rearrangements by polymerase chain reaction analysis on lymph node imprints and fine-needle aspirate smears: a comparison of five different imprint preparations. Diagn Cytopathol. 1999;20(6):333–8.
97. Chen JT, Lane MA, Clark DP. Inhibitors of the polymerase chain reaction in papanicolaou stain. Removal with a simple destaining procedure. Acta Cytol. 1996;40(5):873–7.
98. Jeffers MD, et al. Analysis of clonality in cytologic material using the polymerase chain reaction (PCR). Cytopathology. 1997;8(2):114–21.
99. Vianello F, et al. Detection of B-cell monoclonality in fine needle aspiration by PCR analysis. Leuk Lymphoma. 1998;29(1-2):179–85.
100. Ribera J, et al. Usefulness of IGH/TCR PCR studies in lymphoproliferative disorders with inconclusive clonality by flow cytometry. Cytometry B Clin Cytom. 2014;86(1):25–31.
101. Brozic A, et al. Inconclusive flow cytometric surface light chain results; can cytoplasmic light chains, Bcl-2 expression and PCR clonality analysis improve accuracy of cytological diagnoses in B-cell lymphomas? Diagn Pathol. 2015;10:191.

102. Roepman P, et al. Molecular clonality assessment shows high performance to predict malignant B-cell non-Hodgkin's lymphoma using cytological smears. J Clin Pathol. 2016;69(12):1109–15.
103. Venkatraman L, et al. Role of polymerase chain reaction and immunocytochemistry in the cytological assessment of lymphoid proliferations. J Clin Pathol. 2006;59(11):1160–5.
104. Aiello A, et al. PCR analysis of IgH and BCL2 gene rearrangement in the diagnosis of follicular lymphoma in lymph node fine-needle aspiration. A critical appraisal. Diagn Mol Pathol. 1997;6(3):154–60.
105. Elenitoba-Johnson KS, et al. PCR analysis of the immunoglobulin heavy chain gene in polyclonal processes can yield pseudoclonal bands as an artifact of low B cell number. J Mol Diagn. 2000;2(2):92–6.
106. Davidson B, et al. Evaluation of lymphoid cell populations in cytology specimens using flow cytometry and polymerase chain reaction. Diagn Mol Pathol. 1999;8(4):183–8.
107. Maroto A, et al. A single primer pair immunoglobulin polymerase chain reaction assay as a useful tool in fine-needle aspiration biopsy differential diagnosis of lymphoid malignancies. Cancer. 2003;99(3):180–5.
108. Maroto A, et al. Comparative analysis of immunoglobulin polymerase chain reaction and flow cytometry in fine needle aspiration biopsy differential diagnosis of non-Hodgkin B-cell lymphoid malignancies. Diagn Cytopathol. 2009;37(9):647–53.
109. van Dongen JJ, et al. Design and standardization of PCR primers and protocols for detection of clonal immunoglobulin and T-cell receptor gene recombinations in suspect lymphoproliferations: report of the BIOMED-2 Concerted Action BMH4-CT98-3936. Leukemia. 2003;17(12):2257–317.
110. Langerak AW, et al. EuroClonality/BIOMED-2 guidelines for interpretation and reporting of Ig/TCR clonality testing in suspected lymphoproliferations. Leukemia. 2012;26(10):2159–71.
111. Chen YP, et al. Malignant effusions correlate with poorer prognosis in patients with diffuse large B-cell lymphoma. Am J Clin Pathol. 2015;143(5):707–15.
112. Lobo C, et al. Serous fluid cytology of multicentric Castleman's disease and other lymphoproliferative disorders associated with Kaposi sarcoma-associated herpes virus: a review with case reports. Cytopathology. 2012;23(2):76–85.
113. Mihaescu A, et al. Application of molecular genetics to the diagnosis of lymphoid-rich effusions: study of 95 cases with concomitant immunophenotyping. Diagn Cytopathol. 2002;27(2):90–5.
114. Murphy M, et al. Detection of concurrent/recurrent non-Hodgkin's lymphoma in effusions by PCR. Hum Pathol. 1999;30(11):1361–6.
115. Nepka C, et al. An unusual case of Primary Effusion Lymphoma with aberrant T-cell phenotype in a HIV-negative, HBV-positive, cirrhotic patient, and review of the literature. Cytojournal. 2012;9:16.
116. Philippe B, et al. B-cell pulmonary lymphoma: gene rearrangement analysis of bronchoalveolar lymphocytes by polymerase chain reaction. Chest. 1999;115(5):1242–7.
117. Zompi S, et al. Clonality analysis of alveolar B lymphocytes contributes to the diagnostic strategy in clinical suspicion of pulmonary lymphoma. Blood. 2004;103(8):3208–15.
118. Lovchik J, Lane MA, Clark DP. Polymerase chain reaction-based detection of B-cell clonality in the fine needle aspiration biopsy of a thyroid mucosa-associated lymphoid tissue (MALT) lymphoma. Hum Pathol. 1997;28(8):989–92.
119. Adhikari LJ, Reynolds JP, Wakely PE Jr. Multi-institutional study of fine needle aspiration for thyroid lymphoma. J Am Soc Cytopathol. 2015;5(3):170–6.
120. Chen HI, et al. Restricted kappa/lambda light chain ratio by flow cytometry in germinal center B cells in Hashimoto thyroiditis. Am J Clin Pathol. 2006;125(1):42–8.
121. Zeppa P, et al. Cytologic, flow cytometry, and molecular assessment of lymphoid infiltrate in fine-needle cytology samples of Hashimoto thyroiditis. Cancer. 2009;117(3):174–84.
122. Galindo LM, et al. Fine-needle aspiration biopsy in the evaluation of lymphadenopathy associated with cutaneous T-cell lymphoma (mycosis fungoides/Sezary syndrome). Am J Clin Pathol. 2000;113(6):865–71.

123. Pai RK, et al. Cytologic evaluation of lymphadenopathy associated with mycosis fungoides and Sezary syndrome: role of immunophenotypic and molecular ancillary studies. Cancer. 2008;114(5):323–32.
124. Vigliar E, et al. Lymph node fine needle cytology in the staging and follow-up of cutaneous lymphomas. BMC Cancer. 2014;14:8.
125. Cozzolino I, et al. Fine needle aspiration cytology of lymphoproliferative lesions of the oral cavity. Cytopathology. 2014;25(4):241–9.
126. Rhodes CH, et al. A comparison of polymerase chain reaction examination of cerebrospinal fluid and conventional cytology in the diagnosis of lymphomatous meningitis. Cancer. 1996;77(3):543–8.
127. Ekstein D, et al. CSF analysis of IgH gene rearrangement in CNS lymphoma: relationship to the disease course. J Neurol Sci. 2006;247(1):39–46.
128. Shibata D, et al. Detection of occult CNS involvement of follicular small cleaved lymphoma by the polymerase chain reaction. Mod Pathol. 1990;3(1):71–5.
129. Wildemann B, et al. Rapid distinction of acute demyelinating disorders and central nervous system lymphoma by molecular analysis of cerebrospinal fluid cells. J Neurol. 2001;248(2):127–30.
130. Lobo A, et al. Protocol for the use of polymerase chain reaction in the detection of intraocular large B-cell lymphoma in ocular samples. J Mol Diagn. 2007;9(1):113–21.
131. Gleissner B, et al. CSF evaluation in primary CNS lymphoma patients by PCR of the CDR III IgH genes. Neurology. 2002;58(3):390–6.
132. Sayed D, et al. Immunophenotyping and immunoglobulin heavy chain gene rearrangement analysis in cerebrospinal fluid of pediatric patients with acute lymphoblastic leukemia. Leuk Res. 2009;33(5):655–61.
133. Scrideli CA, et al. Molecular diagnosis of leukemic cerebrospinal fluid cells in children with newly diagnosed acute lymphoblastic leukemia. Haematologica. 2004;89(8):1013–5.
134. Hug A, et al. Single-cell PCR analysis of the immunoglobulin heavy-chain CDR3 region for the diagnosis of leptomeningeal involvement of B-cell malignancies using standard cerebrospinal fluid cytospins. J Neurol Sci. 2004;219(1-2):83–8.
135. Liu L, et al. Detection of malignant B lymphocytes by PCR clonality assay using direct lysis of cerebrospinal fluid and low volume specimens. Int J Lab Hematol. 2015;37(2):165–73.
136. Ranty ML, et al. Improving the cytological diagnosis of intraocular lymphoma from vitreous fluid. Histopathology. 2015;67(1):48–61.
137. Slack GW, Gascoyne RD. Next-generation sequencing discoveries in lymphoma. Adv Anat Pathol. 2013;20(2):110–6.
138. Alizadeh AA, et al. Distinct types of diffuse large B-cell lymphoma identified by gene expression profiling. Nature. 2000;403(6769):503–11.
139. Scott DW, et al. Determining cell-of-origin subtypes of diffuse large B-cell lymphoma using gene expression in formalin-fixed paraffin-embedded tissue. Blood. 2014;123(8):1214–7.
140. Kendrick S, et al. Diffuse large B-cell lymphoma cell-of-origin classification using the Lymph2Cx assay in the context of BCL2 and MYC expression status. Leuk Lymphoma. 2016;57(3):717–20.
141. Swerdlow SH, et al. The 2016 revision of the World Health Organization classification of lymphoid neoplasms. Blood. 2016;127(20):2375–90.
142. Goy A, et al. The feasibility of gene expression profiling generated in fine-needle aspiration specimens from patients with follicular lymphoma and diffuse large B-cell lymphoma. Cancer. 2006;108(1):10–20.
143. da Santos GC, et al. Multiplex sequencing for EZH2, CD79B, and MYD88 mutations using archival cytospin preparations from B-cell non-Hodgkin lymphoma aspirates previously tested for MYC rearrangement and IGH/BCL2 translocation. Cancer Cytopathol. 2015;123(7):413–20.
144. Saieg MA, et al. EZH2 and CD79B mutational status over time in B-cell non-Hodgkin lymphomas detected by high-throughput sequencing using minimal samples. Cancer Cytopathol. 2013;121(7):377–86.

145. Morin RD, et al. Frequent mutation of histone-modifying genes in non-Hodgkin lymphoma. Nature. 2011;476(7360):298–303.
146. Tiacci E, et al. BRAF mutations in hairy-cell leukemia. N Engl J Med. 2011;364(24):2305–15.
147. Tiacci E, et al. Simple genetic diagnosis of hairy cell leukemia by sensitive detection of the BRAF-V600E mutation. Blood. 2012;119(1):192–5.
148. Badalian-Very G, et al. Recurrent BRAF mutations in Langerhans cell histiocytosis. Blood. 2010;116(11):1919–23.
149. Mason EF, et al. Detection of activating MAP2K1 mutations in atypical hairy cell leukemia and hairy cell leukemia variant. Leuk Lymphoma. 2016;58(1):233–6.
150. Waterfall JJ, et al. High prevalence of MAP2K1 mutations in variant and IGHV4-34-expressing hairy-cell leukemias. Nat Genet. 2014;46(1):8–10.
151. Brown NA, et al. High prevalence of somatic MAP2K1 mutations in BRAF V600E-negative Langerhans cell histiocytosis. Blood. 2014;124(10):1655–8.
152. Diamond EL, et al. Diverse and targetable kinase alterations drive histiocytic neoplasms. Cancer Discov. 2016;6(2):154–65.
153. Fernandez V, et al. Genomic and gene expression profiling defines indolent forms of mantle cell lymphoma. Cancer Res. 2010;70(4):1408–18.
154. Hunter ZR, et al. The genomic landscape of Waldenstrom macroglobulinemia is characterized by highly recurring MYD88 and WHIM-like CXCR4 mutations, and small somatic deletions associated with B-cell lymphomagenesis. Blood. 2014;123(11):1637–46.
155. Ngo VN, et al. Oncogenically active MYD88 mutations in human lymphoma. Nature. 2011;470(7332):115–9.
156. Kiel MJ, et al. Whole-genome sequencing identifies recurrent somatic NOTCH2 mutations in splenic marginal zone lymphoma. J Exp Med. 2012;209(9):1553–65.
157. Clipson A, et al. KLF2 mutation is the most frequent somatic change in splenic marginal zone lymphoma and identifies a subset with distinct genotype. Leukemia. 2015;29(5):1177–85.
158. Cornet E, et al. Developing molecular signatures for chronic lymphocytic leukemia. PLoS One. 2015;10(6):e0128990.
159. Scott DW, et al. TBL1XR1/TP63: a novel recurrent gene fusion in B-cell non-Hodgkin lymphoma. Blood. 2012;119(21):4949–52.
160. Vasmatzis G, et al. Genome-wide analysis reveals recurrent structural abnormalities of TP63 and other p53-related genes in peripheral T-cell lymphomas. Blood. 2012;120(11):2280–9.
161. Kucuk C, et al. Activating mutations of STAT5B and STAT3 in lymphomas derived from gammadelta-T or NK cells. Nat Commun. 2015;6:6025.
162. Schwock J, et al. Enteropathy-associated intestinal T-cell lymphoma in cavitating mesenteric lymph node syndrome: fine-needle aspiration contributes to the diagnosis. Diagn Cytopathol. 2015;43(2):125–30.
163. Feldman AL, et al. Discovery of recurrent t(6;7)(p25.3;q32.3) translocations in ALK-negative anaplastic large cell lymphomas by massively parallel genomic sequencing. Blood. 2011;117(3):915–9.
164. Yoo HY, et al. A recurrent inactivating mutation in RHOA GTPase in angioimmunoblastic T cell lymphoma. Nat Genet. 2014;46(4):371–5.
165. Sakata-Yanagimoto M, et al. Somatic RHOA mutation in angioimmunoblastic T cell lymphoma. Nat Genet. 2014;46(2):171–5.
166. Palomero T, et al. Recurrent mutations in epigenetic regulators, RHOA and FYN kinase in peripheral T cell lymphomas. Nat Genet. 2014;46(2):166–70.
167. Zeppa P, et al. Fine-needle cytology and flow cytometry immunophenotyping and subclassification of non-Hodgkin lymphoma: a critical review of 307 cases with technical suggestions. Cancer. 2004;102(1):55–65.
168. Amador-Ortiz C, et al. Combined core needle biopsy and fine-needle aspiration with ancillary studies correlate highly with traditional techniques in the diagnosis of nodal-based lymphoma. Am J Clin Pathol. 2011;135(4):516–24.

Molecular Cytology Application on Thyroid

Esther Diana Rossi and Massimo Bongiovanni

10.1 Introduction

This chapter deals with the evaluation of molecular diagnostic cytopathology applied on thyroid nodules (TN). The application of molecular testing in the diagnostic cytopathology of difficult thyroid cases has paralleled the progress reported in surgical pathology and continues to grow and offer valid results. Recent advances in thyroid and cancer biology have led to the development and marketing of several tests to define whether a TN is benign or malignant [1–3]. In fact, detection of point mutations, loss of heterozygosis analysis, and clonality assays require the isolation of DNA which is more stable than RNA and can be easily isolated also from cytological specimens [1–6]. However, apart from fresh or frozen tissues, formalin-fixed paraffin-embedded (FFPE) specimens, obtained as cell-block also from cytological aspirations, can be successfully adopted with also the additional option to enrich a tumor population with manual or laser capture micro-dissection frequently performed from unstained tissue sections or under the guidance of hematoxylin and eosin (H&E) slides. Given that, FNACs provide good quality of DNA and are more than acceptable for testing. Besides, the analysis of RNA is used for the detection of chromosomal rearrangements (i.e., RET/PTC, PAX8/PPARγ), gene expression profiling, and miRNA profiling [4–7]. One of the major inconveniences in the use of RNA is linked with the fact that it is a less stable molecule than DNA and is easily degraded by a variety of ribonuclease enzymes that are replete within the cell and

E. D. Rossi (✉)
Division of Anatomic Pathology and Histology, Fondazione Universtaria
Policlinico Agostino Gemelli-IRCCS, Rome, Italy
e-mail: esther.rossi@policlinicogemelli.it

M. Bongiovanni
Service of Clinical Pathology, Lausanne University Hospital, Institute of Pathology,
Lausanne, Switzerland
e-mail: Massimo.Bongiovanni@chuv.ch

© Springer International Publishing AG, part of Springer Nature 2018
F. C. Schmitt (ed.), *Molecular Applications in Cytology*,
https://doi.org/10.1007/978-3-319-74942-6_10

environment. For this reason, only freshly collected or frozen tissue and non-fixed FNA samples are considered to be reliable specimens for these techniques [1–3]. As reported in the chapter about miRNAs in thyroid lesions, some good results have been obtained even with conventional (CS) and liquid based cytology (LBC). In fact, RNA isolated from FFPE tissue is of poor quality and has to be used with great caution for clinical testing. When we have FFPE tissue, the best alternative for detection of rearrangements is utilization of fluorescence in situ hybridization (FISH) technique, which provides reliable evaluation in the majority of cases.

10.2 Thyroid Lesions

According to several papers, TNs occur in approximately 50% of the general population and 5–15% result to be malignant [8, 9]. Although the majority of these lesions may be univocally diagnosed as either non-neoplastic or neoplastic entities, there is a number of nodules that are comprised in the controversial grey area of follicular nodules (FNs) which belong to the indeterminate categories according to the Bethesda system for reporting thyroid cytopathology (TBSRTC) [10–15].

The relevance of fine-needle aspiration cytology (FNAC) as the first diagnostic tool for the evaluation of thyroid lesions has been clearly demonstrated and validated in these last decades. Unequivocally, it represents the most commonly used approach in thyroid nodules because of its simplicity, safety, and cost-effectiveness leading to a correct diagnosis in the majority of cases [10–24]. Regardless of the classification system adopted, about 85–90% of TNs are benign and a benign cytological category is diagnosed in 60–70% of all thyroid FNACs with only a minority of them (5–15%) signed out as "malignant" lesions [25–38]. The remaining 20–25% of them are included in an indeterminate result, belonging to the so-called "grey zone of indeterminate neoplasms" among which it is not always possible to specify whether the nodules are benign or malignant entities [25–38]. Driven by these issues, the attempts for a correct diagnosis of these indeterminate lesions resulted in the division into the three subgroups of atypia of undetermined significance/follicular lesions of undetermined significance (AUS/FLUS); suspicious for follicular neoplasm/follicular neoplasm (SFN/FN) and suspicious for malignancy (SM) [10]. These lesions harbor a 24% risk of malignancy (ROM); too high to be ignored, but driving surgery where most nodules are benign. In fact several cases resulted in unnecessary surgical resections and higher health care costs [38]. As expected, this indeterminate category highlights the major morphological flaws and controversies of FNACs. This is also due to the fact that the presence of any vascular and capsular invasion can be univocally established only with a thorough histological evaluation of the nodule. Moreover, this FN category includes several cases of follicular variant of papillary thyroid carcinoma (FVPC) in which the absence of the peculiar nuclear features of PTC may fall short of a definitive malignant diagnosis [39–43]. A new challenge was the recent reclassification of non-invasive-FVPCs as a tumor (noninvasive follicular thyroid neoplasm with papillary-like nuclear features-NIFTP) rather than "carcinoma" which may have a significant impact on the implied

ROM for the indeterminate/follicular proliferations [39]. A large number of growing literatures is trying to address and solve this issue. Accordingly, Strickland et al. studied a series of 655 FNAs with surgical resection specimens demonstrating that the introduction of NIFTPs led to the fact that the ROM for AUS/FLUS, NF, and SM resulted in a significant decrease (between 20 and 48%) [39–42]. Moreover, Maletta et al. showed that NIFTP nodules were found in the diagnosis of "FN/SFN" in 56% of cases, "suspicious for malignancy" in 27%, "AUS/FLUS in 15%, and "malignant" in 2% of cases [40]. However, despite the small number of NIFTPs series, Maletta et al. found that a predominantly follicular pattern may be linked with NIFTPs even if these authors did not find any morphological finding able to discriminate between NIFTPs and invasive FVPCs on FNAC [40]. On the other hand, the presence of nuclear pseudo-inclusions, papillary structures are typical features of PTCs. This new terminology portends significant diagnostic and management implications especially on cytology justifying also the additional support of ancillary techniques [43].

In order to overcome the limitations of morphology, several authors encouraged the application of both immunocytochemistry (ICC) and molecular analysis [25–31] on thyroid FNAC processed with either CS or LBC [44–57]. Additionally, this molecular evaluation is extremely important because thyroid cancer develops and progresses through the accumulation of genetic alterations, which can serve as central diagnostic, prognostic, and predictive biological markers. According to several researches, there are specific common mutations which occur in PTCs and its variants which are the most common thyroid malignancy accounting for the majority of the cases [54–64]. Nevertheless, apart from well-differentiated thyroid carcinoma (WDTC), another promising field of application is the study of other thyroid malignancies including medullary thyroid carcinoma (MTC) involving the parafollicular cells and/or poorly differentiated thyroid cancers [65–83]. In fact follicular cancers (FC) most frequently harbor specific mutations whilst other genetic alterations are also involved in advanced and dedifferentiating tumors. Additional and specific mutations are known to occur in poorly differentiated (PDC) and anaplastic carcinomas (ATC) [79–83].

10.2.1 Molecular Markers

Numerous scientific data have shown that molecular alterations of specific pathways play a pivotal role in different types of thyroid cancer and, importantly, arise early in the tumorigenic process, justifying the use of these as markers of malignancy in the daily practice. The knowledge of the molecular pathology of thyroid disease has emerged with its relevant implications in the last years with also the publication of the Thyroid Cancer Genome Atlas study of PTC in the thyroid gland [84]. It is now clear that PTCs is either a *BRAF V600E* or a *RAS*-driven tumor. However, the most common mutations that occur in these carcinomas are point mutations of the *BRAF* and *RAS* gene and *RET/PTC* rearrangements; all of which are able to activate the mitogenic-activated protein kinase (MAPK) pathway [60,

62–64, 85–91]. This emerging role of molecular diagnostics is being reflected in the revised management guidelines for patients with thyroid nodules and WDTCs, recently published by the American Thyroid Association (ATA) [85]. In fact, these guidelines suggest the analysis of a molecular panel (including *BRAF, RAS, RET/PTC,* and *PAX8-PPARγ*) in patients with FNs. This would represent an additional and possible aid in guiding their management [51] as well as ThyroSeq2, a recently system developed by Nikiforov and colleagues using targeted next generation sequencing (NGS) [92–94].

10.2.1.1 BRAF

An extensive revision of literature provided that mutations of the B-type RAF kinase (*BRAF*) are the most common alteration in thyroid malignancy, resulting in 40–69% of PTCs and one-third of PDCs [62, 95–97]. However, this mutation is not specific of the thyroid, and was previously described in several tumors including melanoma, colorectal, and lung among others [95–97]. It is well documented that the most common mutation results in a valine to glutamate replacement at residue 600 in exon 15 (V600E), activating the MAPK pathway and associated downstream targets [98–100]. The analysis can be performed adopted various methods of detection including colorimetric detection, allele-specific amplifications, pyrosequencing, multiplex PCR, and direct DNA sequencing analysis which can detect mutations in populations as small as 1–10% of total cells [95]. DNA sequencing and PCR assays have demonstrated the greatest sensitivity, even if extremely high sensitivity may increase the potential of false-positive results [95]. The diagnostic role of *BRAF*[V600E] mutation has been studied in several series, including both prospective and retrospective studies, which have demonstrated that this mutation is a strong predictor of cancer with 100% accurate yields mostly in the FNs [62, 54–56, 59, 60] (Fig. 10.1). Nevertheless, the *BRAF* testing should not be performed in every TN so as to nodules with a low pre-test probability (benign ultrasound and cytopathologic findings) are exceedingly unlikely to harbor a mutation [54–56]. Interestingly, some studies have shown that nodules with non-diagnostic results may occasionally show *BRAF* mutation [54–56]. Therefore both nodules with indeterminate/suspicious ultrasound findings and non-diagnostic categories may benefit from *BRAF* testing. It is well documented that *BRAF* gene mutation analysis is the most widely utilized single-gene test. In fact, a positive test, due to high specificity of somatic mutations should

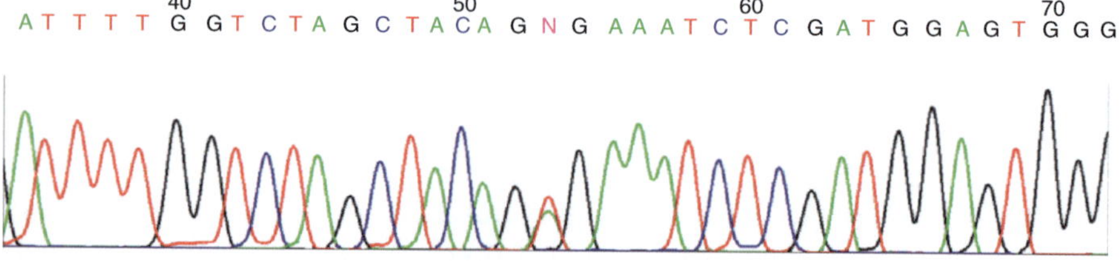

Fig. 10.1 This picture shows the sequence of *p.V600E* in a thyroid lesion diagnosed as positive for malignancy on liquid based cytology (LBC)

not only lead to a total thyroidectomy, but also influence post-operative management because of its prognostic value of a greater risk of lymph node metastases, extra-thyroidal extension, and local recurrence. $BRAF^{V600E}$ mutations may act as a sensitive, although not specific, marker of tumor aggressiveness [62, 63, 83, 86, 89, 90, 101, 102]. Rossi et al. revealed that in the SM category, the detection of a $BRAF^{V600E}$ mutation was linked with 100% histological diagnosis of PTCs ($p = 0.0353$) and also significantly associated with some aggressive parameters including lymph-node metastases ($p < 0.0001$), extra capsular invasion ($p = 0.03$), and multi-focality ($p = 0.0003$) [59]. Hence, Colanta et al. found that 54% of $BRAF^{V600E}$ mutated cases had a clinical stage 2 or higher whereas only 25% of wild-type $BRAF^{V600E}$ cases presented with a similar clinical stage [64]. They also found 42% of the $BRAF^{V600E}$ mutated cases showing some recurrences including four patients who died for the disease [64].

Furthermore, in some papers, $BRAF^{V600E}$ mutation has been highly associated with PTC and more often with the aggressive variants (e.g., tall cell variant and columnar variant) with much lower rate of $BRAF$ mutations in FVPCs [87–89, 101–103]. As largely underlined in literature, FVPCs, mostly diagnosed on FNAC as indeterminate categories (AUS/FLUSs, FNs or SMs) showed an average $BRAF^{V600E}$ expression at around 15% in different studies [104]. As described in limited literature, the detection of other $BRAF$ mutations, such as $BRAF$ K601E mutation as well as the subset of complex and less common $BRAF$ mutations has been observed in FVPCs with less aggressive behavior [104–107].

However, the molecular detection of $BRAF$ mutations has been supported by the easily ICC analysis of the $BRAF$ mutated protein. In fact, although $BRAF^{V600E}$ mutation has been typically performed using DNA-based techniques, the recent introduction of the monoclonal V600E antibody (clone VE1) represents an alternative strategy to detect this mutation in thyroid lesions on cytology. In these last years, two different papers from Zimmerman et al. and Rossi et al. assessed the good sensitivity and specificity ranging from 82 to 86% on cytological samples of thyroid lesions [108–110]. Although its limitation probably due to the limited series published, VE1 antibody represents a feasible first-line approach for evaluating $BRAF^{V600E}$ mutation and might be a valid tool in selecting cases for molecular analysis. Rossi et al. highlighted a statistical significance between molecular and VE1 positivity ($p < 0.0001$) in the comparative analysis of the results obtained from molecular and ICC in PTC [110].

10.2.1.2 RAS

Several papers pointed to the fact that RAS mutations are common in 20–40% of thyroid adenomas as well as in 15% of PTCs (predominately FVPTCs). They have also now been identified in a subset of MCTs [95]. It is well known that three separate genes (*HRAS, NRAS,* and *KRAS*) encode G proteins transmitting signals along the MAPK and PI3K pathways, with several codons having been identified as sources of activating point mutations.

In thyroid tumors, mutations involving NRAS codon 61 (Fig. 10.2) and HRAS codon 61 are by far the most common, although mutations have been found in

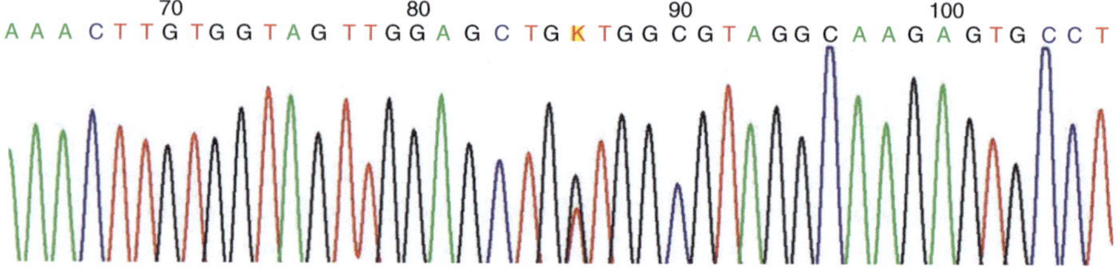

Fig. 10.2 N-*RAS* mutation in a thyroid indeterminate lesion

different hotspots of all three genes. *RAS* mutations are present in benign lesions, but also most *RAS*-positive carcinomas have indeterminate cytology and lack suspicious ultrasound features [111–116]. Additionally *RAS* mutations are also found in 40–50% of follicular carcinomas and 20–40% of follicular adenomas (FA). Specifically in the adenomas, the mutations seemed to be more common in tumors showing a microfollicular pattern. A lower incidence has been reported in oncocytic tumors, in which only 0–4% of adenomas and 15–25% of carcinomas reported to be RAS positive lesions [117–119] As recently studied by Radkay et al. in a series of 204 thyroid fine-needle aspiration cases diagnosed according to the Bethesda system and studied with *RAS* mutations, *KRAS12/13* mutation was associated with a significantly lower prevalence of carcinoma (41.7%) when compared with *HRAS61* (95.5%) and *NRAS61* (86.8%) mutations (*P* < 0.0001) [91].

10.2.1.3 RET/PTC

Different studies found that papillary carcinomas with *RET/PTC* rearrangements are often associated with younger patients, or those with radiation exposure [95, 120–122]. Similar to *BRAF* and *RAS, RET/PTC* gene rearrangements result in activation of the *MAPK* pathway. The two most common rearrangement types, RET/PTC1 and RET/PTC3, are intra-chromosomal inversions with both *RET* and its respective fusion partner genes, H4 and NCOA4 (also known as ELE1), are located on chromosome 10. RET/PTC2 and nine more recently identified types of RET/PTC are all inter-chromosomal translocations [95]. It has been assessed that all the rearrangement types contain the intact tyrosine kinase domain of the RET receptor and enables the RET/PTC chimeric protein to activate the RAS–RAF–MAPK cascade and initiate thyroid tumorigenesis.

A minority (10–20%) of adult sporadic PTCs are found to have RET/PTC rearrangements although its prevalence is highly variable between various observations. This data is due to the difference in sensitivity of the detection methods and also because of some geographical variability [95]. In this perspective, several data demonstrated that *RET/PTC* occurs with higher incidence in patients with the history of radiation exposure (50–80%) and in PTCs from children and young adults (40–70%) [95, 120–122]. In PTCs, RET/PTC1 is the most common comprising 60–70% of all rearrangement types, whereas RET/PTC3 accounts for 20–30% and RET/PTC2 and other novel rearrangement types for 0.5%.

Specifically PTCs with RET/PTC1 rearrangement are more frequently diagnosed in younger age and in cancers with a high rate of lymph node metastases. PCR-based methods are the most common detection methods; however, other techniques including fluorescence in situ hybridization (FISH) have been examined since they may improve overall sensitivity by examining mutations within abnormal-appearing cells.

10.2.2 PAX8/Peroxisome Proliferator-Activated Receptor Gamma (PAX8/PPARγ)

The detection of *PAX8/PPARγ* rearrangement is reported in both adenomas and carcinomas [95]. The exact mechanism of action has not yet been described. However it seems that PAX8/PPARγ rearrangement is a result of translocation between chromosomes 2 and 3, t(2;3)(q13;p25), leading to the fusion between the PAX8 gene coding for the thyroid-specific paired domain transcription factor, and the PPARγ gene. Although *RAS* and *PAX8/PPARγ* are both found in FAs, they seem to be mutually exclusive with only rare reports of both mutations in the same nodule [123]. Furthermore PAX8/PPARγ is found in 30–40% of FC, and with lower prevalence in oncocytic carcinomas (OC) [124–126]. Additionally it can be found in 2–10% of FAs and in some (<5%) FVPTCs [124–126].

10.2.2.1 HMGA2

As described in literature, HMGA2 is a nonhistone chromosomal protein that is usually highly expressed in tumor tissue. In fact, the interaction of HMGA with DNA induces changes in the chromatin structure involving HMGA proteins in the regulation of the expression of a high number of target genes [151, 159]. In order to define the role in thyroid lesions, Jin et al. measured HMGA2 expression levels using RT-PCR in 226 thyroid FNA specimens and found that HMGA2 had 89% sensitivity and 95% specificity in the separation between benign from malignant thyroid tumors on FNA [160]. Despite the valid yields, they did not specify the number of indeterminate FNACs and they did not find an accurate role of HMGA2 as a marker able to differentiate benign from malignant Hurthle cell neoplasms.

10.2.2.2 UbcH10

Another marker was UBE2C (or UbcH10) which seems to be linked with destruction of cell cycle cyclins and facilitation of cell cycle progression [161]. Specifically Guerriero et al. evaluated UbcH10 expression using RT-PCR and immunohistochemistry in 84 thyroid FNA samples. The lesions included only samples of FN or SM (Bethesda IV and V) [161]. The sensitivity and specificity in the correct classification of indeterminate nodules remained fairly low at 72% and 67%, respectively. The study suggested that UbcH10 could, however, be added as a useful adjunct to other gene panels

10.2.3 Diagnostic and Prognostic Involvement of Molecular Alterations in the Different Thyroid Lesions

Molecular diagnosis is the result of the application of molecular techniques and knowledge of molecular mechanisms of thyroid diseases in order to offer a valid aid to their diagnosis, prognosis, and personalized management [1–6]. A large number of information on molecular aspects of thyroid diseases has been developed on cytological samples. Specifically the application of molecular diagnostic cytopathology involves those cases analyzed for routinely cytomorphology and mainly from solid tumors. The majority of the tests are based on the two main approaches available in molecular laboratories including the classical polymerase chain reaction (PCR) technique and also reverse-transcriptase PCR, capillary electrophoresis and conventional sequencing as well as FISH [1–6].

As with other cancers, diagnostic molecular analysis of thyroid samples is not widely utilized routinely. Despite this evidence, recent papers and the ATA guidelines showed the promising role in the diagnosis of the different range and scenario of FNs, WDTCs, and PDCs [11]. In this regard, mutations involving *RET/PTC, TRK, BRAF,* and *RAS* oncogene occur in over 70% of PTC and they are detected by RT-PCR and mutant allele-specific amplification techniques [1–6]. All these mutations arise early in the tumorigenic process, justifying their use as diagnostic markers of malignancy. Several authors have experimented the feasibility and simplicity of the molecular testing for cytological diagnosis of TNs including not only FNs but also SMs as well as its use as a prognostic indicator for the PMs including the different histotypes [44, 51, 54–56, 59, 61, 91–94]. The utility of molecular testing has been extensively studied by Nikiforov et al. in several papers analyzing single or panels of molecular mutations. Analyzing a prospective series of 1056 indeterminate nodules, classified according to the Bethesda system, they reported a 87% and 95% range of malignancy rate in the *BRAF* mutated indeterminate cases [131]. Also Mathur et al. suggested the use of a scoring model including cytology and mutational analysis for the correct classification of follicular lesions with the correct classification as benign or malignant in 91% of the analyzed samples [127].

Apart from the recognition of PTCs and its variants, FCs most frequently harbor other mutations, including *RAS* mutations or *PAX8/PPARγ* rearrangement [91]. Hence, genetic alterations involving the *PI3K/AKT* signaling pathway (*PIK3CA, PTEN, AKT1* mutations) have been found in thyroid tumors, mostly including advanced and dedifferentiating tumors [84]. Additional mutations, comprising the *TP53* and *CTNNB1* genes have been recognized in aggressive histotypes of WDTCs as well as in PDCs and ATCs [84]. On the other hand, MTCs frequently carry point mutations affecting the *RET* and *RAS* genes [65, 67, 68]. Even if somatic mutations of *TSHR* and *GNAS* genes have been frequently occurred in autonomously functioning benign thyroid nodules, *TSHR* mutations, located at specific hotspots and present at high allelic frequency, are also found in FCs [84]. However, other more recently identified point mutations and gene fusions in thyroid cancer include *EIF1AX* mutations and *STRN-ALK and*

ETV6- NTRK3 fusions [132–134]. The growing number of mutations accounts for the recent discovery of additional mutations in the promoter region of the *TERT* gene, either C228T or C250T, which have been reported in PTCs, FCs, and also with higher frequency in PDCs [135, 136]. As previously reported for *BRAF* mutation, also these mutational markers can be used for tumor prognostication. In fact, the presence of *TERT* mutations is associated with tumoral invasiveness at presentation and with a significantly higher risk of distant metastases, disease persistence, and cancer-specific mortality [134–136]. Also *BRAF*^{V600E} mutation has been associated with higher risk of tumor recurrence and cancer-specific survival especially when found in combination with other mutations such as *TERT* [101, 137–139]. In a similar way, the presence of multiple mutations and/or *TP53* mutations may predict more aggressive tumor behavior and predisposition to tumor dedifferentiation in *TP53*-mutant cancers [93].

Additionally the mutational status may also support targeted therapies for advanced thyroid cancer. Accordingly clinical trials with *BRAF* or *MEK* inhibitors to enhance the radioiodine uptake are available for patients with *BRAF*-mutant, RAI-refractory thyroid cancer, and *RAS*-mutant thyroid cancer, and trials with a combination of *BRAF* and MEK inhibitors to treat patients with *BRAF*-mutated ATCs [132, 140, 141]. Some pre-clinical studies and single case reports suggest that patients with advanced thyroid cancer, including ATCs, carrying ALK fusions can benefit from treatment with ALK inhibitors [132, 140, 141].

10.2.4 LBC and Molecular Techniques

The application of ancillary techniques (molecular markers but also ICC) in FNA has encountered two main problems: (1) the difficulties in its application on CS and (2) the nondiagnostic role of a single marker. In order to increase specificity LBC, originally developed for cervical smears, demonstrated to be a valid "alternative" technique for collection and preparation of cytological specimens including thyroid lesions [6, 57–59, 142–144]. The majority of the above-mentioned molecular techniques have been applied also on LBC with feasible and valid results [6, 49, 57–59, 142–144]. LBC is based on the collection of cells into a methanol-based preservative solution, followed by processing with a semi-automated device, leading to an almost complete elimination of the background interference from blood, obscuring background and air-drying artifact [142, 143]. There has been controversial data regarding the efficacy of LBC, however several positive aspects have been highlighting including cost-effectiveness, time-sparing, and most importantly the simple application of ancillary techniques [6, 49, 57–59, 142–147]. In fact several authors stated that the application of ICC and molecular analysis may be more easily performed, pointing out LBC as a promising method for routine use [6, 49, 57–59, 142–147]. According to several authors, LBC provided 100% informative molecular results with cyto-histological concordance [142–145]. Chang et al. studied the application of *BRAF* molecular mutation analysis in a series of PMs on LBC with a resulting 84.9% sensitivity [60].

10.3 The Role of Molecular Testing in Follicular Cell Lesions

According to the fact that increasing knowledge of the molecular pathways involved in thyroid carcinomas led to the recognition of different and specific neoplasms, the application of molecular techniques can have a significant role into the diagnosis, prognosis, and prediction on the " grey zone" of indeterminate proliferations [44, 51, 54–61, 91–94, 127–131, 148–152]. In these last decades, several different studies demonstrated the feasibility and simplicity of molecular testing for their cytological diagnoses involving either single molecular marker or also molecular panels. In 2015, the ATA statement for molecular profiling highlighted that different molecular testing are useful in the evaluation of the three subcategories of FNs. In fact these testing can demonstrate their potentiality to streamline decision making and reduce unnecessary surgery according to the correct prevalence of cancer in the cytologic categories [85]. They may represent an additional support in the choice of the correct treatment (lobectomy versus total thyroidectomy, or more extensive surgical approach) in the different diagnostic categories. Specifically, initially there are two molecular tests commercially available including (a) the 7-gene panel test and (b) the Gene Expression Classifiers (GECs) [85]. In detail, the first analyzes seven different DNA and RNA point mutations and translocations associated with thyroid carcinoma (miRInform, Asuragen, Austin, TX), now modified and commercialized as ThyGenX by Interpace Diagnostics (Parsippany, NJ) [131]. The second assay is based on a microarray in a panel of 167 mRNAs classifying thyroid nodules as "benign" or "suspicious" (Afirma, Veracyte, South San Francisco, CA) [150]. The two tests serve opposite functions: in fact Asuragen assay is performed to confirm malignancy, while the Afirma assay excludes malignancy. These different roles has been highlighted in prospective validation studies [92–94, 131, 150–157]

10.3.1 From the 7-Gene Panel Test to Next Generation Sequencing (NGS) Tests

The first description of a 7-gene panel including somatic mutations and gene rearrangement was done by Nikiforov and confirmed with histological samples. Including a panel of mutations (*BRAF, N-/H-/K-RAS*) and translocations of the *RET/PTC* and *PAX8/PPARγ* genes, they demonstrated that the detection of any mutation rose up a malignancy risk for AUS/FLUS, FN/SFN, and SM of 88%, 87%, and 95%, respectively, compared to 6%, 14%, and 28% in mutation-negative lesions [131]. This was and is a "rule in" test for WDTCs. According to these results, a 7-gene MT positive sample is referred to thyroidectomy regardless of the Bethesda categories [131]. While *BRAF* emerged as the most common mutation detected, *RAS* was the second with 87.5% positive predictive value for malignancy. This test was developed at the University of Pittsburgh and it was then commercialized and offered to outside institutions. Indeterminate cases with mutation-negative panel currently require diagnostic lobectomy; also mutational negative SM are much likely to be treated with an initial lobectomy even if the evaluation should be reasonable taken with the evaluation of the clinical-imaging and estimated risk of malignancy for the category. Then, Nikiforova et al. and Nikiforov et al. experienced the development and implementation of the use of targeted next generation sequencing (NGS) as a simultaneous testing for multiple mutations on FNACs [92–94]. In 2013, Nikiforova et al. adopted a custom panel (ThyroSeq) designed to target 12 cancer genes with 282 hot spots [93]. Sequencing was performed to analyze DNA from 228 thyroid histological samples of neoplastic and non-neoplastic entities and including also 51 FNAC samples composed of all types of thyroid cancer. As stated by their researches, ThyroSeq NGS panel can be performed on DNA and RNA isolated from cytological samples collected into preservative solution, fixed FNA specimens, or FFPE tumor tissue. After that, the analysis can be carried out using next generation, semiconductor-based sequencing. Input DNA and RNA is amplified using the AmpliSeq technology after which the amplicons are modified with adaptors, re-amplified, and subjected to emulsion PCR. The final products are sequenced on a 318 chip. The analytic sensitivity is 3–5% of mutant alleles for detection of mutations and 1% for detection of gene fusions. The input DNA and RNA is about 10 ng [92–94]. In their studies, they obtained successful analysis in 99.6% samples using an amount of 5–10 ng of input DNA. This approach with ThyroSeq allows simultaneous testing for multiple mutations with 100% accuracy with the sensitivity of 3–5% of mutant allele [91]. The most common mutations detected were *BRAF* and *RAS* followed by *PIK3CA, TP53, TSHR, PTEN, GNAS, CTNNB1*, and *RET*. However, in 2014 Nikiforov et al. developed a new NGS-based assay (ThyroSeq2) with a more complete panel of genetic markers which is able to test 91% of known thyroid cancer mutations. This test is conducted simultaneously for point mutations in 13 genes and for 42 types of gene fusions in a series of 143 indeterminate thyroid lesions [93]. The extensive comprehensive genotyping of thyroid nodules, using Thyroseq2, may represent an extraordinary adjunct for the diagnosis of FN/SFN providing a high positive predictive value (PPV) of 83% as well as improving the negative predictive value (NPV) to 96%. This result encouraged the idea that a single test can support both high PPV and NPV. Furthermore, in a recent paper, the same authors reported that ThyroSeqv2.1 multi-gene NGS panel of molecular markers (including 14 genes analyzed for point mutations and 42 types of gene fusions occurring in thyroid cancer) provides both high sensitivity (90.9%) and high specificity (92.1%) for cancer detection in a series of 465 thyroid nodules classified as AUS/FLUS [94].

10.3.2 Gene Expression Classifiers (GECS)

The first description of the amplified transcriptional profile from mRNA of thyroid FNACs was done by Chudova et al. in 2010 when they developed a gene expression test to predict the low risk of malignancy in TNs with surgical follow-up [150]. Additional analyses led to the development of a 142 gene cDNA affymetrix cassette (AFIRMA) gene expression classifier (GEC) [152]. As mentioned above, gene expression profiling, high throughput and computational analyses have provided new methods to identify potential target genes or gene panels to differentiate benign from malignant indeterminate lesions [150–152]. In this perspective RNA-based markers can be divided into single-gene analysis or multiple gene panel analysis. Although in literature several RNA-based markers have been reported to offer valid results, only a few single markers and gene panels have been validated on indeterminate FNACs [152].

Since that the most challenging category is represented by the indeterminate lesions, some authors evaluated the role of GECs mostly in this field of thyroid proliferations [152–157]. A broad GEC was developed as a proprietary method for molecular analysis of thyroid AUS/FLUS and FN mostly with the aim at predicting benign lesions, as a "rule out" test and reducing the unnecessary thyroidectomy which are frequently performed in these categories [152].

The most significant publication and validation of this test has been reported by Alexander et al. in a multicenter validation trial, involving 265 indeterminate lesions out of 4812 FNACs, studying the expression of 167 genes composed of 142 genes in the main classifier (benign or suspicious) and 25 genes to filter out rare neoplasms [152]. Since the beginning, the main purpose of the Afirma test pointed to the improvement of the preoperative risk assessment in the FNs as suggested by the 95% NPV for AUS and 94% for FN with a 62% false-positive rate for the former category [152]. However, the high NPV and sensitivity, which were not found with the "classical" molecular applications, were also counterparted by the low specificity and some false negative results. The valid effect of being a test which is able to propose a more conservative approach for patients with benign Afirma results, does not overcome the expensive economical knock-on effects so that it results apparently simple in super-specialized centers. In fact, some preliminary data about cost analysis underlined that this approach may be cost effective based on the study parameters which need to be confirmed in validation series [151]. As underlined by Faquin and Rossi et al., the potentiality of morphological interpretation supported also by the priceless chance of repeating FNAC was completely under-estimated [128, 129]. Additionally, McIver et al. evaluated the performance of Afirma GEC on 72 nucleic acid samples and demonstrated a lower than expected rate of benign reports in follicular or Hürthle cell neoplasm and a lower than anticipated malignancy rate within GEC-suspicious nodules [153].

Dedhia et al. worked out that the application of GEC was associated with only 7.2% reduction in thyroidectomies especially among AUS/FLUSs and FNs [154]. Wong et al. confirmed that the Afirma test was able to detect the encapsulated-FVPCs and that lobectomy as opposed to total thyroidectomy should be considered for nodules with preceding AUS/FLUS or FN/SFN on cytology and a suspicious Afirma result [158]. This test was designed for the AUS/FLUS and FN categories and it should be adopted for the SM only in specific requested cases. In cases of benign GEC, the most reasonable management should consist in observation especially in the absence of clinical-sonographic suspicious for malignancy.

10.4 The Role of Molecular Testing in Parafollicular Cell Lesions

MCT accounts for 1–2% of thyroid cancer in the United States [162–167]. The diagnosis can be render on cytological samples even though MCT has a variable appearance on aspiration cytology. The MTC cells are usually discohesive or weakly cohesive and may be spindle-shaped, plasmacytoid, or epithelioid [163]. The diagnosis of MTC should be supported by application of ICC showing positivity for Calcitonin, Chromogranin, or CEA and negativity of Thyroglobulin staining, and most importantly by detecting elevated serum CEA and Calcitonin levels in the patient [163]. In these last decades some academic organizations have published guidelines for the management of MTC [164–167]. In 2009 the ATA decided to published and recommended evidence-based guidelines for the diagnosis and management of MTC [162]. This tumor can occur either sporadically, or in a hereditary form as a component of the type 2 multiple endocrine neoplasia (MEN) syndromes, MEN2A, MEN2B, and the related syndrome, familial MTC (FMTC). Takahashi discovered the presence of *RET* oncogene in 1985 [168]. Then, it has been demonstrated that virtually all patients with MEN2A, MEN2B, and FMTC have *RET* germline mutations mostly in codons 609, 611, 618, or 620 of exon 10, or codon 634 of exon 11 and approximately 50% of sporadic MTCs have somatic *RET* mutations [64–74]. Approximately 95% of patients with MEN2B have *RET* germline mutations in exon 16 (codon M918T) and less than 5% have *RET* germline mutations in exon 15 (codon A883F). Another interesting recent discovery was the fact that 18-80% of sporadic MTCs, lacking somatic *RET* mutations, have somatic mutations of *HRAS, KRAS,* or rarely *NRAS* [73, 74]. The additional exomic sequencing studies of MTCs did not detect any other additional common genetic mutations [74]. Specifically Ret germline mutations are crucial for the development of heritable forms of MCT, while somatic mutations of RET may be found in sporadic MCTs (codon M918T mutation) with an aggressive clinical course and metastases [169–172]. Some authors found an association between the prevalence of somatic RET mutation and tumor size which was 60% in patients with tumor larger than 3 cm [169]. A complete tabulation of *RET* germline mutations reported to date, included: single or multiple mutations, duplications, insertions or deletions, and chromosomal rearrangements [169–172]. In patients with hereditary MCT have been identified over 100 mutations, duplications, insertions, or deletions involving *RET* [64–74]. Farndon described familial MTC which is differentiated from MEN2A based on the fact that MCT is identified in at least 4 members of the family without any other manifestations of MEN2A [169]. These members had the RET codon G533C mutation in exon 8. Although some laboratories sequence the entire *RET* coding region, others use another two-tiered approach, starting with the analysis of the most common mutated "hotspot" exons and then sequencing the remaining *RET* exons in cases in which the initial analysis is negative. However rare *RET* double or multiple mutations can be considered and they can only be identified by sequencing the entire *RET* coding sequence. Additionally the presence of multiple *RET* mutations may cause an unusual clinical phenotype compared with the one found in presence of single *RET* mutations. Although the most frequent mutation in MTC is defined by the rearranged during transfection (*RET*) proto-oncogene mutations, the presence of RAS mutations in sporadic MTC is not entirely unexpected, since the evidence of the development of MTC in rascal transgenic mice expressing v-Ha-ras under the control of the calcitonin/calcitonin gene-related peptide promoter [65, 66, 74]. The prevalence of RAS mutations in such cases varies between 0–41.2 and 0–40.9% for HRAS and KRAS, respectively, and between 0 and 1.8% for NRAS. All the above-mentioned mutations can be evaluated on cellular FNAC samples of MCT.

10.5 The Diagnostic Role of miRNAs in Follicular and Parafollicular Neoplasms

Unfortunately, ancillary techniques do not contribute to the correct identification of the nature of 100% of thyroid lesions, particularly among FNs [44–56, 59–61]. In this perspective, some authors have recently investigated the role of microRNAs (miRNAs) defined as small endogenous, non-coding RNAs that mainly act as negative post-transcriptional regulators of coding gene expression whose deregulation is frequently associated with different human cancers [173–195]. Commercially available test comprising miRNA are also available (ThyraMIR, Interpace Diagnostics (Parsippany, NJ)). MicroRNA is a short, single-stranded, non-coding RNA, consisting of 19–23 nucleotides. It regulates messenger RNA by binding to the 30 non-translated regions and can function as tumor suppressor or oncogene. As a small molecule, it is relatively stable in FNA specimens and in formalin-fixed, paraffin-embedded cell-block materials and is, therefore, amenable to detection. Specific microRNA profiles (panels) have been identified in a variety of tumors, and their diagnostic utility has also been explored in TN, including indeterminate lesions. Some authors reported that miR-146b-5p and miR-21deregulation has been associated with progression and metastasis of thyroid cancers. miR-146b-5p and miR-21 have been shown to be upregulated at least tenfold in several studies when comparing PTCs to normal thyroid tissue by quantitative reverse transcription–polymerase chain reaction (qRT-PCR) analysis [186, 191]. miR-21 has also been shown to be upregulated in ATCs and PTCs [196].

Since now, the majority of authors deal with the analysis of miRNAs in malignant and benign thyroid lesions. However an emerging role is the analysis of miRNAs panel as a novel and promising tool in the indeterminate categories [173–192]. Specifically, in two different papers Pallante et al. and Dettmer et al. reported good results from thyroid malignant lesions leading to the conclusion that aberrant expression of miRNAs (i.e. miR-146, 221, 222) is frequently recognized as a marker of thyroid cancers [180, 193]. Hence, in their recent papers, Keutgen et al. and Agretti et al. assessed the evaluation of miRNA expression in 29 FNs and in 53 FNs on CS, respectively [179, 191]. Their analysis can be performed with good results also on LBC material. Rossi et al. documented the feasible evaluation and role of miR-375 in a cyto-histological series of 27 FNs, including AUS/FLUSs and FNs, processed with LBC [178]. As specified in their results, miR-375 was over-expressed in all the FNs associated with a malignant histology. These authors concluded that there has been a perfect correlation between the histological outcome and miR-375 expression in the different categories of indeterminate proliferations. In their paper Rossi et al. defined a higher diagnostic accuracy, sensitivity and specificity than those reported either by Agretti et al. in their 53 FNs or by Shen et al. in their AUS/FLUS cases [178]. According to the high sensitivity (97.1%) and positive predictive value (100%) in the FNs, miR-375 seems to have a concrete role as an additional promising marker in the preoperative discrimination between benign and malignant FNs. Apart from the evaluation of single miRNAs, some authors started to apply an algorithm approach including ICC, somatic mutations, and/or rearrangement and miRNAs. Paskas et al. proposed a predictor model for the FNs through a decision tree which may contribute to correctly define how to classify the patients. Specifically, the first step was based on the *BRAF* mutational analysis followed by Galectin-3 immunostain and then miRNAs. This tree algorithm approach provided a sensitivity of 73.5%; specificity of 89.9% and diagnostic accuracy of 75.7% [197]. Apart from the analysis of single miRNAs, some authors proposed the use of panels of miRNAs which may categorize the lesions. For instance, Shen et al. measured the expression levels of eight miRNAs (miR-146b, miR-221, miR-187, miR-197, miR-346, miR-30d, miR-138, and miR-302c) using RT-PCR in 128 FNA samples [174]. Gene expression analyses and linear discriminant analysis (LDA) were performed in a training set of 60 samples which were adopted to obtain a classification rule that correctly classified FNA cases as benign or malignant. A four-miRNA LDA classification rule (miR-146b, miR-221, miR-187, and miR-30d) had a diagnostic accuracy of 93%, sensitivity of 93%, and specificity of 94% for the training sample set. The application to a validation set of 68 FNA samples led to 85% diagnostic accuracy, 89% sensitivity, and 78% specificity. According to their results, these authors concluded that miRNA study from cytological samples is feasible and that the chosen panel can accurately diagnose PTCs on FNA.

In another study, Kitano et al. analyzed miRNA expression of miR-7, miR-126, miR-374a using RT-PCR in a training set of 95 samples that included 31 indeterminate thyroid FNA samples. The authors found that miR-7 was the best predictor in distinguishing benign from malignant samples, with 100% sensitivity, 29% specificity, 36% PPV, and a 100% NPV, for an overall accuracy of 76% [198]. When applied to indeterminate lesions only, they had an overall accuracy of 37% with 100% sensitivity, 20% specificity, 25% PPV, and 100% NPV. They concluded that the high NPV of miR-7 could induce the clinicians to follow patients with benign results as opposed to perform immediate diagnostic thyroidectomy. The major limitation in this study is the small sample size including only 21 indeterminate lesions. In a recent report by Dettmer et al., 38 FTCs and 10 normal thyroid tissue samples were analyzed for miRNA expression using microarray technology [193]. Differences in miRNA expression between normal thyroid tissue, oncocytic and FCs were demonstrated. A novel miRNA (miR-885-5p) was found to be strongly upregulated (>40-fold) in oncocytic FCs when compared with FCs, FA, and hyperplastic nodules. In this study, a classification and regression tree algorithm applied to 19 indeterminate FNA samples demonstrated that three miR-NAs (miR-885-5p, -221 and -574-3p) allowed A 100% distinction between FCs and hyperplastic nodules. Although only a small number of indeterminate FNAs were analyzed, this report suggested miRNA analysis to differentiate oncocytic and FCs from benign hyperplastic nodules. Specific miRNAs have been demonstrated also in MTCs and PDCs. For the MCTs, several authors found the role of miR21 which is able to regulate the programmed cell death 4 (PDCD4), a tumor suppressor gene involved in tumorigenesis. Another relevant miRNA is represented by miR375. Specifically the expression of the potential downstream targets of miR-375, YAP1 (a growth inhibitor), and SLC16a2 (a transporter of thyroid hormone) was down-regulated in the tumors suggesting that miR-375 is a negative regulator of the expression of these genes. One recent discovery was the role of miR129-5p which is involved in growth and migration in MCTs. Dettmer studied the expression of miRNAs profiles in PDCs including the oxyphilic variant. They found that both tumor types showed upregulation of miR-125a-5p, -15a-3p, -182, -183-3p, -222, -222-5p, and downregulation of miR-130b, -139-5p, -150, -193a-5p, -219-5p, -23b, -451, -455-3p and of miR-886-3p as compared with normal thyroid tissue [194]. In addition, the oxyphilic-PDCs demonstrated upregulation of miR-221 and miR-885-5p. The difference in expression was also observed between miRNA expression in PD and WDTCs

10.6 How to Approach Thyroid Nodules with Ancillary Techniques

According to these novel insights, the management of a thyroid lesion undergoing FNAC might include a different series of sequential steps with are helpful for the correct diagnostic management: (1) Examination of clinical history and serum analysis to rule out the possibility of a toxic adenoma or a Hashimoto's thyroiditis; (2) Evaluation of the nuclear atypia of the follicular cells in order to define the inclusion in the correct diagnostic category according to the different classification systems; (3) Search for the morphological findings (eosinophilic cytoplasms and sickle-shaped nuclei) able to predict $BRAF^{V600E}$ mutation and in those cases $BRAF$ molecular testing is recommended; (4), Evaluation of the expression of HBME-1 and Galectin-3 in the follicular cells, in case the lesion is devoid of the morphological features seen in point 3 and it is likely to be classified as FN. This immunopanel would identify two additional subtypes: low-risk (resulting HBME-1 and Galectin-3 negative) and high-risk (HBME-1 and galectin-3 positive) lesions. In cases with discordant immunomarkers, the authors underlined the relevant role of HBME-1 positivity as a valid marker of malignancy [49, 197]. This identification of two subgroups allows a further discrimination in the risk of malignant neoplasm at histology (76.9% when the concordant panel is positive, 3.2% when the same panel is negative). In those cases with a positive immunopanel, the molecular evaluation of other somatic mutations (including RAS family or $BRAF$ uncommon mutations) might add some diagnostic and prognostic details for the following management.

10.7 The Future of Molecular Thyroid Cytology

Molecular cytology has developed in the last two decades from an academic discipline into a medical specialty with common and routinely application. In several diseases, the application of molecular techniques on cytology is indispensable to establish the correct diagnosis and it may provide additional information for the tailored management of the lesions. According to the quality of DNA material, the cytological sample can represent the most convenient source of tissue. This cytological evaluation may offer the possibility to define a specific tailored therapy in a pre-surgical phase and it may imply the development of alternative management strategies.

The coming years will support the consolidation of molecular cytopathology with the implementation of molecular testing as a cost-efficient operation, with some changes in preparation in order to offer a better preservation of nucleic acids and a training of staff and pathologists in this field.

References

1. Lee V, Ng SB, Salto-Tellez M. New techniques. In: Dabbs I, editor. Diagnostic immunohistochemistry. Theranostic and genomic application. 3rd ed. saunder, elsevier, philadelphia.
2. Salto-Telle M, Koay S. Molecular dignostic cytopathology: definitions, scope, and clinical utility. Cytopathology. 2004;15:252–5.
3. Ng SB, Lee V, Salto-Tellez M. The relevance of molecular diagnostics in the practice of surgical pathology. Expert Opin Med Diagn. 2008;2:1401–14.
4. Srinivassan M, Sedmak D, Jewell S. Effect of fixatives and tissue processing on the content and integraty of nucleic acid. Am J Pathol. 2002;161:1961–71.
5. Sapio MR, Posca D, Raggioli A, et al. Detection of RET/PTC, TRK and BRAF mutations in preoperative diagnosis of thyroid nodules with indeterminate cytological findings. Clin Endocrin. 2007;66:678–83.
6. Rossi ED, Schmitt FC. Pre-analytic steps for molecular testing on thyroid fine-needle aspirations: the goal of good results. Cytojournal. 2013;28:10–24.
7. Da Cunha SG. Standardizing preanalytical variables for molecular cytopathology. Cancer Cytopathol. 2013;121:341–3.
8. Cramer H. Fine-needle aspiration cytology of the thyroid: an appraisal. Cancer. 2000;90:325–9.
9. Gharib H, Papini E, Paschke R. Thyroid nodules: a review of current guidelines, practices and prospects. Eur J Endocrinol. 2008;159:493–505.
10. The Papanicolaou Society of Cytopathology Task Force on Standards of Practice. Guidelines of the Papanicolaou society of cytopathology for the examination of fine needle aspiration-specimens from thyroid nodules. Mod Pathol. 1996;9:710–5.
11. Cooper DS, Doherty GM, Haugen BR, et al. American Thyroid Association (ATA) guidelines taskforce on thyroid nodules and differentiated thyroid cancer. Revised management guidelines for patients with thyroid nodules and differentiated thyroid cancer. Thyroid. 2009;19:1167–214.
12. Gharib H, Papini E, Valcavi R, et al. Aace/ame Task Force on Thyroid Nodules:. American Association of clinical endocrinologists and associazione medici endocrinology and European thyroid association medical guidelines for clinical practice for the diagnosis and management of thyroid nodules. Endocr Pract. 2006;12(63-102):1–43.
13. Lobo C, McQueen A, Beale T, et al. The UK royal college of pathologists thyroid fine-needle aspiration diagnostic classification is a robust tool for the clinical management of abnormal thyroid nodules. Acta Citologica. 2011;55:499–506.

14. Baloch ZW, LiVolsi VA, Asa SL, et al. Diagnostic terminology and morphologic criteria for cytologic diagnosis of thyroid lesions: a synopsis of the National Cancer Institute Fine-needle aspiration state-of-science conference. Diagn Cytopathol. 2008;36:425–37.

15. Cibas ED, Ali SZ. The Bethesda system for reporting thyroid cytopathology. Am J Clin Pathology. 2001;32:658–65.

16. Bongiovanni M, Spitale A, Faquin WC, et al. The Bethesda system for reporting thyroid cytopathology: a meta-analysis. Acta Cytologica. 2012;56:333–9.

17. British Thyroid Association, Royal College of Physicians. Guidelines for the management of thyroid cancer. In: Perros P, editor. Report of the Thyroid Cancer Guidelines Update Group. 2nd ed. London: Royal College of Physicians; 2007.

18. Fadda G, Basolo F, Bondi A, et al. SIAPEC-IAP Italian Consensus Working Group. Cytological classification of thyroid nodules. Proposal of the SIAPEC-IAP Italian consensus working group. Pathologica. 2010;102:405–8.

19. Cochand Priollet B, Schmitt FC, Totsch M, et al. The Bethesda terminology for reporting thyroid cytopathology: from theory to practice in Europe. Acta Cytol. 2011;55:507–17.

20. Nardi F, Basolo F, Crescenzi A, et al. Italian consensus for the classification and reporting of thyroid cytology. J Endocrinol Invest. 2014;37:593–9.

21. Royal College of pathologists of Australasia. Thyroid cytologystructured reporting protocol. https://www.rcpa.edu.au/getattachment/b0545d63-2198-4d39-b190   9624e686404/Protocol-thyroid-FNA-cytology.aspx. Accessed October 9, 2015

22. Raab SS, Vrbin CM, Grzybicki DM, et al. Errors in thyroid gland fine-needle aspiration. Am J Clin Pathol. 2006;125:873–82.

23. Broome JT, Solorzano CC. The impact of atypia/follicular lesion of undetermined significance on the rate of malignancy in thyroid fine-needle aspiration: evaluation of the Bethesda System for Reporting Thyroid Cytopathology. Surgery. 2011;150:1234–9.

24. Ravetto C, Colombo L, Dottorini ME. Usefulness of fine- needle aspiration in the diagnosis of thyroid carcinomas. A retrospective study in 37,895 patients. Cancer Cytopathol. 2000;90:357–63.

25. Poller DN, Ibrahim AK, Cummings MH, et al. Fine-needle aspiration of the thyroid. Importance of an indeterminate diagnostic category. Cancer Cytopathol. 2000;90:239–44.

26. Krane JF, Vanderlaan PA, Faquin WC, et al. The atypia of undetermined significance/follicular lesion of undetermined significance:malignant ratio. Cancer Cytopathol. 2012;120:111–6.

27. Ho AS, Sarti EE, Jain KS, et al. Malignancy rate in thyroid nodules classified as Bethesda category III (AUS/FLUS). Thyroid. 2014;24:832–9.

28. Song JY, Chu YC, Kim L, et al. Reclassifying formerly indeterminate thyroid FNAs using the Bethesda system reduces the number of inconclusive cases. Acta Cytol. 2012;56:122–9.

29. Shi Y, Ding X, Klein M, et al. Thyroid fine-needle aspiration with atypia of undetermined significance: a necessary or optional category? Cancer. 2009;117:298–304.

30. Damiani D, Suciu V, Vielh P. Cytopathology of follicular cell nodules. Endocr Pathol. 2015;26:286–91.

31. Nagarkatti SS, Faquin WC, Lubitz CC, et al. Management of thyroid nodules with atypical cytology on fine-needle aspiration biopsy. Ann Surg Oncol. 2013;20:60–5.

32. Olson MT, Clark DP, Erozan YS, et al. Spectrum of risk of malignancy in subcategories of 'atypia of undetermined significance'. Acta Cytol. 2011;55:518–25.

33. Horne MJ, Chhieng DC, Theoharis C, et al. Thyroid follicular lesion of undetermined significance: evaluation of the risk of malignancy using the two-tier sub-classification. Diagn Cytopathol. 2012;40:410–5.

34. Hyeon J, Ahn S, Shin JH, et al. The prediction of malignant risk in the category "atypia of undetermined significance/follicular lesion of undetermined significance" of the Bethesda System for Reporting Thyroid Cytopathology using subcategorization and BRAF mutation results. Cancer Cytopathol. 2014;122:368–76.

35. Dincer N, Balci S, Yazgan A, et al. Follow-up of atypia and follicular lesions of undetermined significance in thyroid fine needle aspiration cytology. Cytopathology. 2013;24:385–90.

36. Gocun PU, Karakus E, Bulutay P, et al. What is the malignancy risk for atypia of undetermined significance?: Three Years' Experience at a University Hospital in Turkey. Cancer Cytopathol. 2014;122:604–10.
37. Wu HH, Inman A, Cramer HM. Subclassification of "Atypia of Undetermined Significance" in thyroid fine-needle aspirates. Diagn Cytopathol. 2014;42:23–9.
38. Borget I, Vielh P, Leboullex S, et al. Assessment of the cost of fine-needle aspiration cytology as a diagnostic tool in patients with thyroid nodules. Am J Clin Pathol. 2008;129:763–71.
39. Nikiforov YE, Seethala RR, Tallini G, et al. Nomenclature revision for encapsulated follicular variant of papillary thyroid carcinoma: a paradigm shift to reduce overtreatment of indolent tumors. JAMA Oncol. 2016;2(8):1023–9.
40. Maletta F, Massa F, Torregrossa L, et al. Cytological features of "invasive follicular thyroid neoplasm with papillary-like nuclear features" and their correlation with tumor histology. Hum Pathol. 2016;54:134–42.
41. Faquin WC, Wong LQ, Afrogheh AH, et al. Impact of reclassifying noninvasive follicular variant of papillary thyroid carcinoma on the risk of malignancy in the Bethesda system for reporting thyroid cytopathology. Cancer Cytopathol. 2016;124:181–7.
42. Lastra RR, LiVolsi VA, Baloch ZW. Aggressive variants of follicular cell-derived thyroid carcinomas: a cytopathologist's perspective. Cancer Cytopathol. 2014;122:484–503.
43. Strickland KC, Howitt BE, Marquese E, et al. The impact of Noninvasive follicular variant of papillary thyroid carcinoma on rates of malignancy for fine needle aspiration diagnostic categories. Thyroid. 2015;25:987–92.
44. Correia-Rodrigues HG, Nogueira De Pontes AA, et al. Use of molecular markers in samples obtained from preoperative aspiration of thyroid. Endocr J. 2012;59:417–24.
45. Paunovic I, Isic T, Havelka M, et al. Combined immunohistochemistry fro thyroid peroxidase, Galectin-3 and HBME-1 in different diagnosis of thyroid tumors. APMIS. 2012;120:368–79.
46. Chiu CG, Strugnell SS, Griffith OL, et al. Diagnostic utility of galectin-3 in thyroid cancer. Am J Pathol. 2010;176:2067–81.
47. Bartolazzi A, Orlandi F, Saggiorato E, et al. Italian Thyroid Cancer Study Group (ITCSG). Galectin-3 expression analysis in the surgical selection of follicular thyroid nodules with indeterminate fine-needle aspiration cytology: a prospective multicentre study. Lancet Oncol. 2008;9:543–9.
48. Prasad ML, Pellegata NS, Huang Y, et al. Galectin-3, fibronectin-1, CITED-1, HBME-1 and cytokeratin-19 immunohistochemistry is useful for the differential diagnosis of thyroid tumors. Mod Pathol. 2005;18:48–57.
49. Rossi ED. Who was responsible for reaching the Americas-Columbus or his ships?: Focusing on the side of liquid-based cytology: the importance and role of the cytopathologist as opposed to the cytological method used. Cancer Cytopathol. 2014;122:337–9.
50. Herrmann ME, LiVolsi VA, Pasha TL, et al. Immunohistochemical expression of Galectin-3 in benign and malignant thyroid lesions. Arch Pathol Lab Med. 2002;126:710–3.
51. Schmitt FC, Barroca H. Role of ancillary studies in fine needle aspiration from selected tumors. Cancer Cytopathol. 2012;120:145–60.
52. Schmitt FC, Longatto-Filho A, Valent A, et al. Molecular techniques in cytopathology practice. J Clin Pathol. 2008;61:258–67.
53. Longatto-Filho A, Goncalves AE, Martinho O, et al. Liquid based cytology in DNA-based molecular research. Anal Quant Cytol Histol. 2009;31:395–400.
54. Nikiforova MN, Nikiforov Y. Molecular diagnostics and predictors in thyroid cancer. Thyroid. 2009;19:1351–61.
55. Nikiforov YE, Steward DL, Robinson-Smith TM, et al. Molecular testing for mutations in improving the fine needle aspiration diagnosis of thyroid nodules. J Clin Endocrinol Metab. 2009;94:2092–8.
56. Ohori NP, Nikiforova MN, Schoedel KE, et al. Contribution of molecular testing to thyroid fine needle aspiration cytology of "Follicular lesion of undetermined significance/Atypia of undetermined significance". Cancer Cytopathol. 2010;118:17–23.

57. Fadda G, Rossi ED. Liquid based cytology in fine needle aspiration biopsies of the thyroid gland. Acta Cytol. 2011;55:389–400.
58. Rossi ED, Martini M, Capodimonti S, et al. BRAF (v600e) mutation analysis on LBC-processed aspiration biopsies predicts bilaterality and nodal involvement in papillary thyroid microcarcinoma. Cancer Cytopathol. 2013;121:291–7.
59. Rossi ED, Martini M, Capodimonti S, et al. Diagnostic and prognostic value of immunocytochemistry and BRAF mutation analysis on liquid based biopsies of thyroid neoplasms suspicious for carcinoma. Eur J Endocrin. 2013;168:853–9.
60. Chang H, Lee H, Yoon SO, et al. BRAF (V600E) mutation analysis of liquid-based preparation-processed fine needle aspiration sample improves the diagnostic rate of papillary thyroid carcinoma. Human Pathol. 2012;43:89–95.
61. Moses W, Weng J, Sansano I, et al. Molecular testing for somatic mutations improves the accuracy of thyroid fine needle aspiration biopsy. World J Surg. 2010;34:2589–94.
62. Xing M. Braf mutationin papillary thyroid cancer:pathogenic role,molecular bases,and clinical implications. Endocr Rev. 2007;28:742–62.
63. Puxeddu E, Durante C, Avenia N, et al. Clinical implications of BRAF mutation in thyroid carcinoma. Trends Endocrinol Metab. 2008;19:138–45.
64. Colanta A, Lin O, Tafe L, et al. BRAF mutation analysis of fine-needle aspiration biopsies of papillary thyroid carcinoma: impact on diagnosis and prognosis. Acta Cytolog. 2011;55:563–9.
65. Moura MM, Cavaco BM, Leite V. RAS-protooncogene in medullary thyroid carcinoma. Endocr Relat Cancer. 2015;22:R235–52.
66. Tamburrino A, Molinolo AA, Salerno P. Activation of the mTOR pathway in primary medullary thyroid carcinoma and lymph node metastases. Clin Cancer Res. 2012;18:3532–40.
67. Donis-Keller H, Dou S, Chi D, et al. Mutations in the RET proto-oncogene are associated with MEN 2A and FMTC. Hum Mol Genet. 1993;2:851–6.
68. Mulligan LM, Kwok JB, Healey CS, et al. Germ-line mutations of the RET proto-oncogene in multiple endocrine neoplasia type 2A. Nature. 1993;363:458–60.
69. Carlson KM, Dou S, Chi D, et al. Single missense mutation in the tyrosine kinase catalytic domain of the RET protooncogene is associated with multiple endocrine neoplasia type 2B. Proc Natl Acad Sci U S A. 1994;91:1579–83.
70. Hofstra RM, Landsvater RM, Ceccherini I, et al. A mutation in the RET protooncogene associated with multiple endocrine neoplasia type 2B and sporadic medullary thyroid carcinoma. Nature. 1994;367:375–6.
71. Eng C, Smith DP, Mulligan LM, et al. Point mutation within the tyrosine kinase domain of the RET proto-oncogene in multiple endocrine neoplasia type 2B and related sporadic tumours. Hum Mol Genet. 1994;3:237–41.
72. Marsh DJ, Learoyd DL, Andrew SD, et al. Somatic mutations in the RET proto-oncogene in sporadic 97 medullary thyroid carcinoma. Clin Endocrinol. 1996;44:249–57.
73. Moura MM, Cavaco BM, Pinto AE, et al. High prevalence of RAS mutations in RET-negative sporadic medullary thyroid carcinomas. J Clin Endocrinol Metab. 2011;6:E863–8.
74. Boichard A, Croux L, Al Ghuzlan A, et al. Somatic RAS mutations occur in a large proportion of sporadic RET-negative medullary thyroid carcinomas and extend to a previously unidentified exon. J Clin Endocrinol Metab. 2012;97:E2031–5.
75. Ciampi R, Mian C, Fugazzola L, et al. Evidence of a low prevalence of RAS mutations in a large medullary thyroid cancer series. Thyroid. 2013;23:50–7.
76. Agrawal N, Jiao Y, Sausen M, et al. Exomic sequencing of medullary thyroid cancer reveals dominant and mutually exclusive oncogenic mutations in RET and RAS. J Clin Endocrinol Metab. 2013;98:E364–9.
77. Schilling T, Burck J, Sinn HP, et al. Prognostic value of codon 918 (ATG-->ACG) RET proto-oncogene mutations in sporadic medullary thyroid carcinoma. Int J Cancer. 2001;9(5):62–6.
78. Elisei R, Cosci B, Romei C, et al. Prognostic significance of somatic RET oncogene mutations in sporadic medullary thyroid cancer: a 10-year follow-up study. J Clin Endocrinol Metab. 2008;93:682–7.

79. Volante M, Rapa I, Gandhi M, et al. Ras mutation as the predominant nuclear alteration in poorly differentiated thyroid carcinoma and bear prognostic impact. J Clin Endocrinol Metab. 2009;94:4735–41.
80. Volante M, Rapa I, Papotti M. Poorly differentiated thyroid carcinoma: diagnostic features and controversial issues. Endocr Pathol. 2008;19:150–5.
81. Rocha AS, Soares P, Fonseca E, et al. E-cadherin loss rather β-alteration is a common feature of poorly differentiated thyroid carcinomas. Histopathology. 2003;42:580–7.
82. De Falco V, Guarino V, Avilla E, et al. Biological role and potential therapeutic targeting of the chemokine receptor CXCR4 in undifferentiated thyroid cancer. Cancer Res. 2007;67: 1821–9.
83. Nikiforova MN, Kimura ET, Gandhi M, et al. BRAF mutations in thyroid tumors are restricted to papillary carcinoma and anaplastic or poorly differentiated carcinomas arising from papillary carcinomas. J Clin Endocrinol Metab. 2008;88:5399–404.
84. Cancer Genome Atlas Research Network. Integrated genomic characterization of papillary thyroid carcinoma. Cell. 2014;159:676–90.
85. Ferris RL, Baloch ZW, Bernet V, et al. The American Thyroid Association Surgical Affairs Committee. American Thyroid Association Statement on Surgical Application of Molecular Profiling for Thyroid Nodules: Current Impact on Perioperative Decision Making. Thyroid. 2015;25:760–8.
86. Rossi ED, Bizzaro T, Longatto-Filho A, et al. The diagnostic and prognostic role of liquid-based cytology: are we ready to monitor therapy and resistance? Expert Rev Anticancer Ther. 2015;15:911–21.
87. Soares P, Trovisco V, Rocha AS, et al. M.BRAF mutations and RET/PTC rearrangements are alternative events in the ethiopathogenesis of PTC. Oncogene. 2003;22:4578–80.
88. Park SY, Park YJ, Lee YJ, et al. Analysis of differential BRAF (V600E) mutational status in multifocal papillary thyroid carcinoma. Evidence of independent clonal origin in distinct tumor foci. Cancer. 2006;107:1831–8.
89. Soares P, Trovisco V, Rocha AS, et al. Braf mutations typical of papillary thyroid carcinoma are more frequently detected in undifferentiated than in insular and insular-like poorly differentiated carcinomas. Virchows Arch. 2004;444:572–6.
90. Elisei R, Ugolini C, Viola D, et al. BRAF mutation and outcome of patients with papillary thyroid carcinoma: a 15-year median follow-up study. J Clin Endocrinol Metab. 2008;93:3943–50.
91. La R, Chiosea SI, Seethala RR, et al. Thyroid nodules with KRAS mutations are different from nodules with NRAS and HRAS mutations with regard to cytopathologic and histopathologic outcome characteristics. Cancer Cytopathol. 2014;122:873–82.
92. Nikiforov YE, Carry SE, Chiosea SI, et al. Impact of the multigene ThyroSeq next generation sequencing assay on cancer diagnosis in thyroid nodules with atypia of undetermined significance/follicular lesion of undetermined significance cytology. Thyroid. 2015;120:3627–34.
93. Nikiforova MN, Wald AI, Roy S, et al. Targeted next-generation sequencing panel (Thyro Seq) for detection of mutations in thyroid cancer. J Clin Endocrinol Metab. 2013;98:E1852–60.
94. Nikiforov YE, Carty SE, Chiosea SI, et al. Highly accurate diagnosis of cancer in thyroid nodules with molecular tests guide extent of thyroid surgery 767 follicular neoplasm/suspicious for a follicular neoplasm cytology by ThyroSeq v2 next-generation sequencing assay. Cancer. 2014;120:3627–34.
95. Nikiforov YE. Molecular analysis of thyroid tumors. Mod Pathol. 2011;24:534–44.
96. Kimura ET, Nikiforova MN, Zhu Z, et al. High prevalence of BRAF mutations in thyroid cancer: genetic evidence for constitutive activation of the RET/PTC-RAS-BRAF signaling pathway in papillary thyroid carcinoma. Cancer Res. 2003;63:1454–7.
97. Cohen Y, Xing M, Mambo E, et al. BRAF mutation in papillary thyroid carcinoma. J Natl Cancer Inst. 2003;95:625–7.
98. Ardighieri L, Zeppernick F, Hannibal CG, et al. Mutational analysis of *BRAF* and *KRAS* in ovarian atypical proliferative serous (borderline)tumors and associated peritoneal implants. J Pathol. 2014;232:16–22.

99. Hall A, Meyle KD, Lange MK, et al. Dysfunctional oxidative phosphorylation makes malignant melanoma cells addicted to glycolysis driven by the $^{V600E}BRAF$ oncogene. Oncotarget. 2013;4:584–99.

100. Landau MS, Kuan SF, Chiosea S, et al. Braf-mutated microsatellite stable colorectal carcinoma: an aggressive adenocarcinoma with reduced CDX2 and increased cytokeratin 7 immunohistochemical expression. Hum Pathol. 2014;45:1704–12.

101. Xing M, Westra WH, Tufano RP, et al. BRAF mutation predicts a poorer clinical prognosis for papillary thyroid cancer. J Clin Endocrinol Metab. 2005;90:6373–9.

102. Rodolico V, Cabibi D, Pizzolanti G, et al. BRAF V600E mutation and p27 kip1 expression in papillary carcinomas of the thyroid <1 cm and their paired lymph node metastases. Cancer. 2007;110:1218–26.

103. Begum S, Rosenbaum E, Henrique R, et al. BRAF mutations in anaplastic thyroid carcinoma: implications for tumor origin, diagnosis and treatment. Mod Pathol. 2004;17:1359–63.

104. Trovisco V, Vieira de Castro I, Soares P, et al. *BRAF* mutations are associated with some histological types of papillary thyroid carcinoma. J Pathol. 2004;202:247–51.

105. Barollo S, Pezzani R, Cristiani A, et al. Prevalence, tumorigenic role, and biochemical implications of rare *BRAF* alterations. Thyroid. 2014;24:809–19.

106. Santarpia L, Sherman SI, Marabotti A, et al. Detection and molecular characterization of a novel BRAF activated domain mutation in follicular variant of papillary thyroid carcinoma. Hum Pathol. 2009;40:827–33.

107. Barzon L, Masi G, Merante Boschin I, et al. Characterization of a novel complex BRAF mutation in a follicular variant papillary thyroid carcinoma. Eur J Endocrinol. 2008;159:77–80.

108. Capper D, Preusser M, Habel A, et al. Assessment of BRAF V600E mutation status by immunohistochemistry with a mutation-specific monoclonal antibody. Acta Neuropathol. 2001;122:11–9.

109. Zimmermann AK, Camerisch U, Rechsteiner MP, et al. Value of immunohistochemistry in detection of BRAF V600E mutations in fine needle aspiration biopsies of papillary thyroid carcinoma. Cancer Cytopathol. 2014;122:48–58.

110. Rossi ED, Martini M, Capodimonti S, et al. Analysis of immunocytochemical and molecular *BRAF* expression in thyroid carcinomas: a cyto-histological institutional experience. Cancer Cytopathol. 2014;122:527–35.

111. Namba H, Rubin SA, Fagin JA. Point mutations of ras oncogenes are an early event in thyroid tumorigenesis. Mol Endocrinol. 1990;4:1474–9.

112. Karga H, Lee JK, Vickery AL Jr, et al. Ras oncogene mutations in benign and malignant thyroid neoplasms. J Clin Endocrinol Metab. 1991;73:832–6.

113. Hara H, Fulton N, Yashiro T, et al. N-ras mutation: an independent prognostic factor for aggressiveness of papillary thyroid carcinoma. Surgery. 1994;116:1010–6.

114. Basolo F, Pisaturo F, Pollina LE, et al. N-ras mutation in poorly differentiated thyroid carcinomas: correlation with bone metastases and inverse correlation to thyroglobulin expression. Thyroid. 2000;10:19–23.

115. Ezzat S, Zheng L, Kolenda J, et al. Prevalence of activating ras mutations in morphologically characterized thyroid nodules. Thyroid. 1996;6:409–16.

116. Vasko VV, Gaudart J, Allasia C, et al. Thyroid follicular adenomas may display features of follicular carcinoma and follicular variant of papillary carcinoma. Eur J Endocrinol. 2004;151:779–86.

117. Lemoine NR, Mayall ES, Wyllie FS, et al. High frequency of Ras oncogene activation in all stages of human thyroid tumorigenesis. Oncogene. 1989;4:159–64.

118. Suarez HG, du Villard JA, Severino M, et al. Presence of mutations in all three Ras genes in human thyroid tumors. Oncogene. 1990;5:565–70.

119. Esapa CT, Johnson SJ, Kendall-Taylor P, et al. Prevalence of Ras mutations in thyroid neoplasia. Clin Endocrinol (Oxf). 1999;50:529–35.

120. Nikiforov YE, Rowland JM, Bove KE, et al. Distinct pattern of ret oncogene rearrangements in morphological variants of radiation-induced and sporadic thyroid papillary carcinomas in children. Cancer Res. 1997;57:1690–4.

121. Rabes HM, Demidchik EP, Sidorow JD, et al. Pattern of radiation-induced RET and NTRK1 rearrangements in 191 post chernobyl papillary thyroid carcinomas: biological, phenotypic, and clinical implications. Clin Cancer Res. 2000;6:1093–103.
122. Fenton CL, Lukes Y, Nicholson D, et al. The ret/PTC mutations are common in sporadic papillary thyroid carcinoma of children and young adults. J Clin Endocrinol Metab. 2000;85:1170–5.
123. Kroll TG, Sarraf P, Pecciarini L, et al. PAX8-PPARgamma1 fusion oncogene in human thyroid carcinoma [corrected]. Science. 2000;289:1357–60.
124. French CA, Alexander EK, Cibas ES, et al. Genetic and biological subgroups of low-stage follicular thyroid cancer. Am J Pathol. 2003;162:1053–60.
125. Dwight T, Thoppe SR, Foukakis T, et al. Involvement of the PAX8/peroxisome proliferator-activated receptor gamma rearrangement in follicular thyroid tumors. J Clin Endocrinol Metabol. 2003;88:4440–5.
126. Marques AR, Espadinha C, Catarino AL, et al. Expression of PAX8-PPAR gamma 1 rearrangements in both follicular thyroid carcinomas and adenomas. J Clin Endocrinol Metabol. 2002;87:3947–52.
127. Mathur A, Weng J, Moses W. A prospective study evaluating the accuracy of using combined clinical factors and candidate diagnostic markers to refine the accuracy of thyroid fine needle aspiration biopsies. Surgery. 2010;148:1176–7.
128. Faquin W. Can a gene-expression classifier with high negative predictive value solve the indeterminate thyroid fine-needle aspiration dilemma? Cancer Cytopathol. 2013;121:403.
129. Rossi ED, Larocca LM, Fadda G. The first line alternative methods to gene-expression classifier. Cancer Cytopathol. 2013;121:116–9.
130. Rossi ED, Fadda G, Schmitt F. The nightmare of indeterminate follicular proliferations: when liquid-based cytology and ancillary techniques are not a moon landing but a realistic plan. Acta Cytol. 2014;58:543–51.
131. Nikiforov YE, Ohori P, Hodack SP, et al. Impact of mutational testing on the diagnosis and management of patients with cytologically indeterminate thyroid nodules: a prospective analysis of 1056 FNA samples. J Clin Endocrinol Metabol. 2011;96:3390–7.
132. Kelly LM, Barila G, Liu P, et al. Identification of the trasformin STRN-ALK fusion as a potential therapeutic target in the aggressive forms of thyroid cancer. Proc Natl Acad Sci USA. 2014;111:4233–8.
133. Ricarte-Filho JC, Li S, Garcia-Rendueles ME, et al. Identification of kinase fusion oncogenes in post-Chernobyl radiation-induced thyroid cancers. J Clin Invest. 2013;123:4935–44.
134. Landa I, Ganly I, Chan TA, et al. Frequent somatic TERT promoter mutations in thyroid cancers: higher prevalence in advanced forms of the disease. J Clin Endocrinol Metab. 2013;98:E1562–6.
135. Liu X, Bishop J, Shan Y, et al. Highly prevalent TERT promoter mutations in aggressive thyroid cancers. Endocr Relat Cancer. 2013;20:603–10.
136. Melo M, Da Rocha AG, Vinagre J, et al. TERT promoter mutations are a major indicator of poor out come in differentiated thyroid carcinomas. J Clin Endocrinol Metab. 2014;99:E754–65.
137. Xing M, Alzahrani AS, Carson KA, et al. Association between BRAF V600E mutation and mortality in patients with papillary thyroid cancer. JAMA. 2013;309:1493–501.
138. Xing M, Alzahrani AS, Carson KA, et al. Association between BRAF V600E mutation and recurrence of papillary thyroid cancer. J Clin Oncol. 2015;33(1):42–50.
139. Xing M, Liu R, Liu X, et al. BRAF V600E and TERT promoter mutations cooperatively identify the most aggressive papillary thyroid cancer with highest recurrence. J Clin Oncol. 2014;32:2718–26.
140. Demeure MJ, Aziz M, Rosenberg R, et al. Whole-genome sequencing of an aggressive BRAF wild-type papillary thyroid cancer identified EML4-ALK translocation as a therapeutic target. World J Surg. 2014;38:1296–305.
141. Godbert Y, Henriques de Figueiredo B, Bonichon F, et al. Remarkable response to crizotinib in woman with anaplastic lymphoma kinase-rearranged anaplastic thyroid carcinoma. J Clin Oncol. 2015;33:e84–7.

142. Rossi ED, Morassi F, Santeusanio G, et al. Thyroid fine-needle aspiration cytology processed by Thin Prep: an additional slide decreased the number of inadequate results. Cytopathology. 2010;21:97–102.
143. Rossi ED, Raffaelli M, Minimo C, et al. Immunocytochemical evaluation of thyroid neoplasms on thin-layer smears from fine-needle aspiration biopsies. Cancer. 2005;105:87–95.
144. Cochand-Priollet B, Prat JJ, Polivka M, et al. Thyroid fine needle aspiration: the morphological features on ThinPrep slide preparations. Eighty cases with histological control. Cytopathol. 2003;14:343–9.
145. Dabbs D, Abendroth CS, Grenko RT, et al. Immunocytochemistry on the thin-prep processor. Diagn Cytopathol. 1997;17:388–92.
146. Cochand-Priollet B, Dahan H, Laloi-Michelin M, et al. Immunocytochemistry with cytokeratin 19 and HBME-1 increases the diagnostic accuracy of thyroid fine-needle aspirations. Preliminary report of 150 liquid-based fine needle aspirations with histological control. Thyroid. 2011;21:1067–73.
147. Bizzarro T, Martini M, Marrocco C, et al. The role of CD56 in thyroid fine needle aspiration cytology: a pilot study performed on liquid based cytology. PloS One. 2015;17(10):e0132939.
148. Niemeier LA, Kuffner Akatsu H, Song C, et al. A combined molecular-pathologic score improbe risk stratification of papillary micro carcinoma. Cancer. 2011;118:2069–77.
149. Collins J, Rossi ED, Chandra A, et al. Terminology and nomenclature schemes for reporting thyroid cytopathology: an overview. Sem Diagn Pathol. 2015;32:258–63.
150. Chudova D, Wilde JI, Wang ET, et al. Molecular classification of thyroid nodules using high-dimensionality genomic data. J Clin Endocrinol Metab. 2010;95:5296–304.
151. Keutgen XM, Filicori F, Fahey TJ. Molecular diagnosis for indeterminate thyroid nodules on fine needle aspiration. Advances and limitations. Exp Rev Mol Diagn. 2013;13:613–23.
152. Alexander EK, Kennedy GC, Baloch ZW, et al. Preoperative diagnosis of benign thyroid nodules with indeterminate cytology. N Engl J Med. 2012;367:705–15.
153. McIver B, Castro MR, Morris JC, et al. An Independent Study of a Gene Expression Classifier (Afirma) in the evaluation of cytologically indeterminate thyroid nodules. J Clin Endocrinol Metab. 2014;99:4069–77.
154. Dedhia PH, Rubio GA, Cohen MS, et al. Potential effects of molecular testing of indeterminate thyroid nodule fine needle aspiration biopsy on thyroidectomy volume. World J Surg. 2014;38:634–8.
155. Walsh PS, Wilde JI, Tom EY, et al. Analytical performance verification of a molecular diagnostic for cytology-indeterminate thyroid nodules. J Clin Endocrinol Metab. 2012;97:E2297–306.
156. Duick DS, Klopper JP, Diggans JC, et al. The impact of benign gene expression classifier test results on the endocrinologist-patient decision to operate on patients with thyroid nodules with indeterminate cytopathology. Thyroid. 2012;22:996–1001.
157. Li H, Robinson KA, Anton B, et al. Cost-effectiveness of a novel molecular test for cytologically indeterminate thyroid nodules. J Clin Endocrinol Metab. 2011;96:1905–12.
158. Wong KS, Angell TE, Strickland KC, et al. Noninvasive follicular variant of papillary thyroid carcinoma and the afirma gene-expression classifier. Thyroid. 2016;26:911–5.
159. Ma T, Gostissa M, Altamura S, et al. Transcriptional activation of the cicli A gene by the architectural transcription factor HMGA2. Mol Cell Biol. 2003;23:9104–16.
160. Jin L, Lloyd RV, Nassar A, et al. HMGA2 expression analysis in cytological and paraffin-embedded tissue specimens of thyroid tumors by relative quantitative RT-PCR. Diagn Mol Pathol. 2011;20:71–80.
161. Guerriero E, Ferraro A, Desiderio D, et al. UbcH10 expression on thyroid fine-needle aspiration. Cancer Cytopathol. 2010;118:157–65.
162. Wells SA, Asa SL, Dralle H, et al. The American Thyroid Association Guidelines Task Force on Medullary Thyroid Carcinoma. Revised American Thyroid Association Guidelines for the Management of Medullary Thyroid Carcinoma. Thyroid. 2015;25:567–610.

163. Rossi ED, Raffaelli M, Mule A, et al. Relevance of immunocytochemistry on thin-layer cytology in thyroid lesions suspicious for medullary carcinoma: a case-control study. Appl Immunohistochem Mol Morphol. 2008;16:548–53.
164. Hazard JB, Hawk WA, Crile G Jr. Medullary (solid) carcinoma of the thyroid; a clinicopathologic entity. J Clin Endocrinol Metab. 1959;19:152–61.
165. Brandi ML, Gagel RF, Angeli A, et al. Guidelines for diagnosis and therapy of MENtype 1 and type 2. J Clin Endocrinol Metab. 2001;86:5658–71.
166. Tuttle RM, Ball DW, Byrd D, Daniels GH, et al. Medullary carcinoma. J Natl Compr Canc Netw. 2010;8:512–30.
167. Kloos RT, Eng C, Evans DB, Francis GL, et al. Medullary thyroid cancer: management guidelines of the American Thyroid Association. Thyroid. 2009;19:565–612.
168. Takahashi M, Ritz J, Cooper GM. Activation of a novel human transforming gene, ret, by DNA rearrangement. Cell. 1985;42:581–8.
169. Farndon JR, Leight GS, Dilley WG, et al. Familial medullary thyroid carcinoma without associated endocrinopathies: a distinct clinical entity. Br J Surg. 1986;73:278–81.
170. Raue F, Frank-Raue K. Genotype-phenotype correlation in multiple endocrineneoplasia type 2. Clinics (Sao Paulo). 2012;61:69–75.
171. Smith DP, Houghton C, Ponder BA. Germline mutation of RET codon 883 in two cases of de novo MEN 2B. Oncogene. 1997;15:1213–7.
172. Gimm O, Marsh DJ, Andrew SD, et al. Germline dinucleotide mutation in codon 883 of the RET proto-oncogene in multiple endocrine neoplasia type 2B without codon 918 mutation. J Clin Endocrinol Metab. 1997;82:3902–390.
173. Mazeh H, Mizrahi I, Halle D, et al. Development of a microRNA-based molecular assay for the detection of papillary thyroid carcinoma in aspiration biopsy samples. Thyroid. 2011;21:111–8.
174. Shen R, Liyanarachchi S, Li W. MicroRNA signature in thyroid fine needle aspiration cytology applied to "atipia of undetermined significance" cases. Thyroid. et al., 2012;22:9–16.
175. Nikiforova MN, Chiosea SI, Nikiforov YE. MicroRNA expression profiles in thyroid microRNAs in thryoid fine needle aspiration biopsy samples. Thyroid. 2012;22:285–91.
176. Nikiforova MN, Tseng GC, Steward D, et al. MicroRNA expression profiling of thyroid tumors: Biological significance and diagnistic utility. J Clin Endocrinol Metab. 2008;93:1600–8.
177. Mazeh H, Levy Y, Mizrahi I, et al. Differentiating benign from malignant thyroid nodules using micro ribonucleic acid amplification in residual cells obtained by fine needle aspiration biopsy. J Surg Res. 2013;180:216–21.
178. Rossi ED, Martini M, Bizzarro T, et al. The evaluation of miRNAs on thyroid FNAC: the promising role of miR-375 in follicular neoplasms. Endocrine. 2016;54(3):723–32.
179. Keutgen XM, Filicori F, Crowley MJ, et al. A panel of four miRNAs accurately differentiates malignant from benign indeterminate thyroid lesions on fine needle aspiration. Clin Cancer Res. 2012;18:2032–8.
180. Pallante P, Visone R, Ferracin M, et al. MircoRNA deregulation in human thyroid papillary carcinomas. Endocr Rel Cancer. 2006;13:497–508.
182. Weber F, Teresi RE, Broelsch CE, et al. A limited set of human microRNA is deregulated in follicular thyroid carcinoma. J Clin Endocrinol Metab. 2006;91:3584–91.
182. Tetzlaff MT, Liu A, Xu X, Master SR, et al. Differential expression of miRNAs in papillary thyroid carcinoma compared to multinodular goiter using formalin fixed paraffin embedded tissues. Endocr Pathol. 2007;18:163–73.
183. Chen YT, Kitabayashi N, Zhou XK, et al. MicroRNA analysis as a potential diagnostic tool for papillary thyroid carcinoma. Mod Pathol. 2008;21:1139.46.
184. Sheu SY, Grabellus F, Schwertheim S, et al. Differential miRNA expression profiles in variants of papillary thyroid carcinoma and encapsulated follicular thyroid tumors. Br J Cancer. 2010;102:376–82.
185. Peng Y, Li C, Luo DC, et al. Expression profile and clinical significance of microRNAs in papillary thyroid carcinoma. Molecules. 2014;19:11586–99.

186. Chou CK, Chen RF, Chou FF, et al. MiR-146 is highly expressed in adult papillary thyroid carcinoma with high risk features including extrathyroidal invasion and the BRAF (V600E) mutation. Thyroid. 2010;20:489–94.
187. Yip L, Kelly L, Shuai Y, et al. MicroRNA signature distinguishes the degree of aggressiveness of papillary thyroid carcinoma. Ann Surg Oncol. 2011;18:2035–41.
188. Hudson J, Duncavage E, Tamburrino A, et al. Over expression of miR-10a and miR-375 and down regulation of YAP1 in medullary thyroid carcinoma. Exp Mol Pathol. 2013;95:62–7.
189. Yan JW, Lin JS, He XX. The emerging role of miR-375 in cancer. Int J Cancer. 2013;135:1011–8.
190. Jikuzono T, Kawamoto M, Yoshitake H, et al. The miR-221/222 custer, miR-10B and Mir-92a are highly upregulated in metastatic minimally invasive follicular thyroid carcinoma. Int J Oncol. 2013;42:1858–68.
191. Agretti P, Ferrarini E, Rago T, et al. MicroRNA expression profile help to distinguish benign nodules from papillary thyroid carcinomas starting from cells of fine needle aspiration. Eur J Endocrinol. 2012;167:393–400.
192. Zhang Y, Zhong Q, Chen X, et al. Diagnostic value of microRNAs in discriminating malignant thyroid nodules from benign ones on fine needle aspiration samples. Tumor Biol. 2014;35:9343–53.
193. Dettmer M, Perren A, Moch H, et al. Comprehensive microRNA expression profiling identifies novel markers in follicular variant of papillary thyroid carcinoma. Thyroid. 2013;23:1383–9.
194. Dettmer M, Vogetseder A, Durso MB, et al. MicroRNA expression array identifies novel diagnostic markers for conventional and oncocytic follicular thyroid carcinomas. J Clin Endocrinol Metab. 2013;98:E1–7.
195. Paskas S, Jankovic J, Zivalievic V, et al. Malignant risk stratification of thyroid FNA specimens with indeterminate cytology based on molecular testing. Cancer Cytopathol. 2015;123:471–9.
196. Braun J, Hoang-Vu C, Dralle H, et al. Downregulation of microRNAs directs the EMT and invasive potential of anaplastic thyroidcarcinomas. Oncogene. 2010;29:4237–44.
197. Kitano M, Rahbari R, Patterson EE, et al. Expression profiling of difficult-to-diagnose thyroid histological subtypes shows distinct expression profiles and identify candidate diagnostic miRNAs. Ann Surg Oncol. 2011;18:3443–52.
198. Fadda G, Rossi ED, Raffaelli M, et al. Follicular thyroid neoplasms can be classified as low and high risk according to HBME-1 and Galectin 3 expression on liquid based fine needle cytology. Eur J Endocrinol. 2011;165:447–53.

Molecular Cytology Applications on Pancreas and Biliary Tract

11

Rene Gerhard, Roseann I. Wu, and Norge Vergara

11.1 EUS-FNA of Pancreas for Molecular Cytopathology

Endoscopic ultrasound-guided fine-needle aspiration (EUS-FNA) of pancreatic lesions was introduced in the early 1990s [1]. Since then, the technique has become the standard of care for obtaining a tissue diagnosis from the pancreas, particularly pancreatic ductal adenocarcinoma (PDAC). This minimally invasive technique allows for real-time imaging of the pancreatic parenchyma as well as evaluation of peripancreatic lymph nodes. In patients who are not surgical candidates, whether due to comorbidities or advanced disease, samples obtained by EUS-FNA may be the only material available for ancillary testing including molecular studies. Aspiration of cells and/or fluid from solid and cystic pancreatic lesions may yield material for evaluation by a combination of modalities, including cytomorphology, immunocytochemistry, fluid chemistry analysis, and molecular testing.

11.1.1 Molecular Landscape of Solid Pancreatic Neoplasms

The gradual discovery of distinct subtypes of pancreatic cancer has resulted in a new molecular classification of pancreatic neoplasms, and these molecular signatures have been reviewed in the context of histologic subtypes [2–5]. Molecular

R. Gerhard (✉)
Service d'Anatomie Pathologique, Département de Médecine,
Laboratoire National de Santé, Dudelange, Luxemburg
e-mail: rene.gerhard@lns.etat.lu

R. I. Wu · N. Vergara
Department of Pathology and Laboratory Medicine, Hospital of the University of Pennsylvania, Perelman School of Medicine, University of Pennsylvania, Philadelphia, PA, USA
e-mail: roseann.wu@uphs.upenn.edu; norge.vergara@uphs.upenn.edu

© Springer International Publishing AG, part of Springer Nature 2018
F. C. Schmitt (ed.), *Molecular Applications in Cytology*,
https://doi.org/10.1007/978-3-319-74942-6_11

alterations have been described in most solid pancreatic neoplasms, though testing for these alterations has not attained routine use.

Pancreatic ductal adenocarcinoma (PDAC), the most common primary pancreatic malignancy, is believed to progress along a morphologic and molecular pathway from pancreatic intraepithelial neoplasia (PanIN) to invasive carcinoma, given their shared genetic changes. The most commonly associated genetic alterations associated with PDAC are the oncogene *KRAS* and the tumor suppressor genes *TP53*, *p16/CDKN2A*, and *SMAD4* [6]. Somatic (acquired) mutations found in a minority of pancreatic cancers include those in *ARID1A*, *ATM*, *AKT2*, *MAP2K4*, *MLL3*, *TGFβR2*, and *FBXW7*, while germline (inherited) alterations that can predispose to the development of pancreatic cancer include *BRCA2*, *BRCA1*, *PALB2*, *p16/CDKN2A*, *STK11*, *ATM*, *PRSS1*, and the DNA repair genes (such as *MSH2*) [6].

Activating *KRAS* mutations and telomere shortening play an early role in PDAC development, with other gene mutations including *p16/CDKN2A*, *TP53*, and *SMAD4* implicated in progression [7]. Pancreatic neuroendocrine tumors, acinar cell carcinomas, solid pseudopapillary neoplasms, and pancreatoblastomas generally lack the most common abnormalities of PDACs, including mutations in *KRAS*, *TP53*, *DPC4*, and *p16/CDKN2A* [5].

Pancreatic neuroendocrine tumors (PanNETs) have been associated with microsatellite instability and chromosomal losses and gains. In these tumors, loss of 3p, 6pq, and 10pq along with gain of 5q, 12q, 18q, and 20q has been associated with malignant behavior [8]. These tumors may arise in patients with hereditary syndromes including MEN1 and von Hippel-Lindau (VHL) and may show *MEN1* gene mutations and inactivation of the *VHL* gene, respectively [5]. Some factors that are reportedly predictive of more aggressive behavior (at least in univariate analyses) include loss of progesterone receptor expression, aneuploidy, increased Ki67 labeling index, loss of heterozygosity (LOH) of chromosome 17p13, LOH of chromosome 22q, increased fractional allelic loss, upregulated CD44 isoform expression, and immunohistochemical expression of cytokeratin 19 [5]. Somatic mutations of the death-domain-associated protein (*DAXX*) and alpha-thalassemia/mental retardation syndrome X-linked (*ATRX*) genes have been found in sporadic PanNETs, whereas pancreatic neuroendocrine carcinomas (PanNECs) have been shown to have *TP53* and retinoblastoma (*RB-1*) mutations [4].

The development of solid pseudopapillary neoplasms (SPNs) has been linked to Wnt signaling associated with *CTNNB1* mutations, imparting cytoplasmic and nuclear accumulation of β-catenin [9]. Almost all SPNs have a somatic point mutation in exon 3 of the β-catenin gene, implicating the same pathway that is abnormal in acinar neoplasms [5, 10]. Pancreatic acinar cell carcinoma is rare, making it difficult to study. Studies have shown losses on chromosome arm 11p, alterations in *APC*/β-catenin pathway, and loss of DCC expression [11]. *BRAF* mutations may rarely be found, with the most prevalent fusion being *SND1-BRAF*, which may impart sensitivity to treatment with MEK inhibitors [12].

Pancreatoblastoma shows predominantly acinar differentiation and is the most common pediatric pancreatic neoplasm, although it may also occur in adults. These tumors have arisen in patients with Beckwith-Wiedemann syndrome, and a case has been reported in a patient with familial adenomatous polyposis [5]. Molecular alterations are similar to those found in hepatoblastoma and acinar cell carcinoma; the most common genetic alteration is LOH of 11p, but alterations in the *APC*/β-catenin pathway have been reported [5].

Undifferentiated "medullary" carcinoma, defined as pushing borders, syncytial growth, and necrosis, has been shown to demonstrate microsatellite instability and be associated with a better prognosis as compared to classic PDAC [6]. Other genes that have been linked to pancreatic neoplasia include the following: *TGFBR1*, *ACVR1B*, and *RNF43*. Loss of heterozygosity and polysomy has also been identified in pancreatic carcinomas.

11.1.2 Molecular Testing of Solid Pancreatic Neoplasms

EUS-FNA enabled the diagnosis of various solid pancreatic tumors by cytopathologic evaluation, sometimes with rapid on-site evaluation (ROSE) to ensure that adequate material is obtained. In cases of PDAC, only one or two passes could be sufficient for diagnosis, whereas neuroendocrine neoplasms or acinar cell carcinomas may require additional passes to obtain material for immunocytochemical stains. Although cytomorphology is still paramount for the patient's diagnosis and management in cases of solid pancreatic neoplasms, immunocytochemical stains and molecular tests can be used to support the morphologic impression.

If ROSE is requested, the first drop or two of material from each EUS-FNA needle pass may be applied to a glass slide to produce Diff-Quik-stained and/or alcohol-fixed Papanicolaou-stained smears, with the remaining material rinsed into a balanced salt solution. If the needle and device are to be used for subsequent passes, a balanced salt solution is preferable to any alcohol-based preservatives. Molecular testing may be performed using cells from a variety of preparation methods, including cytology smears and touch preps, liquid-based slides, needle rinses, and cell block material. Needle rinses and cell block material are generally preferable to ensure preservation of diagnostic smears or liquid-based slides. Furthermore, molecular testing on needle rinse specimens rather than cell block or surgical material may yield better DNA quality and reduce turnaround time, since this obviates the need to cut additional slides. As with any test, laboratories must run the appropriate validation studies to ensure diagnostic accuracy.

KRAS mutation analysis performed on EUS-FNA specimens combined with cytomorphology does appear to improve overall diagnostic accuracy when distinguishing pancreatic carcinoma and pseudo-tumorous chronic pancreatitis [13, 14]. Indeterminate cytologic specimens obtained by EUS-FNA of pancreatic tumors have been evaluated for tumor suppressor gene-linked microsatellite markers for allelic loss analysis and *KRAS* point mutations to improve diagnostic yield [15]. If material is limited, *KRAS* testing could be prioritized in cases of suspected PDAC. However, multiplex polymerase chain reaction (PCR) "hot spot" mutation testing and next-generation sequencing (NGS) are available in a growing number of laboratories. These tests require a small amount of DNA to query multiple genes of interest. *KRAS* testing could also be performed with a fully automated PCR detection system, which could help streamline testing of EUS-FNA specimens [16].

RNA extraction with real-time gene expression quantification is feasible in EUS-FNA specimens of advanced PDAC, although only samples with high-quality RNA were selected in this study [17]. MicroRNA (miRNA)-based testing in conjunction with cytology can also predict which preoperative pancreatic EUS-FNA specimens contain PDAC, thus reducing the number of indeterminate FNAs and repeat procedures [18]. As with other pancreatobiliary specimens, FISH analysis for loss of 9p21 or changes in copy number for chromosomes 3, 7, and 17 could be considered in cases that are inconclusive or negative by cytology [19].

11.1.3 Immunocytochemistry in Solid Pancreatic Neoplasms

Cell blocks of solid pancreatic neoplasms often suffer from scant cellularity but can be extremely helpful when lesional material is present. A panel of special or immunocytochemical stains can help in differentiating neuroendocrine neoplasms (i.e., chromogranin, synaptophysin, CD56), acinar cell carcinoma (i.e., PAS-D, trypsin, chymotrypsin, lipase), solid-pseudopapillary tumors (i.e., CD10, nuclear β-catenin, cyclin D1), and metastatic malignancies (i.e., differentiation- or organ-specific markers). Loss of SMAD4 immunocytochemical staining has been observed in approximately 55% of PDACs, reflecting genetic inactivation of the *SMAD4* gene [6]. Loss of staining supports a diagnosis of PDAC rather than reactive atypia, suggests a pancreatic primary in cases of metastasis, and is associated with worse prognosis and more widespread metastases [6]. E-cadherin has been used as a marker for poor prognosis in PDAC [20]. Mucin (MUC) expression profiles could also be helpful for diagnosis of PDAC, with MUC16 cytoplasmic expression potentially predicting a poor prognosis [21].

11.1.4 Evaluation of Pancreatic Cystic Lesions

The number of patients diagnosed with pancreatic cysts has increased in the last decades as a result of continuously improving abdominal imaging modalities and their growing use in an increasingly older population [22–24]. The incidence of pancreatic cysts increases with age; some report that pancreatic cysts may be as common as 25% in those older than 70 years. A significant number of cystic lesions in the pancreas are neoplastic. They include a range of benign neoplasms such as serous cystadenomas with almost zero risk of malignant transformation to the other extreme of malignant carcinomas that undergo cystic degeneration. Within this spectrum are low-grade neoplasms such as solid pseudopapillary neoplasms and mucinous neoplasms including mucinous cystic neoplasm (MCN) and intraductal papillary mucinous neoplasm (IPMN), both harboring at least some potential for malignant transformation.

Recent evidence suggests that the great majority of pancreatic cysts are benign on resection. Thanks to a better understanding of the natural history of these lesions, a shift to a more conservative approach has occurred. In contrast to pancreatic surgery, which carries a greater risk of long-term complications and mortality, regular surveillance with imaging studies could be an alternative approach. The overall risk of malignancy in an incidental pancreatic cyst is very low. In some neoplastic lesions such as main duct intraductal papillary mucinous neoplasm (IPMN), a surgical approach may be acceptable.

Although a minority, a proportion of PDACs is known to develop from these preneoplastic mucinous lesions. Early diagnosis of those cysts with early invasive cancer or high-grade dysplasia, along with appropriate surgical management, could reduce mortality from pancreatic adenocarcinomas. It is crucial to correctly triage and manage these patients. Commonly used diagnostic modalities have suboptimal sensitivity and specificity to accurately stratify and manage this population. These modalities include clinical features, CT, MRI, and EUS-FNA for cytologic and chemical analysis. EUS is particularly useful to detect structural alterations of the cyst and evaluate communication with the pancreatic duct, as well as provide the unique opportunity to aspirate fluid in real time for cytologic, biochemical, and molecular analysis.

The role of carcinoembryonic antigen (CEA) levels from pancreatic cyst fluid to determine the mucinous nature of a cyst has been well established. An elevated cyst fluid CEA (>192 ng/mL) is the most accurate (79%) test to distinguish a mucinous cyst [25, 26]. Although this answers an important question in the evaluation of a cyst, mucinous versus non-mucinous, it does not resolve the presence or absence of high-grade dysplasia or malignancy. Cytologic examination appears to be the more specific tool to determine the presence of high-grade dysplasia or malignancy; however, cytology is not very sensitive, mainly due to scarce cellularity in cysts lacking a solid component [26].

11.1.5 Molecular Testing of Pancreatic Cystic Lesions

Molecular analysis, performed on a minimal amount of fluid, smears, or deparaffinized sections of cell blocks, has been proposed to aid in the diagnosis of cystic lesions, based in part on a growing understanding of the molecular mechanisms involved in pancreatic carcinogenesis. As mentioned earlier, common alterations seen in PDAC include mutations in *KRAS*, *p16/CDKN2A*, *TP53*, and *DPC4*. Other molecular changes include those in retinoblastoma-interacting zinc finger (*RIZ*) on 1p36, *VHL* on 3p25-3p26, *APC* on 5q23, *MTS-1* on 9p2, and aberrant expression of the patched gene (*PTCH*) on 9q22 [27–33] (see Table 11.1).

On the assumption that some of these biomarkers may be altered in mucinous cysts with intermediate- to high-grade dysplasia and could be used to identify patients at risk for cancer development, molecular analysis has been proposed to aid in the diagnosis of pancreatic cystic lesions. Tests include mutation analysis (*KRAS*, *GNAS*, *TP53*, *VHL*, *CTNNB1*, and *RNF43*), DNA cyst fluid analysis (quality and quantification), loss of heterozygosity analysis, and microsomal analysis.

Table 11.1 Molecular alterations and testing in pancreatic and biliary neoplasia

Molecular alteration(s)	Molecular test(s)	Diagnostic finding(s)	Neoplasm(s)
KRAS, telomere shortening, *CDKN2A*, *TP53*, *SMAD4*, *BRAF*, *STK11/LKB1* Loss of heterozygosity at microsatellites linked to tumor suppressor gene loci known to be affected in pancreatic carcinogenesis	*KRAS* and other mutation analysis Loss of immunohistochemical staining for the protein product of the SMAD4 gene Loss of heterozygosity analysis	Mutation present in PDCA Loss of IHC staining for protein product of SMAD4 gene supports a diagnosis of ductal adenocarcinoma Losses of chromosome arms 3p, 6pq, and 10pq along with gains of 5q,12q, 18q, and 20q support a diagnosis of adenocarcinoma	PDAC
Selected miRNAs	MicroRNA analysis	Presence of miRNAs such as miR-21 and mi-155 supports a diagnosis of adenocarcinoma	PDAC
VHL (3p) mutation	VHL gene mutation analysis	Mutation present in SCA	SCA
KRAS, *RNF43*, *TP53*, *SMAD4*	Mutation analysis	Mutations seen in both IPMN and MCN	MCN, IPMN
High levels of DNA in cyst fluid, aneuploid, and tetraploid	DNA analysis of cyst fluid	High levels of intact DNA are associated with actively dividing cell; aneuploid and tetraploid favors malignancy	May aid in separation of benign from malignant cysts
GNAS	GNAS mutation analysis	*GNAS* mutation is the second most frequent mutations seen in IPMN, distinguishing it from MCN	IPMN
CTNNB1	*CTNNB1* (beta-catenin) mutation analysis	Mutation present in nearly all SPN	SPN
Polysomy	FISH for polysomy	Copy number abnormalities in CEP3, CEP7, CEP17, and abnormalities of 9p21 favor malignancy	CC
MSI, microsatellite alterations (loss of 3p, 6pq, 10pq, and gain of 5q, 12q, 18q, 20q)	Microsatellite loss analysis	Loss of 3p, 6pq, and 10pq along with the gain of 5q, 12q, 18q, and 20q have been associated with malignant behavior in PanNET	PanNET

PDAC pancreatic ductal adenocarcinoma, *SCA* serous cystadenoma, *MCN* mucinous cystic neoplasm, *IPMN* intraductal papillary mucinous neoplasm, *SPN* solid pseudopapillary neoplasm, *PanNET* pancreatic neuroendocrine tumor, *MSI* microsatellite instability, *CC* cholangiocarcinoma

Activating *KRAS* mutations in codon 12 of exon 1 are common in both intra-ductal papillary mucinous neoplasms and mucinous cystic neoplasms, supporting a mucinous etiology; however, its presence is not specific for malignancy. *KRAS* mutation analysis has an additive value to CEA measurements for distinguishing non-mucinous and mucinous cysts [34]. *RNF43* (ring finger protein 43) encodes a protein with intrinsic E3 ubiquitin ligase activity that promotes cell growth and has recently been linked to the β-catenin pathway. *RNF43* mutations have been shown to occur in MCN and IPMN [35]. The *GNAS* gene encodes for stimulatory G-protein alpha subunit, which is a crucial component of many transduction pathways. In the pancreas, *GNAS* codon 201 mutations appear to be highly specific for intraductal papillary mucinous neoplasms, while *KRAS* and *RNF43* mutations can also be seen in MCNs [36, 37].

Whole exome sequencing of the four most common cystic neoplasms of the pancreas (serous cystadenoma, solid pseudopapillary neoplasm, mucinous cystic neoplasm, and IPMN) has identified a specific mutational profile in each cyst type. *VHL* mutations are seen in serous cystic neoplasms; *CTNNB1* (β-catenin) in solid pseudopapillary neoplasms; *RNF43*, *KRAS*, *TP53*, and *SMAD4* in MCN; and *KRAS*, *RNF43*, *GNAS*, *TP53*, and *SMAD4* in IPMN. It has therefore been suggested that mutational analysis for *GNAS*, *KRAS*, *VHL*, *CTNNB1*, *RNF43*, *TP53*, and *SMAD4* may aid in the differential diagnosis of cystic lesions of the pancreas [35]. The *VHL* tumor suppressor gene is somatically mutated in serous cystadenomas and is not seen in other cystic lesions of the pancreas [36].

DNA analysis may also aid in the separation of nonneoplastic and neoplastic lesions, as well as benign from malignant neoplastic cystic lesions. High levels of intact DNA are associated with actively dividing cells. The concentration of DNA is correlated with optical density (OD) as measured at a wavelength 260/280 nm. The mean concentration of DNA present within a fluid from a pancreatic cystic lesion documented by OD ranges from a low of 6.5 in benign cysts to 16.5 in malignant cysts [34].

Loss of heterozygosity (LOH) analysis identifies loss of heterozygosity at microsatellites linked to tumor suppressor gene loci known to be affected in pancreatic carcinogenesis. An assessment of allelic loss of these tumor suppressor gene-linked microsatellite markers [9p21 (*MTS-1*), 17p (*TP53*), 18q (*DPC4*), 9q22 (*PTCH*), 1p36 (*RIZ*), 3p25-3p26 (*VHL*), 5q23 (*APC*), 10q23 (*PTEN*)] is performed on extracted DNA subjected to polymerase chain reaction (PCR). Products from each PCR are analyzed by capillary electrophoresis on a genetic analyzer. Informative samples with a polymorphic allelic imbalance ratio <0.5 or >2.0 are considered evidence of allelic imbalance and LOH [34]. A buccal brushing sample can be used as a normal control.

MicroRNAs are small (18–24 nucleotide) noncoding RNA molecules whose principal function is to regulate the stability and translation of nuclear mRNA transcripts. Selected panels of dysregulated miRNAs previously identified in invasive pancreatic cancer have also shown aberrant expression in neoplastic mucinous cysts, adding another tool to distinguish mucinous versus non-mucinous cysts [38]. Matthaei et al. [39], using a logistic regression analysis, developed a 9-miRNA model that allowed subclassification of the degree of dysplasia in most instances.

11.1.6 Limitations to Molecular Testing in Pancreatic Lesions

Barriers to implementing molecular analysis include reliance on the presence of substantial diagnostic material (immunohistochemistry, FISH, digital image analysis), imperfect specificity (all tests), and cost (mutation analysis, LOH testing, FISH, digital image analysis), although testing may be helpful in some, usually atypical, cases [40]. While testing for *KRAS* in pancreatic cytology specimens will often yield positive results, the presence of *KRAS* mutations is not entirely specific for malignancy. Although *KRAS* mutation analysis on EUS-FNA samples can support the diagnosis of PDAC and is often associated with worse prognosis, no significant clinical benefits have been derived from therapies targeting KRAS in PDAC [41]. Multiple molecularly targeted therapies have been tested in metastatic pancreatic cancer but have not achieved widespread use in clinical practice [42]. Although there is insufficient evidence of clinical utility at this time to support widespread adoption of molecular testing in solid and cystic pancreatic neoplasms, active investigation may someday offer more targeted therapeutic options.

11.1.7 Recommendations

Overall, cytomorphology is still critical to the diagnosis of solid pancreatic neoplasms, and there is insufficient evidence to indicate that any molecular test should be used as a definitive method of evaluating these neoplasms. Loss of *SMAD4* and positive staining for mesothelin support a diagnosis of PDAC, nuclear staining for beta-catenin supports a diagnosis of solid pseudopapillary neoplasm, and immunocytochemistry for endocrine and exocrine differentiation are helpful for diagnostic purposes in solid pancreatic tumors [8]. FISH for copy number abnormalities can be used to support a cytologic impression of adenocarcinoma. Outside of these general guidelines, molecular testing does not currently have a routine clinical role for diagnostic, prognostic, or therapeutic purposes. Loss of heterozygosity and the presence of certain microRNAs could be used to support the diagnosis of adenocarcinoma, but the clinical utility of these tests remains to be seen. As the diagnosis can usually be made by cytomorphology alone, the addition and costs of these tests may not be warranted.

A multidisciplinary approach for pancreatic lesions with incorporation of all relevant ancillary data to arrive at a cytologic diagnosis is recommended [43–45]. In terms of molecular analyses for predicting malignancy in a mucinous cyst, there are commercially available assays with promising results but which may not be as accurate in classifying smaller (<3 cm), uncomplicated cysts. There is currently insufficient data to warrant their usage in routine practice [45–47].

Once molecular results are obtained, reporting of the results may be issued as an addendum to the cytopathology case and/or reported separately. The advantage of issuing an addendum to the cytopathology case is an opportunity to integrate the molecular findings with the cytomorphology and any other ancillary tests.

11.1.8 Future Directions

There are very few molecular alterations that will change patient management or inform prognosis, and molecular testing is not commonly applied to solid pancreatic neoplasms. Despite limited clinical utility, the hope of personalized medicine and targeted therapies continues to drive research in this area. Testing for certain molecular alterations could enable patients to enroll in clinical trials with targeted therapy, particularly when other therapeutic options have been exhausted. As our understanding of the molecular landscape improves, there may be opportunities to alter the tumor microenvironment. Genes overexpressed in the desmoplastic stroma of PDAC could be a target for chemotherapeutic agents [6]. Patient genetic factors could also influence the effectiveness of therapeutic regimens.

There is still a need for ancillary biomarkers in cyst fluid material that can reliably provide additional distinction between clinically insignificant cystic lesions and mucinous cysts with high-grade dysplasia. Examination of miRNAs could provide the needed test to identify malignant potential in cystic neoplasms of the pancreas. One of the advantages of the short mature miRNAs is the lack of propensity for degradation in biospecimens. Validation with prospective studies of large series with clinical or surgical follow-up is needed before adoption in clinical practice. Looking toward the future, cytopathologists could and should take an active interest in advancing the forefront of molecular cytopathology with regard to solid and cystic pancreatic neoplasms.

11.2 Biliary Tract Sampling for Molecular Cytopathology

The main indication for morphologic evaluation of the biliary tree is a duct stricture as the result of inflammatory or neoplastic disorders. Epithelial tumors originating from the biliary tree usually present a longitudinal growth pattern along the biliary duct rendering their detection more difficult by noninvasive imaging techniques such as ultrasound or computed tomography. On the contrary, the assessment of the biliary tree by endoscopic procedures allows tissue collection for cytologic or histologic diagnosis. Endoscopic retrograde cholangiopancreatography (ERCP), coupled with brush cytology or forceps biopsy, is routinely performed to detect malignancy in patients with biliary strictures [48, 49].

Brush cytology performed during ERCP is simple and safe. Contrary to the simple aspiration of the bile juice, the brush scrapes different sites of the biliary tract mucosa retrieving a cellular material [50]. Usually the samples are well preserved, providing an adequate specimen for cytologic examination. Indeed, the rate of unsatisfactory samples is low, around 5%, and mainly related to air-drying artifact if the samples are not properly fixed [49, 51].

11.2.1 Evaluation of Biliary Tract Specimens

A cytologic diagnosis of malignancy achieved by brush cytology is reliable, and the literature shows a very high specificity for this method, reaching 100% in several series [49, 52–54]. This means that brush cytology has a high positive predictive value and a low rate of false-positive results. In a large series of 406 patients with pancreaticobiliary strictures, Stewart et al. [51] detected only three false-positive cases. Most of the false-positive results are attributed to misinterpretation of atypia in degenerated or reactive epithelial cells, mainly in the context of primary sclerosing cholangitis (PSC), a chronic liver disease causing inflammatory changes and fibrosis of the biliary tract [51, 55].

Despite the reported high specificity, the main limitation of brush cytology is the low sensitivity for detecting malignancy of the biliary tract. In their series of 406 patients, Stewart et al. [51] demonstrated that brush cytology correctly identified neoplastic diseases in 59.8% of the cases. Other series showed sensitivity rates varying from 48% [56] and 54.7% [49] to 68% [52] and 68.6% [54]. The main cause of false-negative results is due to sampling error, probably related to cases where the tumor spreads predominantly to the submucosa of the biliary duct or when the biliary stricture is secondary to an extrinsic compression.

Furthermore, some series reported an atypical or equivocal diagnostic category for which a conclusive cytologic diagnosis is not possible, varying from 4.9% [49] to 10.1% [51] of the cases. According to the terminology proposed by the Papanicolaou Society of Cytopathology, the "atypical" category includes a large spectrum of cytologic or architectural abnormalities that are not compatible with benign reactive changes but, on the other hand, are insufficient to be classified as suspicious or positive for malignancy [44]. Of the 41 cases reported as "atypical" by Stewart et al. [51], 29 were proved to be malignant on clinicopathologic follow-up, while 12 were benign, corresponding mostly to chronic pancreatitis and calculous disease.

Because of the limitations of biliary tract cytology, different complementary approaches have been developed to improve the diagnosis of biliary tract disease. The application of ancillary procedures such as in situ hybridization techniques or gene mutation analysis can improve the accuracy for detection of malignancy in biliary tract brush specimens [8].

11.2.2 Molecular Testing of Biliary Tract Specimens

The commercially available UroVysion FISH probe set (Abbott Molecular, Des Plaines, IL), originally developed for detecting urothelial carcinoma, has been applied to biliary tract specimens, including bile fluid, brushings, and aspirates of the pancreaticobiliary tree [57]. The FISH test can detect chromosome copy number gains and/or chromosome deletions. Aiming to detect cells with chromosome copy number gains (polysomic cells), which can have an association with malignancy, the FISH test employs probes to target the centromeric regions of the chromosomes 3, 7, and 17. According to Kipp et al. [57], a diagnosis suggestive of malignancy is obtained with a polysomic result, defined as five or more cells showing gains in at least two or more FISH probes. The detection by FISH of 9p21 loss (which results in the loss of the tumor suppressor p16) is another criterion that favors a diagnosis of malignancy in pancreatobiliary cytology specimens [58, 59]. Accordingly, 12 or more cells with deletions of 9p21 should be interpreted as a positive FISH result [59] (see Fig. 11.1).

Currently, FISH is considered the most reliable complementary technique to cytology for the detection of biliary tract malignancies [8]. Using biliary brush specimens for the detection of malignancy in 131 patients with biliary tract

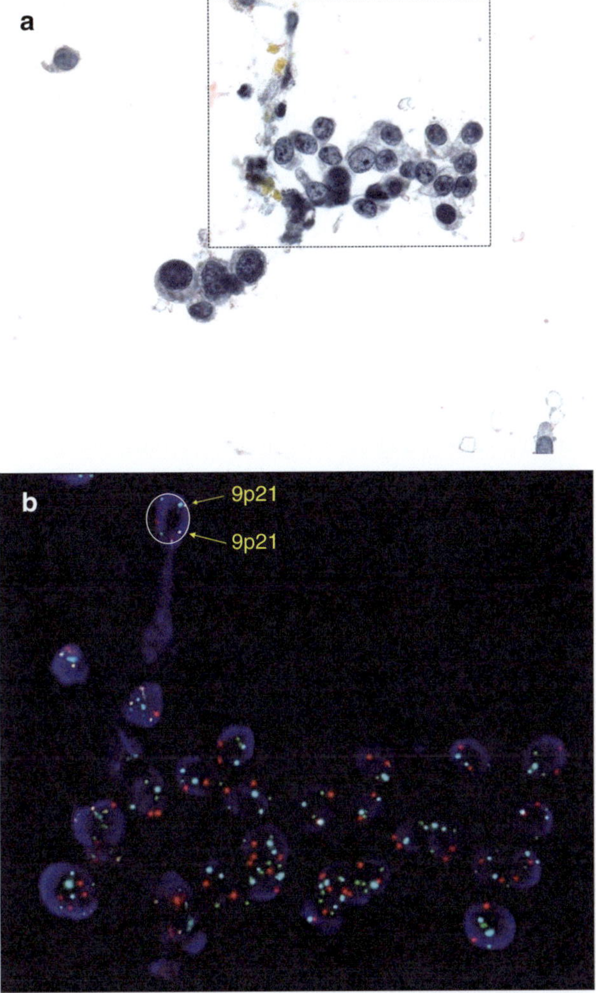

Fig. 11.1 (a) Micrograph shows an example of a biliary brush cytology specimen from a 30-year-old female patient. One cluster of mildly atypical epithelial cells are mixed with rare small lymphocytes (Papanicolaou stain, 400×). (b) The same cells (inset of a) are shown after multi-target fluorescent in situ hybridization (FISH) UroVysion (magnification 600×). The atypical cells demonstrate a complete loss of the 9p21 (FISH-positive). These cells show 2–4 signals for the centromeric probes of chromosomes 3, 7, and 17. The encircled cell correspond to a small lymphocyte with normal two 9p21 signals (yellow signals). Courtesy of Dr Spasenija Savic from the Institute of Pathology of the University Hospital Basel, Switzerland

strictures, Kipp et al. [60] observed that the FISH test was significantly more sensitive in comparison to cytology alone. An analysis of 498 patients with pancreaticobiliary strictures corroborated the results of Kipp et al. [60], demonstrating that FISH testing had a significantly higher sensitivity compared to cytology alone (42.9 vs 20.1%) while retaining the same specificity as cytology (99.6%). Interestingly, the authors showed that the probability of having carcinoma was 77 times higher for patients with polysomic FISH results as compared to patients with normal FISH, whereas the probability of having carcinoma was six times higher for patients with suspicious cytology in comparison to patients with normal cytology [61].

In a small series of 50 patients with biliary strictures, a sensitivity of 89% was achieved when 9p21 loss detected by FISH was added to FISH polysomy + cytology as compared to FISH polysomy + cytology (58%) or cytology alone (21%) [58]. Using the FISH technique to analyze a series of 90 cases of pancreas and extrahepatic biliary tract cytology, Vlajnic et al. [59] found an overall sensitivity of 79% and an overall specificity of 100%. For cases with inconclusive (atypical or suspicious) cytology, sensitivity and specificity of 61.3 and 100% were achieved, respectively. In their study, the authors observed that 74% of FISH-positive results comprised both chromosome copy number gains and 9p21 loss, while 14% corresponded only to copy number gains and 12% consisted only of 9p21 deletion [59].

Patients with PSC may develop strictures of the biliary tract. Based on their symptoms (abdominal pain, jaundice, weight loss), laboratory tests (elevated levels of CA 19-9 and serum liver markers), and a high risk for developing cholangiocarcinoma, ERCP and brushing cytology are frequently applied for the evaluation of biliary tract strictures in such patients. However, cellular abnormalities as a result of inflammatory changes may pose difficulties in the interpretation of the cytologic specimens, resulting in equivocal (atypical, suspicious) or false-positive diagnoses [51, 55]. In a study that evaluated 102 patients with PSC and equivocal brush cytology, 76% of the patients with polysomy detected by FISH developed a pancreaticobiliary tract malignancy within 2 years [62]. The authors also demonstrated that patients with a combination of polysomy and elevated serum levels of CA 19-9 had a 10.92 times higher probability for developing cancer of the pancreaticobiliary tract in comparison to patients without polysomy and low levels of CA 19-9 [62].

The *KRAS* gene mutation is a common genetic alteration in pancreaticobiliary tumors, especially in carcinomas of the pancreas and, less frequently, in cholangiocarcinomas. Most of the *KRAS* mutations occur in codon 12 of exon 2 of the *KRAS* gene [6] (see Fig. 11.2). In an attempt to improve the detection of malignancy of the pancreaticobiliary tract, several studies have investigated the role of molecular techniques in detecting *KRAS* mutations in biliary brush specimens.

Using a PCR-based method to detect mutations of codon 12 in the *KRAS* gene, Sturm et al. [63] compared the sensitivity of brush cytology and molecular testing in a series of 312 patients with bile duct stenosis. Although the sensitivity of both methods were quite similar (36% for cytology and 42% for the molecular testing), it increased to 62% when cytology and *KRAS* mutation analysis were combined. In another study where the same series of patients were evaluated with real-time and quantitative PCR, a sensitivity of 71% was obtained with the combination of

KRAS mutation in IGV

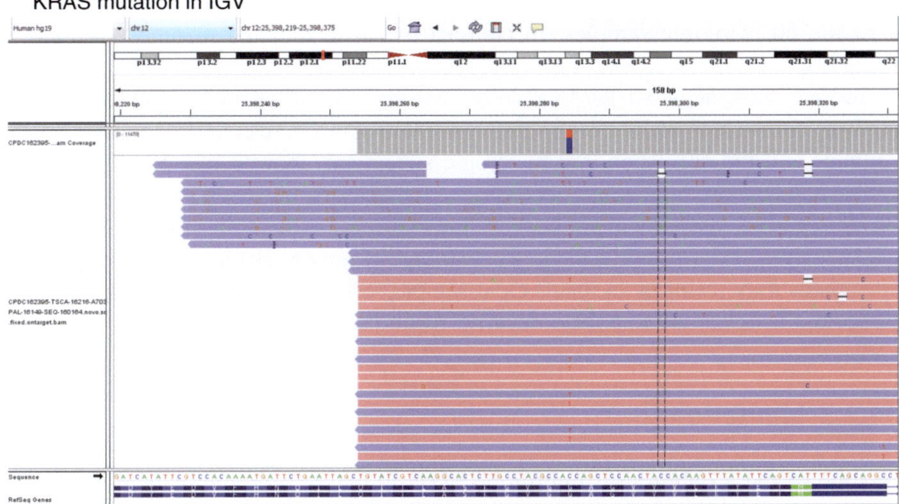

Fig. 11.2 Representative example of the molecular output showing a KRAS G12D mutation detected in a cytologic specimen from the pancreas. Courtesy of Jennifer Morrissette, PhD, from the Department of Pathology and Laboratory Medicine, Hospital of the University of Pennsylvania, Perelman School of Medicine at the University of Pennsylvania, Philadelphia, Pennsylvania, USA

cytology and molecular testing [64]. In a study that analyzed 129 pancreaticobiliary brushings and pancreatic fine-needle aspirations with an indeterminate (atypical or suspicious) cytologic diagnosis, the sensitivity and specificity for the detection of malignancy based on the presence of *KRAS* mutations were 57% and 94%, respectively [65].

Molecular techniques to identify *KRAS* mutations can detect pancreaticobiliary cancers not established by FISH. Kipp et al. [66] studied a series of 132 benign and malignant cytologic brush specimens assessed by FISH and a quantitative PCR-based method for *KRAS* mutations: out of 58 patients with FISH-negative results, 7 had *KRAS* mutations, and 6 of these had a carcinoma in the final histologic diagnosis. Out of 33 patients with FISH-equivocal results, 9 had *KRAS* mutations, including 8 patients with proven malignancy by histology. Although the sensitivity of the molecular technique (47%) and the FISH test (50%) were similar, the combination of both methods increased overall sensitivity to 68% [66].

In these studies, most of the detected *KRAS* mutations in the brush specimens involved codon 12 of the *KRAS* gene. More specifically, the G12D and G12V mutations were the two most prevalent, both resulting in a change from a glycine to an aspartic acid (G12D) or a valine (G12V) amino acid. These are followed in frequency by the G12R mutation, which changes a glycine to an arginine amino acid. Mutations in codon 13 of the *KRAS* gene were also found and resulted from the change of a glycine to an aspartic acid amino acid [63, 64, 66]. In a detailed analysis of 60 cases of brush cytologic samples and the corresponding carcinomas on histology, Sturm et al. [63] verified that when present, all detected mutations were identical in both specimens. However, no mutation was found (wild-type *KRAS*) in 7 of the 60 cytologic samples, in contrast to *KRAS*-mutated matched histologic samples.

Indeed, false-negative *KRAS* results have been reported in the literature. In a study by Sturm et al. [63], a comparison of *KRAS* status between the cytologic brush samples and the corresponding histologic specimens showed that 53 of 60 cases (88%) had concordant results. According to the authors, the discrepant results could be the result of sampling error, because the cytologic evaluation of these cases was also negative [63]. Certainly, the low percentage of tumor cells in some biliary brush specimens may result in an insufficient sample, below the limit of detection of the molecular test, leading to a false-negative result [66].

11.2.3 Limitations

In spite of the reliability of multiprobe FISH in diagnosing malignancy in biliary tract brush specimens, there are some limitations that can result in equivocal and false-positive results. For instance, misinterpretation of FISH signals can lead to false-positive results. According to Kipp et al. [57], cells with weak or absent signals secondary to poor hybridization may be misinterpreted as having a deletion of 9p21. In a study by Barr Fritcher et al. [62], 6 of the 25 patients with FISH-positive results were not found to have a pancreaticobiliary tract malignancy on clinico-pathologic follow-up. The authors postulated that some false-positive FISH results may result from detection of chromosomal abnormalities in dysplastic cells that do not progress to cancer [62]. Finally, we have to consider that a negative FISH result does not exclude a malignancy of the biliary tract. Vlajnic et al. [59] stated that if not correctly pre-evaluated, FISH slides with no or few tumor cells may result in false-negative results.

Furthermore, tumor cells with chromosomal abnormalities other than those potentially detected by the UroVysion FISH test may occur [59]. Indeed, other types of chromosomal abnormalities such as tetrasomy (four copies of all four probes) and trisomy (single probe gains) are considered equivocal FISH results and do not contribute to the diagnosis [57]. In their series of 102 patients with PSC, Barr Fritcher et al. [62] detected 33 cases (32% of the total) with non-polysomic FISH results comprising 3 cases with tetrasomy, 29 cases with trisomy 7, and just 1 case with trisomy 3. The majority of these abnormalities (88%) were found in patients without cancer on follow-up, suggesting that these patients may have a similar outcome as compared to patients with FISH-negative results. However, in their study, there were four patients (12%) with non-polysomic FISH abnormalities that developed biliary tract malignancy within 2 years of follow-up [62].

Unfortunately, *KRAS* mutations can occur in nonneoplastic pancreaticobiliary diseases. In one study, *KRAS* mutations were detected in brush specimens from 8 of 74 patients with histologically proven benign bile duct stenosis, including 3 cases of chronic pancreatitis, 3 cases of PSC, and 2 cases of "post-surgical stenosis" [63]. In another study with surgical follow-up, *KRAS* mutations were found in brush specimens from patients with chronic pancreatitis (1 of 8 cases) and with "unremarkable histology" (1 of 28 cases) [65]. In a study by Kipp et al. [66], the *KRAS* test was negative for mutations in 50 of 52 patients with benign diseases of the pancreaticobiliary tract, corresponding to a specificity of 96%. Two patients had false-positive *KRAS* results: one patient with PSC and one patient with ulcerative colitis [66]. It has been speculated that *KRAS* mutations can precede overt histologic changes of malignancy [65] and that increased or uncontrolled RAS activity as a result of an inflammatory process can induce genetic changes leading to tumorigenesis [66].

11.2.4 Recommendations

In general, *KRAS* mutation analysis has a fair sensitivity for the identification of malignancy in the pancreaticobiliary tree, as demonstrated by the studies described above. Currently, there is no consensus to support the use of *KRAS* testing as an ancillary technique for the diagnosis of biliary duct strictures [8].

11.2.5 Future Directions

Recent advances in molecular techniques, such as next-generation sequencing (NGS), could provide a more comprehensive knowledge of the molecular genetics underlying pancreaticobiliary tumors and may result in the discovery of potential biomarkers. A recent study evaluated the role of targeted NGS in pancreaticobiliary brushing specimens in a series of 74 patients who underwent ERCP [67]. Among the 24 cases that had a positive NGS result, the most commonly mutated gene was *KRAS* (21 cases), followed by *TP53* (14 cases), *SMAD4* (6 cases), and *p16/CDKN2A* (4 cases). In this study, the NGS technique was the most sensitive test with a sensitivity of 74% when compared to cytology (67% sensitivity) and FISH (55% sensitivity). Adding the FISH test to cytology increased the sensitivity to 76%. When NGS was added to cytology, the sensitivity increased to 85%. This sensitivity (85%) remained the same when FISH was added to NGS and cytology, meaning that the FISH test had no impact on the sensitivity of NGS + cytology. Considering these results and that FISH is a labor-intensive and challenging technique, the authors concluded that NGS could be an alternative to FISH as an ancillary test for pancreaticobiliary brushing specimens [67].

References

1. Vilmann P, Jacobsen GK, Henriksen FW, et al. Endoscopic ultrasonography with guided fine needle aspiration biopsy in pancreatic disease. Gastrointest Endosc. 1992;38:172–3.
2. Shi C, Daniels JA, Hruban RH. Molecular characterization of pancreatic neoplasms. Adv Anat Pathol. 2008;15:185–95.
3. Hong SM, Park JY, Hruban RH, et al. Molecular signatures of pancreatic cancer. Arch Pathol Lab Med. 2011;135:716–27.

4. Reid MD, Saka B, Balci S, et al. Molecular genetics of pancreatic neoplasms and their morphologic correlates: an update on recent advances and potential diagnostic applications. Am J Clin Pathol. 2014;141:168–80.

5. Klimstra DS. Nonductal neoplasms of the pancreas. Mod Pathol. 2007;20(Suppl 1):S94–112.

6. Hruban RH, Klimstra DS. Adenocarcinoma of the pancreas. Semin Diagn Pathol. 2014;31:443–51.

7. Cowan RW, Maitra A. Genetic progression of pancreatic cancer. Cancer J. 2014;20:80–4.

8. Layfield LJ, Ehya H, Filie AC, et al. Utilization of ancillary studies in the cytologic diagnosis of biliary and pancreatic lesions: the Papanicolaou Society of Cytopathology guidelines for pancreatobiliary cytology. Diagn Cytopathol. 2014;42:351–62.

9. Tanaka Y, Kato K, Notohara K, et al. Frequent beta-catenin mutation and cytoplasmic/nuclear accumulation in pancreatic solid-pseudopapillary neoplasm. Cancer Res. 2001;61:8401–4.

10. Abraham SC, Klimstra DS, Wilentz RE, et al. Solid-pseudopapillary tumors of the pancreas are genetically distinct from pancreatic ductal adenocarcinomas and almost always harbor beta-catenin mutations. Am J Pathol. 2002;160:1361–9.

11. La Rosa S, Sessa F, Capella C. Acinar cell carcinoma of the pancreas: overview of clinicopathologic features and insights into the molecular pathology. Front Med. 2015;2:41.

12. Chmielecki J, Hutchinson KE, Frampton GM, et al. Comprehensive genomic profiling of pancreatic acinar cell carcinomas identifies recurrent RAF fusions and frequent inactivation of DNA repair genes. Cancer Discov. 2014;4:1398–405.

13. Bournet B, Gayral M, Torrisani J, et al. Role of endoscopic ultrasound in the molecular diagnosis of pancreatic cancer. World J Gastroenterol. 2014;20:10758–68.

14. Bournet B, Souque A, Senesse P, et al. Endoscopic ultrasound-guided fine-needle aspiration biopsy coupled with *KRAS* mutation assay to distinguish pancreatic cancer from pseudotumoral chronic pancreatitis. Endoscopy. 2009;41:552–7.

15. Khalid A, McGrath K, Pal R, et al. Microdissection based genotyping improves the accuracy of EUS guided FNA of pancreatic tumors. Gastrointest Endosc. 2004;59:94.

16. de Biase D, de Luca C, Gragnano G, et al. Fully automated PCR detection of *KRAS* mutations on pancreatic endoscopic fine-needle aspirates. J Clin Pathol. 2016. https://doi.org/10.1136/jclinpath-2016-203696.

17. Bournet B, Pointreau A, Souque A, et al. Gene expression signature of advanced pancreatic ductal adenocarcinoma using low density array on endoscopic ultrasound-guided fine needle aspiration samples. Pancreatology. 2012;12:27–34.

18. Brand RE, Adai AT, Centeno BA, et al. A microRNA-based test improves endoscopic ultrasound-guided cytologic diagnosis of pancreatic cancer. Clin Gastroenterol Hepatol. 2014;12:1717–23.

19. Kubiliun N, Ribeiro A, Fan YS, et al. EUS-FNA with rescue fluorescence in situ hybridization for the diagnosis of pancreatic carcinoma in patients with inconclusive on-site cytopathology results. Gastrointest Endosc. 2011;74:541–7.

20. Winter JM, Ting AH, Vilardell F, et al. Absence of E-cadherin expression distinguishes noncohesive from cohesive pancreatic cancer. Clin Cancer Res. 2008;14:412–8.

21. Higashi M, Yokoyama S, Yamamoto T, et al. Mucin expression in endoscopic ultrasound-guided fine-needle aspiration specimens is a useful prognostic factor in pancreatic ductal adenocarcinoma. Pancreas. 2015;44:728–34.

22. Carpizo DR, Allen PJ, Brennan MF. Current management of cystic neoplasms of the pancreas. Surgeon. 2008;6:298–307.

23. Laffan TA, Horton KM, Klein AP, et al. Prevalence of unsuspected pancreatic cysts on MDCT. Am J Roentgenol. 2008;191:802–7.

24. Lee KS, Sekhar A, Rofsky NM, et al. Prevalence of incidental pancreatic cysts in the adult population on MR imaging. Am J Gastroenterol. 2010;105:2079–84.

25. Brugge WR, Lewandrowski K, Lee-Lewandrowski E, et al. The diagnosis of pancreatic cystic neoplasms: a report of the cooperative pancreatic cyst (CPC) study. Gastroenterology. 2004;126:1330–6.

26. Cizginer S, Turner B, Bilge AR, et al. Cyst fluid carcinoembryonic antigen is an accurate diagnostic marker of pancreatic mucinous cysts. Pancreas. 2013;40:1024–8.
27. Jimenez RE, Warshaw AL, Z'graggen K, et al. Sequential accumulation of *KRAS* mutations and p53 overexpression in the progression of pancreatic mucinous cystic neoplasms to malignancy. Ann Surg. 1999;230:501–9.
28. Z'graggen K, Rivera JA, Compton CC, et al. Prevalence of activating *KRAS* mutations in the evolutionary stages of neoplasia in intraductal papillary mucinous tumors of the pancreas. Ann Surg. 1997;226:498–500.
29. Biankin AV, Biankin SA, Kench JG, et al. Aberrant p16(INK4A) and DPC4/Smad4 expression in intraductal papillary mucinous tumors of the pancreas is associated with invasive ductal adenocarcinoma. Gut. 2002;50:861–8.
30. Iacobuzio-Donahue CA, Wilentz RE, Argani P, et al. Dpc4 protein in mucinous cystic neoplasms of the pancreas: frequent loss of expression in invasive carcinomas suggests a role in genetic progression. Am J Surg Pathol. 2000;24:1544–8.
31. Lapkus O, Gologan O, Liu Y, et al. Determination of sequential mutation accumulation in pancreas and bile duct brushing cytology. Mod Pathol. 2006;19:907–13.
32. Caldas C, Hahn SA, da Costa L, et al. Frequent somatic mutations and homozygous deletions of the p16 (MTS1) gene in pancreatic adenocarcinoma. Nat Genet. 1994;8:27–32.
33. Shao J, Zhang L, Gao J, et al. Aberrant expression of PTCH (patched gene) and SMO (smoothened gene) in human pancreatic cancerous tissues and its association with hyperglycemia. Pancreas. 2006;33:38–44.
34. Khalid A, Zahid M, Finkelstein SD, et al. Pancreatic cyst fluid DNA analysis in evaluating pancreatic cysts: a report of the PANDA study. Gastrointest Endosc. 2009;69:1095–102.
35. Macgregor-Das AM, Iacobuzio-Donahue CA. Molecular pathways in pancreatic carcinogenesis. J Surg Oncol. 2013;107:8–14.
36. Wu J, Jiao Y, Dal Molin M, et al. Whole-exome sequencing of neoplastic cysts of the pancreas reveals recurrent mutations in components of ubiquitin-dependent pathways. Proc Natl Acad Sci U S A. 2011;27:21188–93.
37. Wu J, Matthaei H, Maitra A, et al. Recurrent GNAS mutations define an unexpected pathway for pancreatic cyst development. Sci Transl Med. 2011;3:92ra66.
38. Ryu JK, Matthaei H, dal Molin M, et al. Elevated microRNA miR-21 levels in pancreatic cyst fluid are predictive of mucinous precursor lesions of ductal adenocarcinoma. Pancreatology. 2011;11:343–50.
39. Matthaei H, Wylie D, Lloyd MB, et al. miRNA biomarkers in cyst fluid augment the diagnosis and management of pancreatic cysts. Clin Cancer Res. 2012;17:4713–24.
40. Bellizzi AM, Stelow EB. Pancreatic cytopathology: a practical approach and review. Arch Pathol Lab Med. 2009;133:388–404.
41. Bournet B, Buscail C, Muscari F, et al. Targeting KRAS for diagnosis, prognosis, and treatment of pancreatic cancer: Hopes and realities. Eur J Cancer. 2016;54:75–83.
42. Zagouri F, Sergentanis TN, Chrysikos D, et al. Molecularly targeted therapies in metastatic pancreatic cancer: a systematic review. Pancreas. 2013;42:760–73.
43. Pitman MB, Layfield LJ. Guidelines for pancreaticobiliary cytology from the Papanicolaou Society of Cytopathology: a review. Cancer Cytopathol. 2014;122:399–411.
44. Pitman MB, Centeno BA, Ali SZ, et al. Standardized terminology and nomenclature for pancreatobiliary cytology: the Papanicolaou Society of Cytopathology guidelines. Diagn Cytopathol. 2014;42:338–50.
45. Layfield LJ, Ehya H, Filie AC, et al. Utilization of ancillary studies in the cytologic diagnosis of biliary and pancreatic lesions: the Papanicolaou Society of Cytopathology guidelines. Cytojournal. 2014;11(suppl 1):4.
46. Gillis A, Cipollone I, Cousins G, et al. Does EUS-FNA molecular analysis carry additional value when compared to cytology in the diagnosis of pancreatic cystic neoplasm? A systematic review. HPB. 2015;17:377–86.
47. Panarelli NC, Sela R, Schreiner AM, et al. Commercial molecular panels are of limited utility in the classification of pancreatic cystic lesions. Am J Surg Pathol. 2012;36:1434–43.

48. Weber A, Schmid RA, Prinz C. Diagnostic approaches to cholangiocarcinoma. World J Gastroenterol. 2008;14:4131–6.
49. Sethi R, Singh K, Warner B, et al. The impact of brush cytology from endoscopic retrograde cholangiopancreatography (ERCP) on patient management at a UK teaching hospital. Frontline Gastroenterol. 2016;7:97–101.
50. Brugge W, Dewitt J, Klapman JB, et al. Papanicolaou Society of Cytopathology. Techniques for cytologic sampling of pancreatic and bile duct lesions. Diagn Cytopathol. 2014;42:333–7.
51. Stewart CJR, Mills PR, Carter R, et al. Brush cytology in the assessment of pancreatico-biliary strictures: a review of 406 cases. J Clin Pathol. 2001;54:449–55.
52. Govil H, Reddy V, Kluskens L, et al. Brush cytology of the biliary tract: retrospective study of 278 cases with histopathologic correlation. Diagn Cytopathol. 2002;26:273–7.
53. Eiholm S, Thielsen P, Kromann-Andersen H. Endoscopic brush cytology from biliary duct system is still valuable. Dan Med J. 2013;60:A4656.
54. Mehmood S, Loya A, Yusuf MA. Biliary brush cytology revisited. Acta Cytol. 2016;60:167–72.
55. Layfield LJ, Cramer H. Primary sclerosing cholangitis as a cause of false positive bile duct brushing cytology: report of two cases. Diagn Cytopathol. 2005;32:119–24.
56. Logrono R, Kurtycz DF, Molina CP, et al. Analysis of false-negative diagnoses on endoscopic brush cytology of biliary and pancreatic duct strictures: the experience at 2 university hospitals. Arch Pathol Lab Med. 2000;124:387–92.
57. Kipp BR, Barr Fritcher EG, Pettengill JE, et al. Improving the accuracy of pancreatobiliary tract cytology with fluorescence in situ hybridization: a molecular test with proven clinical success. Cancer Cytopathol. 2013;121:610–9.
58. Gonda TA, Glick MP, Sethi A, et al. Polysomy and p16 deletion by fluorescence in situ hybridization in the diagnosis of indeterminate biliary strictures. Gastrointest Endosc. 2012;75:74–9.
59. Vlajnic T, Somaini G, Savic S, et al. Targeted multiprobe fluorescence in situ hybridization analysis for elucidation of inconclusive pancreatobiliary cytology. Cancer Cytopathol. 2014;122:627–34.
60. Kipp BR, Stadheim LM, Halling SA, et al. A comparison of routine cytology and fluorescence in situ hybridization for the detection of malignant bile duct strictures. Am J Gastroenterol. 2004;99:1675–81.
61. Barr Fritcher EG, Kipp BR, Halling KC, et al. A multivariable model using advanced cytologic methods for the evaluation of indeterminate pancreaticobiliary strictures. Gastroenterology. 2009;136:2180–6.
62. Barr Fritcher EG, Voss JS, Jenkins SM, et al. Primary sclerosing cholangitis with equivocal cytology: fluorescence in situ hybridization and serum CA 19-9 predict risk of malignancy. Cancer Cytopathol. 2013;121:708–17.
63. Sturm PD, Rauws EA, Hruban RH, et al. Clinical value of K-ras codon 12 analysis and endobiliary brush cytology for the diagnosis of malignant extrahepatic bile duct stenosis. Clin Cancer Res. 1999;5:629–35.
64. van Heek NT, Clayton SJ, Sturm PD, et al. Comparison of the novel quantitative ARMS assay and an enriched PCR-ASO assay for K-ras mutations with conventional cytology on endobiliary brush cytology from 312 consecutive extrahepatic biliary stenoses. J Clin Pathol. 2005;58:1315–20.
65. Cai G, Mahooti S, Lipata FM, et al. Diagnostic value of K-ras mutation analysis for pancreaticobiliary cytology specimens with indeterminate diagnosis. Cancer Cytopathol. 2012;120:313–8.
66. Kipp BR, Fritcher EG, Clayton AC, et al. Comparison of KRAS mutation analysis and FISH for detecting pancreatobiliary tract cancer in cytology specimens collected during endoscopic retrograde cholangiopancreatography. J Mol Diagn. 2010;12(6):780.
67. Dudley JC, Zheng Z, McDonald T, et al. Next-generating sequencing and fluorescence in situ hybridization have comparable performance characteristics in the analysis of pancreaticobiliary brushings in malignancy. J Mol Diagn. 2016;18:124–30.

Molecular Cytology Applications in Soft Tissue

12

Kossivi E. Dantey and Sara E. Monaco

12.1 Introduction

Soft tissue tumors are relatively rare neoplasms that arise in any of the mesenchymal tissues of the extremities, trunk/retroperitoneum, or head and neck [1]. They display a wide range of behavior in the way they grow, recur, or metastasize. Some tumors are benign and rarely recur or metastasize, whereas others are rapidly aggressive in their dissemination. The relative scarcity of these neoplasms, as well as the diversity of tumor subtypes, makes their diagnosis an extreme challenge to many pathologists, especially those without expertise in bone and soft tissue pathology. Thankfully, between 20 and 30% of such neoplasms are estimated to harbor specific chromosomal abnormalities, which can assist in diagnosis and offer potential targets for future therapies [2, 3]. Due to their wide range of behavior, the treatment plans can range from a simple excision to a team-oriented, multidisciplinary, individualized treatment plan. Hence it is crucial to have the correct diagnosis and to start the appropriate treatment as soon as possible.

Fine needle aspiration (FNA) is a well-recognized diagnostic tool for the evaluation of soft tissue and bone lesions that are clinically and radiologically suspicious for a primary or secondary malignancy. Recent studies have shown a very high accurate diagnostic rate [4]. It is quick, simple, reliable, and safe with low risk of complications. The two main advantages of FNA in the evaluation of suspected soft tissue tumors is to obtain a definitive diagnosis prior to treatment planning (is the lesion a primary or metastatic soft tissue tumor? is the lesion benign or malignant?) and to help in the investigation of suspected tumor recurrences or metastases. Some of the disadvantages of using FNA as a primary diagnostic modality for soft tissue tumors include problems with obtaining sufficient material for diagnosis and ancillary studies, in addition to the issue of not having architectural features to evaluate [5].

K. E. Dantey · S. E. Monaco (✉)
University of Pittsburgh Medical Center, Pittsburgh, PA, USA
e-mail: monacose@upmc.edu

© Springer International Publishing AG, part of Springer Nature 2018
F. C. Schmitt (ed.), *Molecular Applications in Cytology*,
https://doi.org/10.1007/978-3-319-74942-6_12

However, the use of FNA with trained and experienced clinicians performing and interpreting the biopsies, sometimes with image guidance and/or in combination with core biopsy, can usually minimize nondiagnostic cases and maximize diagnostic yield. In large academic centers, FNA cytology has been shown to have a sensitivity and specificity greater than 95% [6, 7], with less than 5% of cases inadequate for diagnosis [6]. This success in diagnosing and subtyping soft tissue tumors is due to the fact that immunohistochemical and molecular techniques (like RT-PCR and FISH) can be easily applied to cytology specimens and the increasing number of characteristic chromosomal abnormalities that have been discovered in specific soft tissue tumors. In fact, this has also made FNA cytology preferable over intraoperative frozen section in some settings, given that ancillary studies cannot be applied intraoperatively [6].

12.2 Overview of Molecular Testing in Soft Tissue Tumors

Recent advances have determined that mechanisms that drive some soft tissue tumors can be divided into three broad categories: transcriptional dysregulation owing to aberrant fusion proteins resulting from genomic translocation, somatic mutations in key genes and signaling pathways, and DNA copy number abnormalities (amplifications) [8] (Table 12.1). Real-time polymerase chain reactions (RT-PCR) and fluorescence in situ hybridization (FISH) studies can detect some of the genetic abnormalities characteristic of soft tissue tumors and allow for accurate rapid diagnoses in small specimens. These molecular techniques can be applied to almost any soft tissue cytopathology specimens, including aspirate smears, cytospins, ThinPrep, and cell block, thereby making them easy to incorporate into the work flow. These molecular tests currently play an important integral part in the FNA diagnosis of soft tissue lesions. In addition, there is a growing use of next-generation sequencing and more in-depth molecular techniques to look for new, undiscovered genetic abnormalities and to look for actionable biomarkers for treatment.

12.2.1 Fluorescence In Situ Hybridization (FISH)

Fluorescence in situ hybridization (FISH) is a technique that utilizes fluorescently labeled DNA probes to detect chromosomal alterations in cells. FISH can detect various types of genetic anomalies like duplication, amplification, deletion, or translocation. Given that an increasing number of soft tissue tumors can be characterized

Table 12.1 Main molecular mechanisms involved in soft tissue tumorigenesis

1. Transcriptional dysregulation with aberrant fusion proteins resulting from genomic translocations
2. Somatic mutations in genes or signaling pathways
3. DNA copy number alterations due to gene amplification

by chromosomal alterations, FISH can help reach a more definitive diagnosis by detecting these characteristic abnormalities in tumor cells from exfoliative and aspiration cytology specimens. In fact, cytology aspirate smears and cytospins are ideal specimens given that the entire cell nucleus is present in the preparation without the truncation artifact that is seen with five micron sections of a cell block or tissue section, which leads to more accurate signal enumeration. In addition, FISH is advantageous because a fresh specimen is not required, unlike flow cytometry, which makes it amenable to apply to fixed tissue that may not have a fresh specimen available.

There are three basic types of probe sets used in FISH: break-apart, fusion, and gene probe sets [9]. Break-apart probes are those in which DNA probes bind to the opposite ends of one gene or chromosomal region. One probe is labeled with a red/orange fluorescent chromophore, while the other is labeled in green. In an intact (normal) chromosome, the signals are close together, and the resulting overlapping signal appears as a yellow dot. In a rearranged locus, one signal remains on the parent chromosome, while the second signal has been translocated to a distant location, usually on a different chromosome, but occasionally on the same chromosome. In this abnormal situation, the red/orange and green signals are separated from each other and are visualized as distinct separate dots. The break-apart probes tend to be more sensitive than fusion probes given that it is simply looking for a split in the gene of concern, but does not determine what the partner gene is. In addition, break-apart probes can be more cost effective in that they can be used for a wide range of tumors that each shares an abnormality in a common gene. The best example is the *EWSR1* gene on chromosome 22, which is seen in a wide variety of tumors [10] (Table 12.2). Instead of laboratories having different fusion probes for specific translocations involving chromosome 22, they can simply use the chromosome 22 break-apart probe to say that there is a rearrangement of chromosome 22. This, in combination with the morphology and immunophenotype, is usually sufficient for a diagnosis, but if more specific analysis to find the fusion partner were required, then fusion probes or PCR could be used. As with other ancillary tests, one should be aware of the pitfalls including the fact that FISH studies do not detect other chromosomal abnormalities that may be seen with classical cytogenetics, and other genetic alterations can lead to false positive findings. A recent example is the findings that *SMARCB1*-deficient tumors (e.g., rhabdoid tumors, epithelioid sarcoma) with INI1 protein loss can appear to have an *EWS* gene rearrangement by FISH due to the juxtaposition of *SMARCB1* and *EWSR1* on chromosome 22 [11].

Table 12.2 Tumors that share chromosome 22 (*EWSR1* gene) rearrangements	
	1. Ewing sarcoma/primitive neuroectodermal tumor (EWS/PNET)
	2. Desmoplastic small round cell tumor
	3. Clear cell sarcoma
	4. Extraskeletal myxoid chondrosarcoma
	5. Angiomatoid fibrous histiocytoma
	6. Soft tissue myoepithelial tumors
	7. Myxoid-round cell liposarcoma (rare)
	8. Osteosarcoma, small cell variant (rare)

Fusion or dual-color translocation probes are used to detect specific translocations associated with tumors. The two genes involved in the translocation are labeled in different colors, usually one red and one green chromophore are used, with one corresponding to the 5′ (upstream) fusion partner and the other corresponding to the 3′ (downstream) partner. A positive result consists of three signals, a fused yellow signal, as well as one red and one green signal from each of the uninvolved alleles. A negative result is four split signals (two each red and green). Chromosomal aneuploidy can complicate these results due to changes in chromosomal copy number. This test is more specific than the break-apart probe, but is not as sensitive, as a negative result does not exclude the presence of a different fusion partner.

Some soft tissue tumors are associated with amplification of a gene, and in these cases, enumeration probes are helpful to detect the relative copy number. One probe corresponds to the gene locus in question, while a second probe labels the centromere of the chromosome that the target gene locus is on. In a normal cell, the ratio between target and centromere probes is 1–2:1. However, in the amplified state, the ratio is greatly increased. The centromere probe serves as an ideal internal control to demonstrate that the chromosome is present and not amplified and that it is simply the gene locus that is amplified.

Some of the limitations of FISH include requirement for adequate tissue fixation without decalcification, as decalcifying agents and ceratin fixatives with harsh acids or heavy metals may impact interpretation of FISH results, causing indeterminate results. FISH testing also requires technical expertise and typically results in a longer turnaround time than immunohistochemical stains. Given the need for a longer turnaround time, cytopathologists need to decide whether to sign out their biopsy results with a pattern-based diagnosis and differential diagnosis, followed by an addendum incorporating the ancillary study findings, or to wait and incorporate all findings when complete. This can be difficult as clinicians are demanding faster answers with smaller tissue biopsies. Another limitation is that most FISH laboratories have the more commonly used break-apart probes, so characteristic translocations are not specifically identified in some cases. As mentioned before, FISH testing does not detect all genetic abnormalities, such as mutations and other chromosomal abnormalities that may require other testing, such as next-generation sequencing and classical cytogenetics. This emphasizes the need for cytopathologists who can tie all the ancillary testing results together to reach a specific diagnosis and optimize patient care.

12.2.2 Real-Time PCR (RT-PCR)

Polymerase chain reaction (PCR) allows amplification and analysis of nucleic acid target. PCR can be used to detect genetic abnormalities (e.g., translocations or mutations) in tumors. As an ancillary technique, PCR can help confirm the cytologic diagnosis of soft tissue tumors by confirming the actual fusion transcripts or mutations present.

Real-time PCR (RT-PCR) is a PCR technique where the amplified DNA product or amplicon product is measured as the reaction progresses, in real time, with product quantification after each cycle. Real-time PCR results can either be qualitative (e.g., the presence or absence of a sequence) or quantitative (e.g., copy number). RT-PCR is rapid, accurate with a high sensitivity and specificity, and feasible with small samples (e.g., fluids, direct smears, cytospins), which makes them useful to apply to cytology specimens. For example, RT-PCR was shown to be highly sensitive and 100% specific for the diagnosis of synovial sarcoma [12]. Limitations include poor nucleic acid quality, sampling errors, and cross contamination. In addition, cytological samples with scant viable cells, abundant necrosis, or cellular debris may fail testing.

FISH and RT-PCR are complementary, and sometimes both tests will be performed given the advantages of the different techniques. For example, FISH testing may be used initially with break-apart probes, given that they are more widely available and cost-effective. Then, if FISH is positive and there is a need to determine the particular partner gene, RT-PCR could be used to identify that partner gene and thereby provide relevant diagnostic and prognostic information.

12.2.3 Next-Generation Sequencing (NGS)

Next-generation sequencing (NGS) is also gaining popularity in solid tumors, including soft tissue sarcomas, due to its ability to screen for a multitude of different actionable biomarkers in very small tissue samples that may impact treatment choices with the numerous targeted therapies available. Recently, ion torrent sequencing was applied to a small series of patients with Ewing sarcoma and discovered some novel mutations in cancer-related genes, including some linked to targeted therapies, that may help in determining a personalized treatment plan for these patients [13]. Furthermore, NGS is also helping us to understand soft tissue tumors better, which may lead to improved diagnosis and developments of targeted therapies. One example is the detection of mutations in *p53* and *ATRX* (alpha-thalassemia/mental retardation X-linked) in 35% and 17% of leiomyosarcomas, respectively, based on NGS testing [14]. The advantages of NGS testing are that it can be performed on very small samples in a variety of different fixatives (e.g., fresh, nucleic acid preservatives, alcohol fixed, or formalin fixed) and has a very high sensitivity. The disadvantages include cases with inadequate preservation or insufficient cellularity, in addition to the requirement for a high complexity laboratory to perform the testing and the increased cost.

12.3   Handling and Triage of Cytology Specimens

There are some critical questions the cytopathologist has to be able to answer in the evaluation of a suspected soft tissue tumor. These questions include: Is the lesion benign or malignant? Is the lesion low grade or high grade? What is the tumor origin? Is an excisional biopsy or resection required for diagnosis or treatment? Is there sufficient material for ancillary studies? What ancillary studies should be ordered?

The cytologic features of some soft tissue tumors have been well documented [6, 7, 15], but in a subset of cases, core biopsies or tissue blocks might be obtained for proper evaluation (e.g., tumor differentiation, necrosis, and mitosis) [16, 17]. In bone and soft tissue cytology, which includes both adult and pediatric patients, in addition to FNAs and touch preparations, on-site evaluation can be helpful for the appropriate real-time triage of the case and lead to more accurate diagnoses [6, 7, 15–20]. On initial inspection of the aspirates, the overall cellularity is important to determine adequacy, as hypocellular or bloody specimens are typically nondiagnostic or inadequate for morphological diagnosis and ancillary studies. An exception to this rule of thumb would include hypocellular, cystic lesions like ganglion or synovial cysts, which typically yield thick proteinaceous fluid without significant cellularity but truly explain a mass lesion (Fig. 12.1). Then, under high-power magnification, the relationship of the cells (e.g., cohesive or discohesive), shape of the cells (e.g., round or spindle), and background material (e.g., myxoid or necrotic) can help in formulating a differential diagnosis (Table 12.3). Based on the differential diagnosis, the aspirate material can be triaged for microbial cultures if infectious and immunostains and FISH studies if neoplastic, in addition to flow cytometry if suspicious for a lymphoid neoplasm. Cytology is fortunate in that there are multiple different types of cellular preparations that can be used for immunostains and FISH studies, if properly validated. This includes unstained aspirate smears, cytospins, liquid-based cytology preparations, and cell block sections. The choice of material depends on what is available and what yields the optimal cellularity. In some settings, a cell block may be insufficient, so extra aspirate smears prepared from the best pass may be helpful in order to ensure sufficient material for FISH studies without the dilutional effect seen with the cell block prepared from the needle rinse in multiple passes [6, 18]. In other scenarios, particularly in soft tissue and bone lesions with suboptimal cellularity at on-site assessment, a core biopsy may be helpful in obtaining tissue.

When evaluating the aspirates or touch preparations, it is also important for the cytopathologist to be able to morphologically categorize the findings in an FNA into a broad category based on morphological pattern and then to generate a differential diagnosis and appropriately triage the aspirates to obtain a complete and definitive diagnosis. A summary of the main differential diagnosis for different morphological patterns and the associated molecular abnormalities are summarized in Table 12.3. This is a constantly changing list, as new molecular genetic research and next-generation sequencing discover novel genetic abnormalities and lead to the discovery of distinct neoplasms.

A soft tissue lesion sampled by FNA or core biopsy is affected by similar issues. Some of the problems with cytological specimens and small biopsies include the issue of nondiagnostic or insufficient samples and the fact that the small sample may not be entirely representative. Furthermore, accurate subtyping and

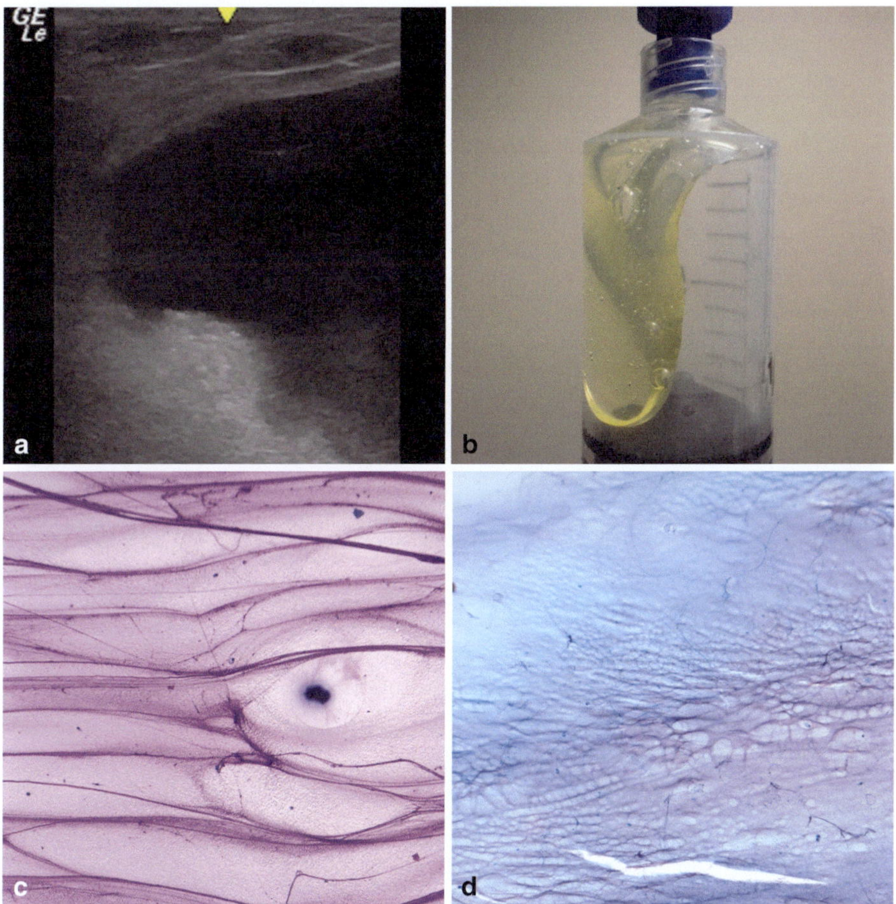

Fig. 12.1 FNA cytology of ganglion cyst. (**a**) Ultrasound image showing an anechoic rounded mass with posterior acoustic enhancement, which is typical for cystic lesions. (**b**) Aspirates from the mass were thick and gelatinous on gross inspection in the syringe. (**c**, **d**) The aspirate slides revealed abundant proteinaceous fluid with rare bland-appearing cells (**c** DQ stain, low power; **d** Pap stain, low power)

classification can be challenging in FNA specimens. In articles looking at the ability of FNA and core needle biopsies to accurately grade soft tissue tumors, only about 70% were accurately graded as high grade or low grade when the small biopsy was compared to the resection, and most of the underestimated grading on small biopsies occurred with lipogenic tumors given heterogeneity and sampling issues [16, 17]. In addition, grading is typically more accurate for high-grade or malignant tumors than for low-grade tumors on small samples [17]. However, both FNA and image-guided core needle biopsies are advantageous in that they alleviate the need for an open excisional biopsy under anesthesia and may enhance operative planning for resectable tumors after the biopsy and ancillary studies are complete [6, 17].

Table 12.3 Pattern-based approach to soft tissue cytomorphology highlighting entities with characteristic molecular findings

a. "Small" round blue cell tumors

Tumor	Translocation/other	Fusion genes/other
Alveolar rhabdomyosarcoma	t(2;13)(q35;q14)	*PAX3-FKHR*
Embryonal rhabdomyosarcoma	LOH at the 11p15 locus of the *IGF2* gene 1p deletion	*IGF2 gene*
Ewing sarcoma/PNET	t(11;22)(q24;q12)	*EWSR1-FLI1*
Desmoplastic small round cell tumor	t(11;22)(p13;q12)	*EWSR1-WT1*
Undifferentiated round cell sarcoma	t(4;19)(q35;q13) t(10;19)(q26;q13)	*CIC-DUX4*
Malignant lymphoma	B-cell or T-cell gene rearrangements or characteristic translocations	*IgH gene rearrangements* *TCR gene rearrangements*

b. Epithelioid cell neoplasms

Tumor	Translocation/other	Fusion genes/other
Epithelioid sarcoma	22q11.2 anomalies	*SMARCB1*
Alveolar soft part sarcoma	der(17)t(X;17)(p11;q25)	*ASPSCR1-TFE3*

c. Spindle cell neoplasms

Tumor	Translocation/other	Fusion genes/other
Inflammatory myofibroblastic tumor	t(1;2)(q22;p23)	*TPM3-ALK*
Giant cell fibroblastoma/dermatofibrosarcoma protuberans	t(17,22)(q21.3;q13)	*COL1A1-PDGFB*
Congenital/infantile fibrosarcoma	t(12;15)(p13;q25)	*ETV6-NTRK3*
Synovial sarcoma	t(X;18)(p11.2;q11.2)	*SS18-SSX1* *SS18-SSX2*
Extraskeletal mesenchymal chondrosarcoma	inv(8)(q13q21)	*HEY1-NCOA2*
Solitary fibrous tumor	12q13 rearrangements	*NAB2-STAT6*
Low-grade fibromyxoid sarcoma/sclerosing epithelioid fibrosarcoma	t(7;16)(q33;p11) t(11;16)(p11;p11)/MUC4 immunohistochemical stain positive	*FUS-CREB3L2* *FUS-CREB3L1*
Myxoinflammatory fibroblastic sarcoma/atypical myxoinflammatory fibroblastic tumor	t(1;10)(p22;q24)	*TGFBR3-MGEA5*

d. Myxoid neoplasms

Tumor	Translocation/other	Fusion genes/other
Nodular fasciitis	t(17;22)(p13;q13.1)	*MYH9-USP6*
Lipoblastoma	8q11-13 rearrangements	*PLAG1*
Myxoid liposarcoma	t(12;16) (q13;p11) t(12;22)(q13;p11)	*FUS-DDIT3* *EWSR1-DDIT3*
Extraskeletal myxoid chondrosarcoma	t(9;22)(q22;q12)	*EWSR1-NR4A3*

Table 12.3 (continued)

e. Adipocytic neoplasms

Tumor	Translocation/other	Fusion genes/other
Lipoblastoma	8q11-13 rearrangements	*PLAG1*
Myxoid liposarcoma	t(12;16) (q13;p11) t(12;22)(q13;p11)	*FUS-DDIT3* *EWSR1-DDIT3*
Dedifferentiated liposarcoma	Chromosome 12 amplifications	*MDM2*

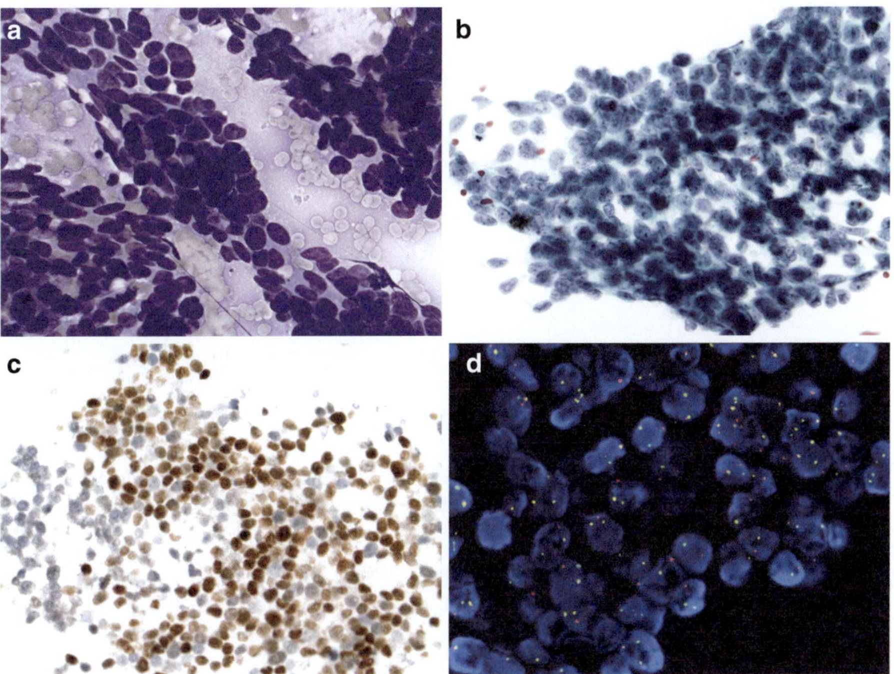

Fig. 12.2 Alveolar rhabdomyosarcoma. (**a**, **b**) Cytomorphology of small round blue cell tumor showing some alveolar type spaces (**a** DQ stain, high power; **b** Pap stain, high power). (**c**) Immunostaining for myogenin performed on the cell block material is positive. (**d**) FISH studies confirming a *FKHR* gene rearrangement using the *FKHR* break-apart probe

12.4 Summary of Molecular Alterations in Different Morphological Patterns of Soft Tissue Tumors

12.4.1 Small Round Blue Cell Tumors

Small round cell tumors are neoplasms composed of hyperchromatic, small-to-intermediate-sized round cells that are slightly larger than the size of lymphocytes. They include sarcomas, such as alveolar rhabdomyosarcoma, embryonal rhabdomyosarcoma, Ewing sarcoma/PNET, desmoplastic small round cell

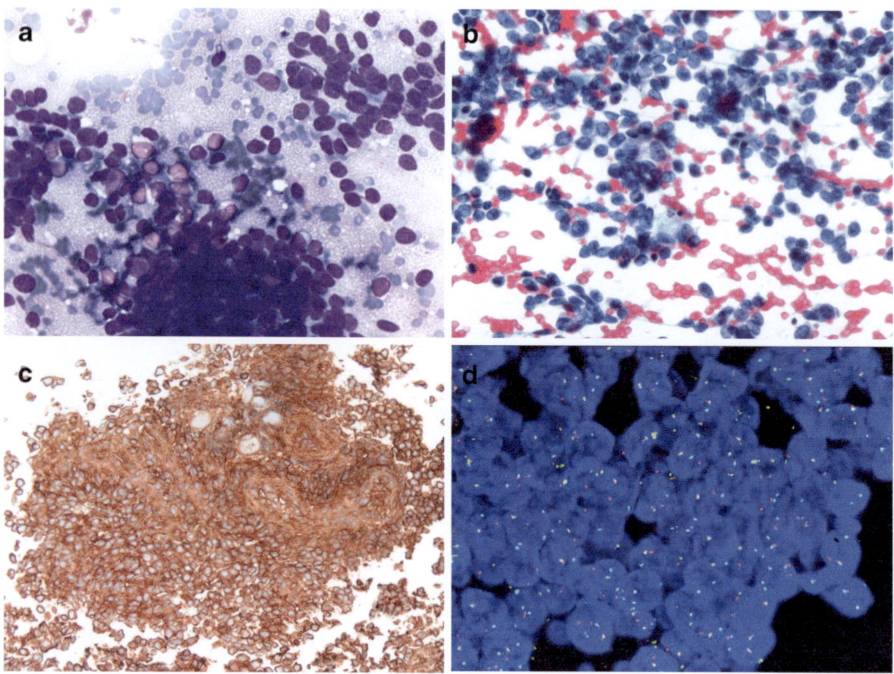

Fig. 12.3 Ewing sarcoma. (**a**, **b**) Aspirate smears show a small round blue cell tumor with light and dark cells, in addition to a tigroid background on the Diff-Quik-stained smears (**a** DQ stain, high power; **b** Pap stain, high power). (**c**) CD99 positivity in tumor cells on the cell block. (**d**) FISH showing an *EWS* gene rearrangement with the break apart probe for *EWSR1* on chromosome 22

tumor, and undifferentiated round cell sarcoma (Figs. 12.2 and 12.3). The non-sarcomatous tumors in this category include lymphoma, neuroblastoma, meta-static small cell carcinoma, and Merkel cell carcinoma. Morphological features, in conjunction with ancillary techniques, can usually subtype these small round blue cell tumors. However, in a subset of cases, a definitive diagnosis may not be possible due to technical difficulties (e.g., inadequate sampling), lack of characteristic phenotypic or molecular profile, or lack of material (e.g., insuffi-cient fresh tissue for flow cytometry). In addition, one should remember benign mimics of small round blue cell malignancies, such as pilomatricoma (Fig. 12.4).

12.4.1.1 Rhabdomyosarcoma

Rhabdomyosarcoma is the most common pediatric sarcoma [21, 22]. The inter-national classification of rhabdomyosarcomas subdivides these sarcomas into five types with different clinical behaviors: embryonal, spindle, embryonal bot-ryoid, alveolar, mixed alveolar/embryonal, and rhabdomyosarcoma, not other-wise specified or sarcoma, not otherwise specified [23]. This chapter will only review the alveolar and embryonal type, sometimes referred to as *FKHR* fusion-positive or *FKHR* fusion-negative cases, respectively.

Fig. 12.4 Pitfall of small round blue cell tumors. (**a**, **b**) Pilomatricomas can morphologically resemble small round blue cell malignancies, but in addition to the basaloid cells, there should also be ghost cells and multinucleated giant cells. On cell block, tissue fragments can show the abrupt keratinization in these lesions as well (**a** DQ stain, high power; **b** H&E stain, low power)

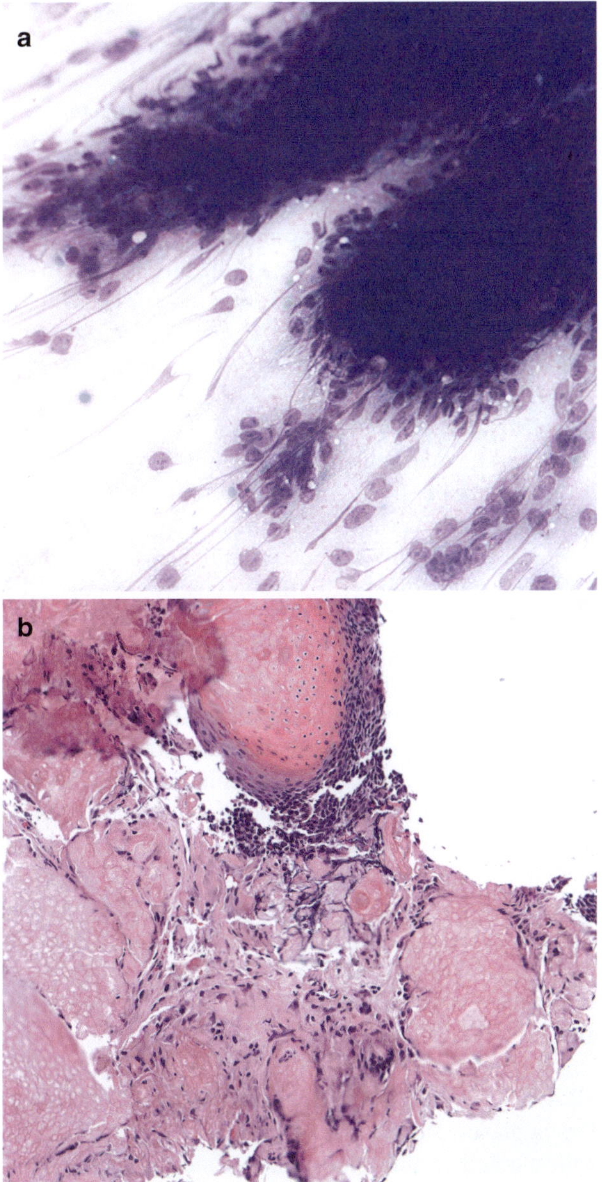

Alveolar Rhabdomyosarcoma

Alveolar rhabdomyosarcoma (ARMS) occurs at all ages but is most often seen in adolescents and young adults. It typically involves the extremities, trunk, and head and neck region. Cytological findings include cellular smears with apoptotic bodies in the background and lack of lymphoglandular bodies. The cells are arranged in loose clusters of uniform small round blue cells with fine chromatin, inconspicuous nucleoli, and vacuolated cytoplasm. Occasional spaces can be seen in the larger clusters on cytological aspirates due to the alveolar pattern (Fig. 12.2). There can be a variable number of rhabdomyoblasts and occasional multinucleated tumor giant cells with wreath-like nuclei [24, 25]. Genetic studies usually demonstrate a t(2;13) (q35;q14) resulting in the *PAX3-FKHR* gene fusion in 70% of cases and a t(1;13) (p36;q14) resulting in *PAX7-FKHR* in 10–20% of cases (Fig. 12.2d).

Embryonal Rhabdomyosarcoma

Embryonal rhabdomyosarcoma is the most common subtype of rhabdomyosarcoma in children [21, 22]. The most common affected sites are the head and neck region and the genitourinary system. Aspirates are cellular and composed of primitive round to larger rhabdomyoblastic cells. Binucleated, multinucleated (strap cells), "tadpole," or "racket cells" can be seen. The cells have fine granular chromatin and cytoplasmic vacuoles [25]. Cytogenetic analyses do not show recurrent structural chromosome rearrangements, which is helpful and can be important in distinguishing these tumors from ARMS, given that the treatment can vary and there can be morphological overlap. In fact, some suggest that if you have a RMS in a child, the most important feature in determining treatment is the presence or absence of the *FKHR* rearrangement (e.g., fusion positive or negative).

12.4.1.2   Ewing Sarcoma/PNET

Ewing sarcoma/PNET is a small round cell tumor accounting for 6–8% of primary malignant bone tumor and typically affects children and young adults [1]. It present as a rapidly enlarging mass. Pain is the most common clinical symptom. The smears are highly cellular and show discohesive or loose cluster of monomorphic small round cells. A dimorphic population of tumor cells is characteristic, smaller, and darker cells mixed with lighter cells. The lighter cells have pale chromatin and small nucleoli, while the darker cells have condensed chromatin and scarce cytoplasm. Nuclear molding can be prominent (Fig. 12.3). Occasionally, rosettes and tigroid background can be seen, particularly on air-dried Romanowsky stained preparations [26]. Approximately 90% of cases harbor a t(11;22)(q24;q12) rearrangement resulting in the fusion between *EWSR1* and *FLI1*; however, alternative rearrangements also exist (Fig. 12.3d).

12.4.1.3   Desmoplastic Small Round Cell Tumor

Desmoplastic small round cell tumor is a malignant soft tissue tumor associated with marked stromal desmoplasia and polyphenotypic profile. It typically affects children and young adults. Most tumors arise in the abdominal cavity [1]. The smears are variably cellular and composed of single or loose clusters of round cells with high N/C ratio. The nuclei have irregular membrane clefts and finely granular chromatin. The cytoplasm is usually scant. The background displays fragments of hypervascular desmoplastic stroma [27, 28]. Immunohistochemical staining shows positive dot-like staining for desmin and positive staining for cytokeratin, vimentin, NSE, and WT1.

Genetic studies reveal a t(11;22)(p13;q12) resulting the gene fusion *EWS-WT1*.

12.4.2 Epithelioid Neoplasms

Epithelioid soft tissue neoplasms are characterized by large, round to polygonal cells with moderate to abundant cytoplasm.

12.4.2.1 Epithelioid Sarcoma

Epithelioid sarcoma is a rare soft tissue tumor that typically occurs in the distal extremities of young adults as a slow-growing nodule within the dermis and subcutis or in the deep soft tissues. Two clinicopathological subtypes are recognized: the classic "distal" form (distal extremities) and the proximal type (trunk). Cytological smears are variably cellular and composed of discohesive cells with occasional loose clusters. The cells are round with large eccentric nuclei with mild to moderate nuclear pleomorphism and prominent nucleoli. There are well-delineated cytoplasmic borders with moderate to abundant dense cytoplasm [29]. Loss of nuclear staining for INI1 occurs in both subtypes and can be helpful as a clue. The loss of INI1 nuclear staining is related to the chromosome 22 deletions seen in the *SMARCB1* gene. Although loss of staining for INI1 is helpful, it can be seen in other tumors, including extrarenal rhabdoid tumors, myoepithelial carcinomas, and other tumors. Cytogenetic studies do not show recurrent structural chromosome rearrangements. However, there are frequently chromosome 22 deletions in the *SMARCB1* gene, which is located near the *EWSR1* gene, and may therefore show *EWSR1* gene abnormalities by FISH [11].

12.4.2.2 Alveolar Soft Part Sarcoma

Alveolar soft part sarcoma is a slow-growing painless soft tissue tumor most commonly seen in between ages 15 and 35 years [1]. It involves in the majority of cases the deep soft tissue of the lower extremities in adults and the head and neck region in children. Cytological findings are low to moderate cellularity composed of sheets or single large cells with a vague acinar arrangement. The cells have markedly enlarged nuclei/nucleoli. Numerous bare nuclei are seen in the background.

The cytoplasm is finely granular and vacuolated. Nuclear pseudo inclusions and extracellular crystalloids are occasionally noted. Genetic studies demonstrate a t(X;17)(p11;q25) resulting in the *ASPSCR1-TFE3* fusion gene [30].

12.4.3 Spindle Cell Neoplasms

Cytological diagnosis of spindle cell tumors is challenging due to the difficulty in distinguishing benign and malignant tumors. The presence of high cellularity, dispersed cells, necrosis, and increased mitotic activity would favor a malignant lesion. However, for definitive answers to the question of benign versus malignant, low grade versus high grade, and tumor line of differentiation, ancillary techniques are usually needed.

12.4.3.1 Inflammatory Myofibroblastic Tumor

Inflammatory myofibroblastic tumor is a rare spindle cell neoplasm of children and young adults primarily involving soft tissue and viscera. It is composed of myofibroblastic and fibroblastic cells associated with an inflammatory infiltrate.

The smears are mildly to moderately cellular with bland, uniform oval-to-spindle cells intermixed with inflammatory cells (plasma cells, lymphocytes, and/or eosinophils). The cells are plump with oval or bipolar nuclei with vesicular chromatin. The cytoplasm is slightly dense and amphophilic with tapered ends [31]. The immunohistochemical stain for ALK is positive in tumor cells (cytoplasmic). Genetic studies in children and young adults show a t(1;2)(q22;p23) resulting in the *TPM3-ALK* fusion gene.

12.4.3.2 Giant Cell Fibroblastoma/Dermatofibrosarcoma Protuberans

Giant cell fibroblastoma/dermatofibrosarcoma protuberans are locally aggressive superficial low-grade soft tissue tumors. Giant cell fibroblastoma is a variant of dermatofibrosarcoma protuberans that primarily affects children and is characterized by multinucleated giant cells and pseudovascular channels.

The cytological smears are moderately cellular and composed of mononuclear oval-to-spindle cells. Occasional floret-like giant cells can be noted. The nuclei are vesicular with minimal cytological atypia. The background contains fragments of dense metachromatic stroma [32] (Fig. 12.5). By immunohistochemical staining, the tumor cells are positive for CD34. They are cytogenetically characterized by a t(17,22)(q21.3;q13) resulting in the *COL1A1-PDGFB* fusion gene.

12.4.3.3 Congenital/Infantile Fibrosarcoma

Congenital/infantile fibrosarcoma is a soft tissue tumor usually found in children less than 1 year of age [1]. It presents as a rapidly enlarging mass most often seen in the distal extremities. Cytological examination demonstrates cellular smears with loose cluster of spindle cells with elongated nuclei and evenly distributed chromatin [33]. Genetic studies demonstrate a t(12;15)(p13;q25) resulting in the *ETV6-NTRK3* fusion gene, which has also been seen in a subset of secretory carcinomas of the breast, mammary analog secretory carcinoma of the salivary gland, and some leukemias.

12.4.3.4 Synovial Sarcoma

Synovial sarcoma is a mesenchymal tumor typically found in adolescents and young adults. It variably displays epithelial differentiation. Every location on the body can be involved, but most tumors arise in the deep soft tissue of the lower and upper extremities [1]. By histology it can be monophasic, biphasic, or poorly differentiated.

The smears are cellular and show clusters, branching tissue fragments, and discohesive cells. The cells are small to medium sized and spindle shaped. The nuclei are ovoid, round to fusiform with bland chromatin [34, 35]. The biphasic form can show occasional acinar arrangement. Immunohistochemical staining reveals tumor cells staining positive for bcl2, CD99, vimentin, AE1/ AE3 cytokeratin, EMA, and

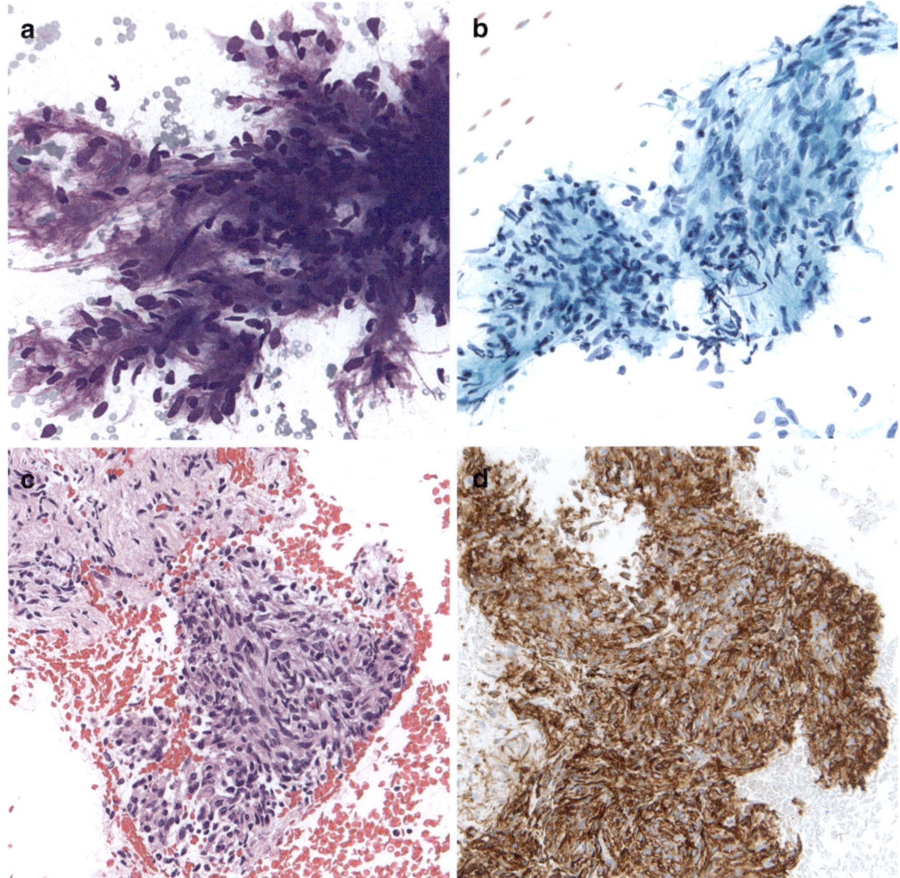

Fig. 12.5 Dermatofibrosarcoma protuberans (DFSP) in a young patient with a superficial soft tissue mass. (**a–c**) Aspirates in these lesions will typically show cellular spindle cell lesions with a background of fibrillary or metachromatic material that appears eosinophilic on cell block (**a** DQ stain, high power; **b** Pap stain, high power; **c** H&E stain, medium power). (**d**) CD34 immunostaining is positive in these tumors

TLE1. Genetically the lesions have a specific t(X;18)(p11.2;q11.2) leading to the formation of a *SS18-SSX* fusion gene (Fig. 12.6).

12.4.3.5 Spindle Cell Melanoma

The possibility of melanoma should also be considered when a spindle cell neoplasm is seen in cytology. This is the reason that most immunohistochemistry panels for spindle cell neoplasms include melanoma markers, such as S100 protein, MelanA, and SOX10. HMB45 can be negative in these tumors. In addition, a pitfall is that S100 protein and SOX10 will also be positive in neurogenic tumors, such as schwannoma. Morphologically, spindle cell melanomas are cellular but can be quite bland without the obvious binucleation, prominent nucleoli, and intranuclear inclusions

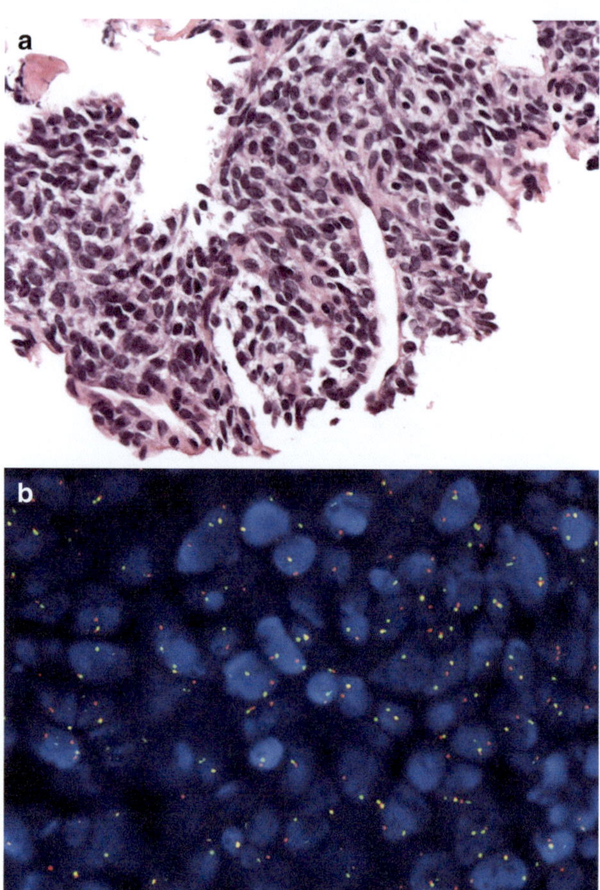

Fig. 12.6 Synovial sarcoma. (a) FNA showing a cellular spindle cell neoplasm with nuclear atypia that was positive for EMA, CD99, TLE3, and bcl2. (b) FISH studies confirmed an *SS18 or SYT* gene rearrangement using a chromosome 18q11.2 break-apart probe

seen with the epithelioid melanomas (Fig. 12.7). A diagnosis of melanoma is critical given that most FNAs are of metastatic lesions, which should undergo mutational testing for *BRAF* and *RAS* mutations given that they impact treatment.

12.4.4 Myxoid Neoplasms

Myxoid soft tissue tumors are mesenchymal lesions with a "myxoid" background, composed of mucopolysaccharide substances. They are a heterogeneous group composed of benign and malignant tumors. Cytologically, myxoid-type material is usually easy to identify on Romanowsky-stained slides.

12.4.4.1 Nodular Fasciitis

Nodular fasciitis is a self-limiting soft tissue lesion composed of undulating bundles of loosely arranged fibroblasts and myofibroblasts that display a culture-like growth pattern. The smears have moderate to high cellularity with a metachromic myxoid stroma in the background. The cells are arranged in a loosely cohesive to

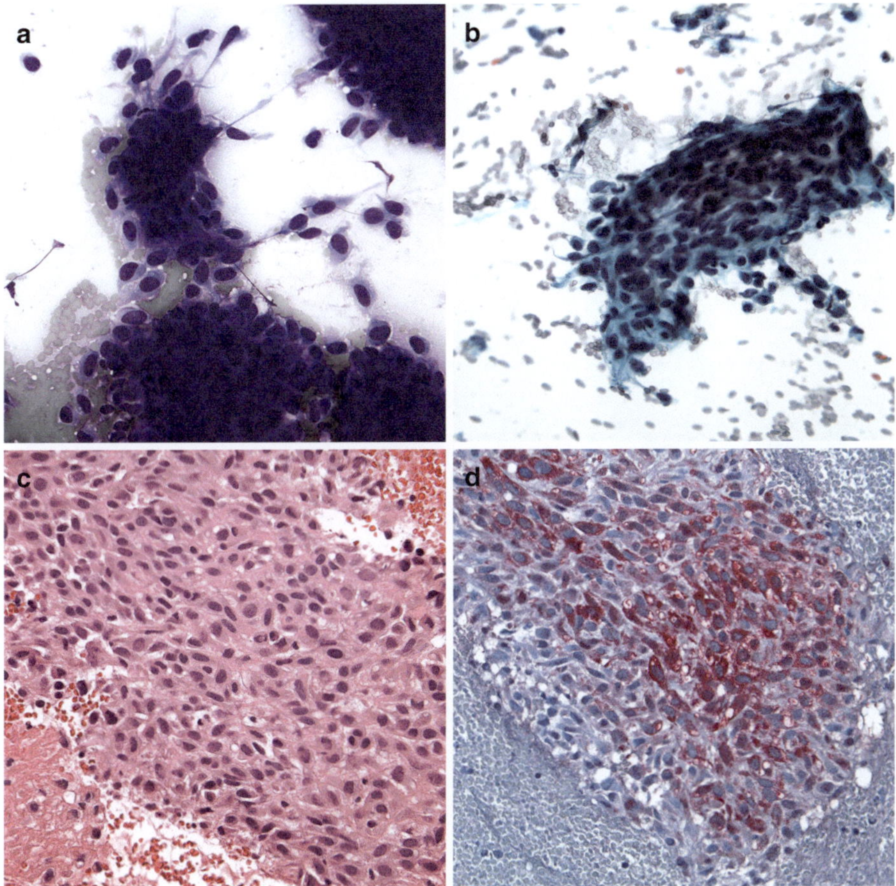

Fig. 12.7 Spindle cell melanoma. (**a–c**) The possibility of a melanoma should always be considered in a spindle cell neoplasm. The aspirates show a monotonous appearing spindle cell neoplasm with atypia but without pigment. The tumor cells lack the characteristic features seen in epithelioid melanomas (**a** DQ stain, high power; **b** Pap stain, high power; **c** H&E stain, medium power). (**d**) S100 protein staining on the cell block is positive, confirming the diagnosis. These cases should be sent for *BRAF* mutational testing in the metastatic setting

cohesive manner. Individual tumor cell are oval-to-spindle shaped and bland looking; however, the presence of mitoses can be alarming and lead to an overdiagnosis of sarcoma. Inflammatory cells (neutrophils, lymphocytes, histiocytes, multinucleated giant cells, and occasionally eosinophils) are also present in the background (Fig. 12.8). The t(17;22)(p13;q13.1) resulting in *MYH9-USP6* gene fusion is a recurrent event, and there is a FISH probe commercially available for *USP6* [36].

12.4.4.2   Extraskeletal Myxoid Chondrosarcomas

Extraskeletal myxoid chondrosarcomas is believed to be an intermediate-grade soft tissue tumor with high rate of recurrence and metastasis. These lesions affect young adults and often arise from the extremities [1]. The smears are paucicellular to

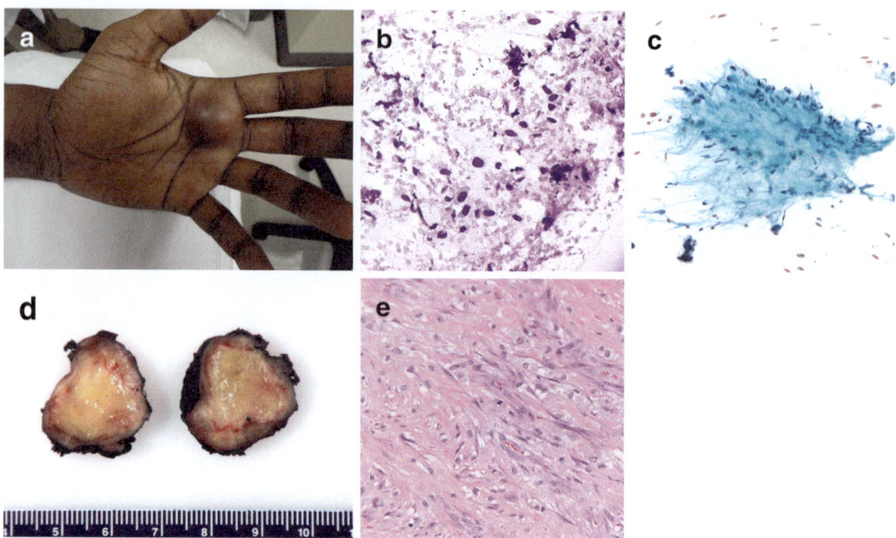

Fig. 12.8 Nodular fasciitis on the palmar surface of the hand in a young chef. (**a**) Clinical image of the patient's hand with the mass, prior to FNA biopsy. (**b**, **c**) Aspirates show mild-to-moderate cellularity with bland-appearing cells that have oval-to-round nuclei within a background with some myxocollagenous material (**b** DQ stain, high power; **c** Pap stain, high power). (**d**) Surgical excision of the lesion showing a gelatinous soft tissue lesion that is relatively well circumscribed. (**e**) Histology of the lesion showing a moderately cellular spindle cell lesions with mitosis (central) and a collagenous type background with scattered inflammatory cells (**e** H&E stain, high power)

cellular smears with a bright magenta fibrillary stroma. The tumor cells have a cord and lacelike arrangement and are embedded in background matrix. The cells are bland, uniform, fusiform, and round to oval. The nuclei have fine granular chromatin with small prominent nucleoli [38]. The genetic hallmark is a t(9;22)(q22;q12) resulting in the *EWSR1-NR4A3* gene fusion.

12.4.5 Adipocytic Neoplasms

Adipocytic neoplasms are mesenchymal lesions with lipogenic differentiation. This group includes very common lesions like benign lipomas to highly malignant lesions like pleomorphic liposarcomas. One of the most helpful FISH studies in these tumors is the *MDM2* amplification test, which can help to solidify a diagnosis of a dedifferentiated liposarcoma that can mimic other pleomorphic spindle cell neoplasms (Fig. 12.9) [37, 39, 40].

12.4.5.1 Myxoid Liposarcoma

Myxoid liposarcoma (MLPS) is a subtype of liposarcoma most commonly affecting young adults and usually located in the deep soft tissue of the extremities (e.g., the thigh). Cytological examination demonstrates cellular smears with single cells and/

Fig. 12.9 Dedifferentiated liposarcoma with *MDM2* amplification. (**a**) FNA cytology in dedifferentiated liposarcoma will show moderately cellular aspirates with pleomorphic spindle cells. Definitive lipoblasts are often not seen (**a** DQ stain, high power). (**b**) FISH studies confirm the presence of an *MDM2* gene amplification, which can help confirm that the tumor is a dedifferentiated liposarcoma, opposed to another high-grade sarcoma

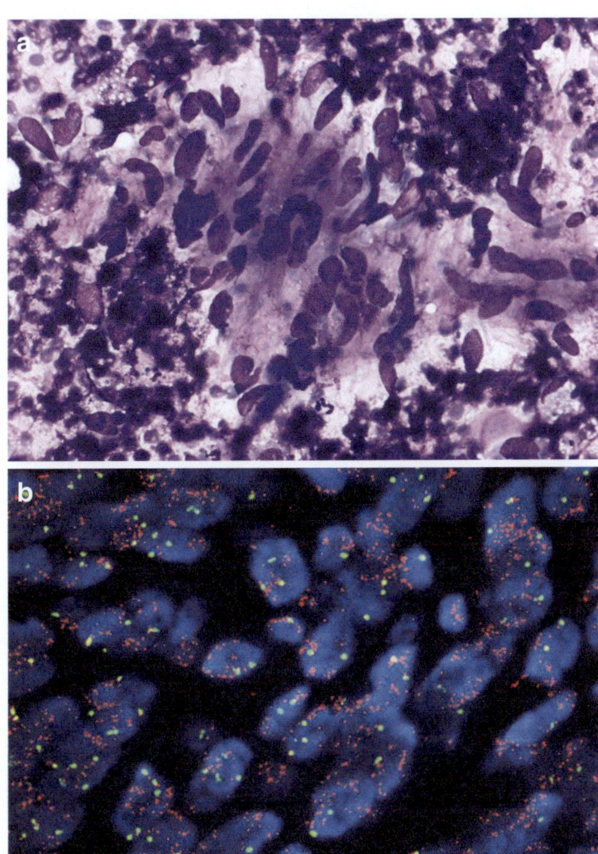

or cells clusters. The background reveals branching, delicate thin-walled capillaries in myxoid stroma, and thus, the presence of increased vascularity in myxoid material should raise suspicion for MLPS (Fig. 12.10). Lipoblasts in various stages of differentiation (small round cells to well-differentiated lipoblasts) are easily noted. Uniform, round, small tumor cells with occasional lipid vacuoles (round cell component) can also be present [40]. Genetic studies demonstrate the rearrangement t(12;16) (q13;p11) *FUS-DDIT3* (Fig. 12.10c).

12.4.6 Pediatric Soft Tissue Neoplasms

The diagnostic approach to soft tissue tumors arising in the pediatric population are similar to that involving adult patients, whereby a small biopsy or FNA can help in the preoperative setting to determine the appropriate management. This is particularly important in pediatrics given that there is a high level of anxiety for young patients and

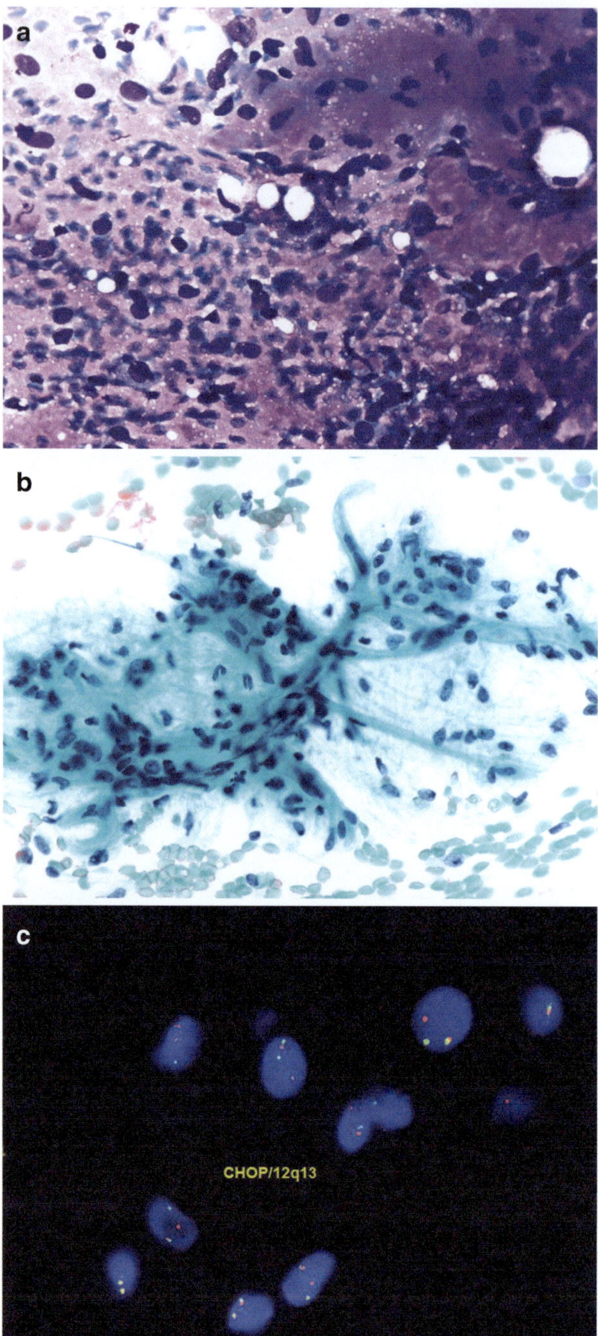

Fig. 12.10 Myxoid liposarcoma. (**a**, **b**) Aspirates show paucicellular myxoid material with increased thin-walled chicken-wire type vasculature (**a** DQ stain, high power; **b** Pap stain, high power). (**c**) FISH testing confirmed the presence of a chromosome 12 gene rearrangement, which is typical for these tumors

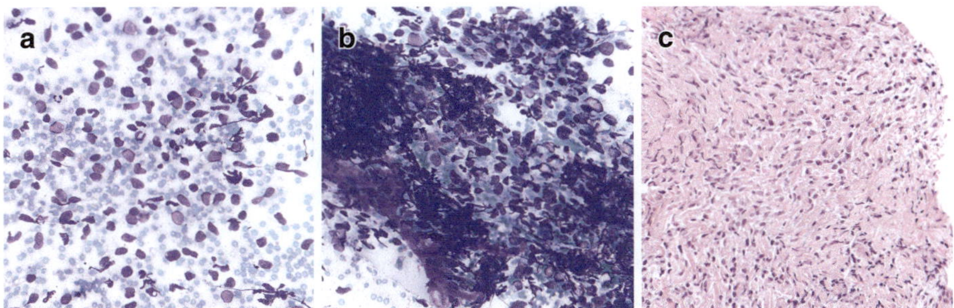

Fig. 12.11 Cytology and core biopsy of small cell osteosarcoma in a 15-year-old boy. (**a**, **b**) The cytological findings show features of a small round blue cell tumor with some nuclear pleomorphism and rare metachromatic material that appears more dense than typical myxoid material (**a**, **b** DQ stain, high power). Histological features of the core biopsy include areas of tumor cells with eosinophilic osteoid matrix, confirming the diagnosis of an osteosarcoma (**c** H&E stain, medium power). FISH studies for *EWS* and *SS18* were negative in this case, excluding a Ewing sarcoma and synovial sarcoma, respectively

their families when a mass lesion is identified. In addition, when planning the approach to biopsying these lesions, the patient age and maturity is crucial in order to determine if the biopsy can be safely done without sedation or anesthesia, as many young children may have difficulty sitting still for an FNA biopsy, necessitating immobilization devices (e.g., papoose), sedation, or general anesthesia [19]. In the United States, FNA biopsy is typically used more often for benign, superficial pediatric lesions (e.g., reactive lymph nodes), opposed to malignant lesions due to the need for histological sampling for many tumors in order for children to be candidates for clinical trials or oncology groups. This differs from other countries that use FNA biopsy for first-line diagnoses of tumors, leading to potential neoadjuvant treatment prior to surgery [20].

On the interpretation side, pediatric soft tissue lesions conjure up a slightly different differential diagnosis than in the adult population, as small round blue cell tumors will outnumber other morphological patterns and certain tumors will be more common than in adults (e.g., neuroblastoma). Furthermore, some tumors that we don't typically consider in a small round blue cell tumor differential can have a small round blue cell pattern in rare subtypes, which makes cytogenetic studies important. An example is a challenging case of a young patient with a bone lesion, showing a small cell variant of osteosarcoma, where negative *EWS* gene rearrangement studies and a core biopsy showing osteoid helped to solidify the diagnosis (Fig. 12.11). In addition, metastatic carcinomas and small B-cell lymphomas are very unlikely in young children, moving the differential diagnosis more toward either high-grade lymphomas or sarcomas. Overall, benign soft tissue tumors are more common than malignant soft tissue tumors (sarcomas) in both the adult and pediatric populations and can be treated with simple excision. This is why an accurate preoperative diagnosis is crucial in order to avoid more aggressive surgery and associated morbidity. In contrast, malignant nonlymphoid tumors usually require resection and a team-oriented, multidisciplinary treatment plan, whereas malignant lymphomas can be treated nonsurgically. Thus, accurate diagnosis of lymphoid tumors is crucial on small biopsies to spare young patients from unnecessary surgical excision.

12.5 Summary

Many bone and soft tissue tumors in adults and children are characterized by specific genetic abnormalities, and detection of these genetic changes with molecular techniques (FISH, RT-PCR, and NGS) can greatly enhance diagnostic accuracy. Understandably, there is a great need to obtain adequate material for proper patient evaluation. FNA procedures are safe and cost-effective in providing adequate samples for molecular studies; hence molecular pathology is nowadays an integral part of cytopathology in the evaluation of soft tissue tumors.

References

1. Fletcher K, Christopher DM. WHO classification of tumours of soft tissue and bone. Lyon: IARC; 2013.
2. Ducimetiere F, Lurkin A, Ranchere-Vince D, et al. Incidence of sarcoma histotypes and molecular subtypes in a prospective epidemiological study with central pathology review and molecular testing. PLoS One. 2011;6:e20294.
3. Mitelman F. Recurrent chromosome aberrations in cancer. Mutat Res. 2000;462:247–53.
4. Zhang S, Gong Y. From cytomorphology to molecular pathology: maximizing the value of cytology of lymphoproliferative disorders and soft tissue tumors. Am J Clin Pathol. 2013;140:454–67.
5. Dodd LG, Bedrossian CW. Sarcoma redux: past, present, and future. Diagn Cytopathol. 2012;40(Suppl 2):E81–5.
6. Khalbuss WE, Teot LA, Monaco SE. Diagnostic accuracy and limitations of fine-needle aspiration cytology of bone and soft tissue lesions. Cancer. 2010;118:24–32.
7. Layfield LJ, Anders KH, Glasgow BJ, Mitra JM. Fine-needle aspiration of primary soft tissue lesions. Arch Pathol Lab Med. 1986;110:420–4.
8. Taylor BS, Barretina J, Maki RG, Antonescu CR, Singer S, Ladanyi M. Advances in sarcoma genomics and new therapeutic targets. Nat Rev Cancer. 2011;11:541–57.
9. Lazar A, Abruzzo LV, Pollock RE, Lee S, Czerniak B. Molecular diagnosis of sarcomas: chromosomal translocations in sarcomas. Arch Pathol Lab Med. 2006;130:1199–207.
10. Romeo S, Dei Tos AP. Soft tissue tumors associated with EWSR1 translocation. Virchows Arch. 2010;456:219–34.
11. Huang SC, Zhang L, Sung YS, Chen CL, Kao YC, Agaram NP, Antonescu CR. Secondary EWSR1 gene abnormalities in SMARCB1-deficient tumors with 22q11-12 regional deletions: potential pitfalls in interpreting EWSR1 FISH results. Genes Chromosomes Cancer. 2016;55(10):767–76.
12. Guillou L, Coindre J, Gallagher G, Terrier P, Gebhard S, de Saint Aubain Somerhausen N, Michels J, Jundt G, Vince DR, Collin F, Trassard M, Le Doussal V, Benhattar J. Detection of the synovial sarcoma translocation t(X;18) (SYT;SSX) in paraffin-embedded tissues using reverse transcriptase-polymerase chain reaction: a reliable and powerful diagnostic tool for pathologists. A molecular analysis of 221 mesenchymal tumors fixed in different fixatives. Hum Pathol. 2001;32:105–12.
13. Zhang N, Liu H, Yue G, Zhang Y, You J, Wang H. Molecular heterogeneity of ewing sarcoma as detected by ion torrent sequencing. PLoS One. 2016;11:e0153546.
14. Yang CY, Liau JY, Huang WJ, Chang YT, Chang MC, Lee JC, Tsai JH, Su YN, Hung CC, Jeng YM. Targeted next-generation sequencing of cancer genes identified frequent TP53 and ATRX mutations in leiomyosarcoma. Am J Transl Res. 2015;7:2072–81.
15. Khalbuss WE, Parwani AV. Cytopathology of soft tissue and bone lesions. New York: Springer; 2011.

16. Lin X, Davion S, Bertsch EC, Omar I, Nayar R, Laskin WB. FNCLCC grading of soft tissue sarcomas on needle core biopsies using surrogate markers. Hum Pathol. 2016;56:147–54.
17. Kaur I, Handa U, Kundu R, Garg SK, Mohan H. Role of fine-needle aspiration cytology and core needle biopsy in diagnosing musculoskeletal neoplasms. J Cytol. 2016;33:7–12.
18. Monaco SE, Teot LA, Felgar RE, Surti U, Cai G. Fluorescence in situ hybridization studies on direct smears: an approach to enhance the fine-needle aspiration biopsy diagnosis of B-cell non-Hodgkin lymphomas. Cancer. 2009;117:338–48.
19. Khalbuss WE, Monaco SE, Pantanowitz L. Quick compendium of cytopathology. Chicago: ASCP Press; 2013. p. 576.
20. Monaco SE, Teot LA. Cytopathology of pediatric malignancies: where are we today with fine-needle aspiration biopsies inpediatric oncology? Cancer Cytopathol. 2014;122:322–36.
21. Pohar-Marinsek Z, Anzic J, Jereb B. Topical topic: value of fine needle aspiration biopsy in childhood rhabdomyosarcoma: twenty-six years of experience in Slovenia. Med Pediatr Oncol. 2002;38:416–20.
22. Klijanienko J, Caillaud JM, Orbach D, et al. Cyto-histological correlations in primary, recurrent and metastatic rhabdomyosarcoma: the Institut Curie experience. Diagn Cytopathol. 2007;35:482–7.
23. Parham DM. Pathologic classification of rhabdomyosarcomas and correlations with molecular studies. Mod Pathol. 2001;14:506–14.
24. Das K, Mirani N, Hameed M, Pliner L, Aisner SC. Fine-needle aspiration cytology of alveolar rhabdomyosarcoma utilizing ThinPrep® liquid-based sample and cytospin preparations: a case confirmed by FKHR break apart rearrangement by FISH probe. Diagn Cytopathol. 2006;34:704–6.
25. De Almeida M, Stastny JF, Wakely PE, Frable WJ. Fine-needle aspiration biopsy of childhood rhabdomyosarcoma: reevaluation of the cytologic criteria for diagnosis. Diagn Cytopathol. 1994;11:231–6.
26. Sanati S, Lu DW, Schmidt E, Perry A, Dehner LP, Pfeifer JD. Cytologic diagnosis of Ewing sarcoma/peripheral neuroectodermal tumor with paired prospective molecular genetic analysis. Cancer. 2007;111:192–9.
27. Ferlicot S, Coue O, Gilbert E, et al. Intraabdominal desmoplastic small round cell tumor: report of a case with fine needle aspiration, cytologic diagnosis and molecular confirmation. Acta Cytol. 2001;45:617–21.
28. Presley AE, Kong CS, Rowe DM, Atkins KA. Cytology of desmoplastic small round-cell tumor. Cancer. 2007;111:41–6.
29. Cardillo M, Zakowski MF, Lin O. Fine-needle aspiration of epithelioid sarcoma. Cancer. 2001;93:246–51.
30. Wakely PE Jr, McDermott JE, Ali SZ. Cytopathology of alveolar soft part sarcoma: a report of 10 cases. Cancer. 2009;117:500–7.
31. Stoll LM, Li QK. Cytology of fine-needle aspiration of inflammatory myofibroblastic tumor. Diagn Cytopathol. 2011;39:663–72.
32. Davis JL, Mathes E, Berry AB. FNA diagnosis of giant cell fibroblastoma: a case report of an unusual pediatric soft tissue tumor. Diagn Cytopathol. 2015;43:325–8.
33. Koss LG, Melamed MR, Koss LG. Chapter 35 soft tissue lesions. In: Koss' diagnostic cytology and its histopathologic bases. Philadelphia: Lippincott Williams & Wilkins; 2006. p. 1309.
34. Klijanienko J, Caillaud JM, Lagace R, et al. Cytohistologic correlations in 56 synovial sarcomas in 36 patients: the Institut Curie experience. Diagn Cytopathol. 2002;27:96–102.
35. Akerman M, Domanski HA. The complex cytological features of synovial sarcoma in fine needle aspirates, an analysis of four illustrative cases. Cytopathology. 2007;18:234–40.
36. Kong CS, Cha I. Nodular fasciitis: diagnosis by fine needle aspiration biopsy. Acta Cytol. 2004;48:473–7.
37. Dodd LG. Update on Liposarcoma: a review for cytopathologists. Diagn Cytopathol. 2012;40:1122–31.

38. Gaudier F, Khurana JS, Dewan S, Shen T. Fine-needle aspiration cytology of intra-abdominal wall extraskeletal myxoid chondrosarcoma: a case report and review of the literature. Arch Pathol Lab Med. 2003;127:1211–3.
39. Kloboves-Prevodnik VV, Us-Krasovec M, Gale N, Lamovec J. Cytological features of lipoblastoma: a report of three cases. Diagn Cytopathol. 2005;33:195–200.
40. Szadowska A, Lasota J. Fine needle aspiration cytology of myxoid liposarcoma; a study of 18 tumours. Cytopathology. 1993;4:99–106.

Molecular Cytology Applications in Metastases

13

Francisco Beca and Fernando C. Schmitt

13.1 Why Study Metastatic Disease?

Cancer is the second most common cause of death in the USA and in most of western countries, only to be exceeded by heart disease. Survival statistics vary greatly by cancer type and stage at diagnosis, but there has been a global improvement in survival reflecting both earlier diagnosis and improvements in treatment [1]. Still, in 2016, 595,690 patients are expected to die of cancer in the USA alone, and in Europe 1.75 million deaths from cancer were estimated in 2012 [1, 2]. Independently of the developed country or year considered, approximately 90% of cancer deaths were due to metastatic disease. With the exception of the tumors of the CNS, only rarely mortality is due to local invasion.

Historically, achieving locoregional control of cancer was the first milestone of cancer treatment achieved, followed by reduction of local relapse. Presently, in several cancer types, as breast and colon cancer, prevention of local relapse has been perfected. Successful treatments of these cancer types are measured in long intervals of time after diagnosis and only interrupted by the diagnosis of metastatic disease. More than ever, understanding the complexity of metastatic disease is essential. Advanced cancer treatment is rapidly evolving and focusing on prevention and control of metastatic disease. Cytopathology as a fundamental field of oncologic

F. Beca
Department of Pathology, Stanford University School of Medicine, Stanford, CA, USA

F. C. Schmitt (✉)
Department of Pathology, Medical Faculty of Porto University, Porto, Portugal

I3S, Instituto de Investigação e Inovação em Saúde, Universidade do Porto, Porto, Portugal

IPATIMUP, Institute of Molecular Pathology and Immunology of Porto University, Porto, Portugal
e-mail: fschmitt@ipatimup.pt

© Springer International Publishing AG, part of Springer Nature 2018
F. C. Schmitt (ed.), *Molecular Applications in Cytology*,
https://doi.org/10.1007/978-3-319-74942-6_13

pathology should logically follow to adapt to this new paradigm in cancer treatment.

Until recently, progression to metastatic disease has been viewed as linear process in which cancer cells pass through multiple successive rounds of mutation and selection for competitive fitness in the context of the primary tumor. These successive rounds of selection would then lead to cell clones with a more invasive and metastatic phenotype. After a number of such rounds, these tumor cell clones would expand and leave the primary site to seed secondary growths. As such, the development of metastasis was considered a late consequence of the evolution of the primary tumor and would be expected to recapitulate much of the genetic landscape of the primary tumor with the differences observed attributed to epigenetic regulation/variation induced by local selective pressures [3].

But for a number of decades now, this linear progression model has been challenged. The first evidence questioning the linear progression model was presented in studies comparing proliferation rate of the primary and the metastatic sites [4, 5]. According to these early studies, most of the observed metastases were simply too large to be initiated only at the late stages of primary tumor development. The alternative hypothesis the authors proposed was that given the metastases growth rate, the metastatic seeding would have to have occurred long before the first symptoms appeared (or the primary tumor was diagnosed). During the last decades, this alternative progression model has been gaining acceptance based on a growing body of supporting evidence [3, 6]. This model was named parallel progression, and the cornerstone of this progression model is that the metastatic potential/phenotype occurs in the early stages of the disease, in theory, even before diagnosis.

Independently of the model considered, tumor evolution occurs because of intrinsic and extrinsic selective pressures exerted. At each tumor location, and due to the different selective pressures, a unique complex clonal landscape can potentially develop (Fig. 13.1). This possibility leads to important clinical implications, being the most obvious that tumors will have differential and evolving responses to treatment. Examples from studies of breast cancer and colorectal cancer strongly support this possibility [7–9]. However, while this variability may be explained by the emergence of genomically distinct clones, most genomic profiling to date has relied on bulk tumor and therefore only reflects the broad mutational landscape of the majority of cells in the primary tumors [10]. Another consequence of relying on initial analyses of tumors is that evolutionary pathways are not monitored, which then leaves us unable to account for the emergence of different phenotypes with different therapeutic susceptibility during the course of the disease as a result of natural tumor progression and selective therapeutic pressures [11].

Despite the clinical challenges presented by tumor heterogeneity and evolution, this natural selection phenomenon can present significant opportunities. Clonal heterogeneity may be considered a "molecular phenotype" and used as a prognostic marker [12, 13]. Clonal diversity measures such as the Shannon diversity index, adapted from ecology and evolution, have been shown to predict progression to adenocarcinoma in patients with Barrett's esophagus and be associated with response to neoadjuvant breast cancer chemotherapy [14, 15]. Additionally, by constituting a source of variability, intratumor heterogeneity can lead to the emergence of targetable oncogenic alterations for which approved targeted therapies may

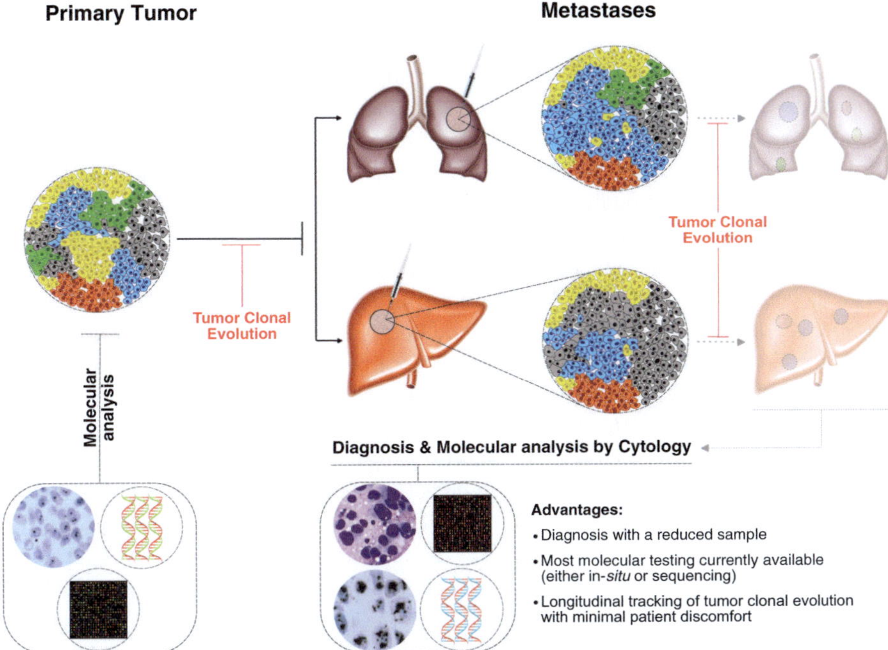

Fig. 13.1 Tumor evolution leads to a diverse clonal architecture. Due to the local selective pressures and therapy-induced selective pressure, metastases can display a diverse clonal architecture. This can lead to different phenotypes and resistance to therapy. By using cytopathology techniques as FNA combined with molecular techniques, it is possible to better understand the tumor landscape, and longitudinally track the complexity of metastatic foci, to make better therapeutic decisions

already exist, thus creating new therapeutic opportunities that did not exist or were not relevant at the time of initial diagnosis [16].

In summary, while the exact mechanisms on the origin metastatic disease are not yet well-understood, metastatic disease is the cause of death by cancer for a large majority of patients and therefore should be a priority for research and patient care. Intratumor heterogeneity and evolution are added challenges still mostly neglected when considering metastatic disease care, and we believe cytology can have a transformative role in pathology practice by simplifying the monitoring of metastatic disease. Over the next section of this chapter, we will explore some of the ancillary studies performed in metastatic disease using cytological samples and explore the modern role of cytology in metastatic disease monitoring and ultimately patient care.

13.2 Molecular Techniques Applied to Metastatic Disease Study

In the previous chapters of this book, molecular tests and applications in cytological material were discussed for a variety of cancer types and locations. In this section, we will highlight some of the most recent and thought-provoking studies performed focusing on metastatic disease and potentially of great impact in clinical practice in a near future.

Like what happened in the past with the application of immunohistochemistry, molecular techniques in routine pathological examination are changing practice paradigms. Cytological samples present several advantages with regards to performing ancillary molecular studies when comparing to FFPE samples, including the ability to check the quality/quantity of the sample immediately after harvesting and better preservation of DNA and RNA for archiving [17–19].

As discussed in detail in Chap. 3, a wide array of molecular techniques are nowadays successfully used in cytology ranging from PCR-based methods to massive parallel sequencing. Briefly, PCR-based methods can be used to detect chromosomal alterations such as deletions and translocations or point mutations in individual genes that are currently used in cytology for detecting gene mutations, for clonal gene rearrangements, and for the detection of viral sequences. Other techniques, such as in situ hybridization (ISH), with either fluorescent or chromogenic markers, have also been extensively applied in cytology to detect numerical or structural aberrations of chromosomes; in addition to its reliability, this technique is particularly useful for analyzing cytological material, as it can be applied to samples directly. ISH techniques are routinely used to detect gene amplifications, for example, of the HER2 gene in breast carcinoma or of NMYC in neuroblastomas [18]. These techniques can also be easily applied to cytological samples obtained from metastatic sites, allowing a comparison of the characteristics of these cells with those of the primary tumor. Other techniques as PCR or conventional comparative genomic hybridization have been used in combination with DNA extracted from cytological slides proving they can be successfully used in routine cytology specimens [20, 21].

More recently, sequencing techniques, mostly targeted sequencing, have been employed in many studies in cytology and are making its way to the clinical setting. To this, the advent of new nucleic acid extraction protocols as well as new sequencing platforms requiring reduced nucleic acid quantity requirements have contributed tremendously, allowing the use of cytological specimens for high-throughput analysis. Several recent studies have been published showing the feasibility of conducting next-generation sequencing, both targeted and whole-exome sequencing in cytological samples [22–26]. For this purpose, Shah et al. used effusion fluid samples from patients with high-grade serous ovarian carcinomas (HGSCs), whose frozen tumors had been previously extensively characterized as part of The Cancer Genome Atlas (TCGA) [25]. In this study, copy number variation (CNV) profiles were similar independently of the sample type, and for mutation profiling, smear samples had a better performance probably due to the higher tumor concentration in these cytological samples of ovarian HHSCs [25]. In fact, cytological samples are increasingly recognized as performing even better than FFPE samples for sequencing analysis, especially in defined clinical settings as the analysis of bone metastasis from lung and colon cancers and melanoma [26].

Another important step for both clinical care and oncologic pathology research was also taken by proving the feasibility of the use of archival cytological samples for both targeted and whole-exome sequencing (WES). Piqueret-Stephan et al. compared cytological material collected from archival smears processed for routine diagnosis, many of them from pleural and peritoneal effusions, with matched frozen samples [27]. Not only cytological samples proved to be a reliable source of nucleic acids for targeted sequencing but also WES and for SNP array-based analysis [27]. Importantly, by using archival cytological samples, this study unlocked the use of the cytological samples stored in pathological archives and previously processed and used for routine diagnostic, offering new opportunities for cytopathologists and oncologists.

In recent years, other types of nuclear acids and other DNA and messenger RNA (mRNA) have been investigated in cytological samples as microRNAs (miRNA). While quantification of miRNAs in FFPE samples is frequently challenging, due to the stability of miRNAs in fluids and the possibility of being quantified in very low amounts of sample material, cytological samples have proven to be the best source for routine miRNA quantification in the clinical setting. In fact many of today's commercially available mutational panels to use with cytological samples are based on miRNA analysis as the ThyraMIR™ and RosettaGX™ for thyroid lesions with other panels clamming clinical usefulness in frequently overlooked areas as small-cell lung cancer (SCLC) [28, 29]. As with miRNAs, lncRNAs seem to be highly tissue and phenotype specific, allowing accurate tumor type and subtype classification [30, 31]. As such, we also expect in the near future this (and other) type of RNAs will make their way into clinical applications coupled with cytology techniques.

Additional proof-of-principle and validation studies are also being taken to extend the use in molecular applications of cytological samples for both clinical and research applications. One curious recent application was the use of routine cytological techniques and samples to monitor in patient-derived 3D tumor organoids in vitro using WGS and for the use in functional studies, as pharmacologic screening and tumor drug resistance studies [32]. Other application in molecular cytopathology that currently is largely investigational, but showing great potential for more routine applications, is the characterization and establishment of patient-derived xenografts or PDXs. These mouse models are based on the transfer of primary tumors directly from the patient into a mouse and allow the growth of the tumor for deep characterization, evolutionary analysis, and multiple pharmacological screenings. Of course, this is only a possibility as many of the PDX models have shown to replicate much of the characteristics of the tumor in the human "host," namely, histology, gene expression profiles, and CNVs [33–35]. The transfer of tumors from the patient into a mouse is usually performed by obtaining fresh tumor tissue from surgery, at which point part of the tumor is mechanically or chemically digested, with a small portion saved as a primary stock, and established in a mouse. One major advance in a clinical PDX program would be the establishment of the tumor using FNA and/or effusion samples as it would present numerous advantages. With FNA and/or effusion samples, the sample handling would be less challenging as no digestion would be required, tumor purity could be promptly evaluated, and it would make the establishment of PDX models of tumor metastasis easier, which are potentially more useful to tailored therapeutic selection in the setting of progression and resistance.

In summary, the quantity and quality of nucleic acids extracted from cytological samples are usually adequate for modern protocols of molecular techniques, and it is frequently superior to traditional FFPE samples in sequencing studies, either targeted or WES. Newer sequencing technologies have also allowed an easier analysis of emerging nucleic acids in cytological samples. Finally, as newer molecular applications and models to study metastatic disease are emerging, as the generation of PDX models for clinical applications, we believe the role of cytology will continue to expand in both the research setting and the clinical management of metastatic cancer.

13.3 Role of Cytology in the Management of Metastatic Cancer

Presently the usefulness of molecular cytology applications on metastatic sites and disease is highly dependent on the existence of molecular classification systems and/or of molecularly targeted therapies that often depend on the identification of a distinct genomic abnormality; examples of these include (1) monoclonal antibodies (trastuzumab and cetuximab) in HER2-positive breast cancer and wild-type KRAS colorectal cancer; (2) tyrosine kinase inhibitors (TKIs) such as imatinib, gefitinib, or crizotinib in non-small-cell lung cancers; and (3) intracellular agents (as vemurafenib) in metastatic malignant melanoma. When only considering solid malignancies, five areas or organs/systems emerge as the most promising and important fields in which cytology combined with molecular assessment can be effectively applied [36]. These areas are metastatic breast, colorectal, lung, and ovarian carcinomas as well as metastatic melanoma.

Metastatic breast cancer (MBC) complexity is only now being understood. Recent data suggests that the molecular signature of each breast cancer is unique, even when compared with other breast cancers of the same molecular classification and more so if we also consider metastatic disease [37]. MBC is frequently diagnosed by combining clinical features, namely, medical history and imaging data. Once diagnosed, in MBC patients, the choice of systemic therapy is usually made based on the ER, PR, and HER2 status of the dominant clone in the primary tumor, often diagnosed several years before. Biopsy of suspected metastatic lesions is rarely undertaken, and repeated collection of biopsy tissue during the course of the disease is exceptional and presently reserved for an investigational setting. However, discrepancies between the pathology report for the primary tumor and for the metastatic lesions are as high as 30–40% for MBCs that are hormone receptor (ER and PR) positive and are up to 10% for HER2-overexpressing carcinomas [38–40]. More importantly, the discrepancies between primary tumor and metastatic biopsies have been shown to be responsible for a therapy regimen change in 14–20% of patients [38, 40]. Even if not considering more sophisticated therapeutic regimens, these results highlight the need for resampling metastasis in MBC [41]. We consider that in MBC the need for longitudinal sampling of metastatic disease will only increase as therapy becomes more personalized and concepts as tumor clonal evolution are translated to the therapeutic regimens/schemes [42].

In metastatic colorectal carcinomas, KRAS gene mutations in patients with metastatic colorectal cancer are possible molecular diagnostic markers that predict sensitivity to anti-EGFR therapeutics [43]. Anti-EGFR agents, as cetuximab and panitumumab in combination with conventional chemotherapy, are effective in colorectal cancer [44, 45]. However, sensitivity to these agents is highly dependable on KRAS mutation status with a significant percentage of primarily KRAS-WT patients not responding at some point [46, 47]. One of the reasons for this fact is the discrepancy in KRAS mutation status between the primary tumor and the metastasis. In a study of 250 patients with sporadic colorectal cancer, a discrepancy of up to 17% was reported between the KRAS and BRAF mutation status between the primary tumor and a metastasis [48]. Additionally, Despite the routine use of colonoscopy for diagnosis and screening, a significant number of patients (approximately 11% even in a prescreened with colonoscopy population [49]) are still diagnosed with metastatic colorectal carcinoma at presentation. As cytological specimens are a reliable source of sample material for KRAS and BRAF mutation analysis [50], the acquisition of metastatic colorectal samples by FNA, either during the evolution of established disease or at presentation, should always be considered in metastatic colorectal carcinoma patients as a suitable alternative to more invasive methods.

Another area where cytological patient samples are frequently used for molecular testing is lung cancer. In primary lung cancer, specifically non-small-cell lung cancer (NSCLC), EGFR and KRAS gene mutation status analyses are frequently conducted in cytological samples and more recently ALK gene rearrangements [51, 52]. NSCLC patients are frequently diagnosed solely by cytology, with only about a third displaying indication for curative surgery and many presenting with solid metastasis and pleural effusions. Therefore, several studies were conducted early on to show the feasibility of routine molecular testing in cytological samples of primary and metastatic NSCLC [53–57]. While many of these studies confirm the feasibility of molecular testing in cytological samples of NSCLC metastasis, including metastasis to bone, adrenal gland, soft tissues, and liver, some discrepancies are to be expected in molecular testing of the metastasis in these patients. Discrepancies in these cases seem to occur more frequently between different metastatic sites and as time between primary tumor analysis and the metastasis analysis is increased [54], occasionally resulting in emergence of new mutations (due to the earlier mentioned considerations about tumor evolution and metastatic spread model). Taken together, these studies strongly reinforce the feasibility and clinical usefulness of cytological samples for molecular assays in NSCLC, as well as the feasibility and need of biopsying metastatic sites at diagnosis or during the course of disease.

Ovarian cancer and in particular ovarian carcinomas is another area where it is believed that molecular applications coupled with cytology can make a difference, particularly in the metastatic setting. Like in the areas already mentioned, obtaining cytological samples from metastatic ovarian carcinomas and ovarian peritoneal effusions is feasible and informative. More than 10 years ago, it was shown by Centeno et al. that FNA samples from ovarian carcinoma contained high percentage of tumor cells and quality RNA for gene expression profiling using microarray technology [58]. More recently, other authors confirmed the feasibility of analysis of ovarian carcinoma metastasis by targeted NGS using residual FNA rinse [59]. Therefore, there is no question about the feasibility of molecular tool application in metastatic ovarian carcinoma cytological samples or effusions. Nevertheless, there is an extensive work to be done regarding discovery and validation of molecular biomarkers in metastatic ovarian carcinoma using cytological samples. Much due to the more aggressive surgical techniques aimed at optimal cytoreduction, the survival of women with ovarian carcinoma has been improving. Yet, approximately 60% of patients with advanced disease at primary diagnosis will experience a recurrence within 5 years of diagnosis, and many will develop resistance to chemotherapy [60]. Aimed at improving theses outcomes, several new drugs are being evaluated and used in ovarian carcinomas, including agents that target VEGF, VEGF receptor, EGFR, PARP and PTEN [61]. However, biomarkers of response aimed at identifying groups of patients that would benefit from these therapies are limited. The use of cytological samples coupled with molecular techniques could help in the clinical comprehensive profiling of metastatic ovarian carcinomas and in the near future contribute to the development of clinical useful biomarkers of both prognosis and response in ovarian metastatic carcinoma.

The last area reviewed in this chapter where there is substantial evidence for a central role of molecular cytology applications on metastatic sites is melanoma. Melanoma is a highly aggressive tumor with generally poor prognosis. Approximately 30% of melanoma patients recur, and the 5-year survival rate for patients with metastatic melanoma is less than 15% with a median overall survival of 8–10 months [62]. Mutations in BRAF are the most frequent actionable abnormality encountered in melanoma. The majority of these mutations are characterized by the substitution of valine by glutamic acid at residue 600 (BRAF V600E), which activates mitogen-activated protein kinase (MAPK) signal transduction cascade and leads to uncontrolled melanoma cell growth [63]. Vemurafenib and dabrafenib, two selective inhibitors of BRAF Val600, have been shown to produce a clinical response, with the addition of trametinib, which targets MEK downstream of BRAF, adding a clear benefit over monotherapy [62, 64]. Other mutations, in NRAS and c-KIT, are of potential therapeutic value, and the development of new targeted therapies is currently in progress [65]. Presently, it is imperative that all metastatic melanomas are tested for BRAF mutations and, in the near future, probably for other mutations as well. FNA has been more commonly used for the diagnosis of multiple recurrences and restaging of melanoma than core biopsy or excision specimens [66] and recurrently shown to be suitable for BRAF mutation testing in metastatic melanoma [67, 68]. Consequently, FNA biopsies are suitable for establishing diagnosis and for identifying patients with metastatic melanoma in whom targeted therapy is most likely to be effective.

It is clear in all of the abovementioned examples that cytological samples are feasible for the molecular analysis currently needed for targeted therapy patient selection in five areas briefly reviewed. It is also clear that specifically considering metastatic disease, cytological samples offer a number of advantages (Fig. 13.1). First, the use of FNA makes the sample collection easier, especially in cases when the use of large-core biopsy needles is not possible or, simply, too traumatic. Second, it allows the analysis of molecular abnormalities in patients with a malignant effusion (either at presentation or a recurrent malignant effusion). Third, it allows the easy resampling of the metastasis, which is increasingly needed due to the recognition of potential genetic evolution and/or the occurrence of new genetic abnormalities during the course of treatment that may determine acquisition of resistance (or susceptibility to a new drug) during the course of treatment

13.4 Conclusions and Future Directions

In contemporary oncology and pathology practice, therapy selection based on different biomarkers is a reality for many cancer types, especially in the context of primary disease. In the context of metastatic disease and much due to the increase in recognition of tumor evolution and heterogeneity, it is becoming more frequent to biopsy (or re-biopsy) metastases. This practice is fundamental to achieve a comprehensive profile of the several metastatic sites in a given patient as well as the clonal evolution at each of the metastatic sites. The use of cytologic samples (either FNAs or effusions) offers a better alternative to core needle or surgical biopsies for frequent biopsy of metastatic sites: it is minimally invasive, causes marginal discomfort for the patients, and allows use of most clinically relevant molecular studies. Coupled with modern interventional radiology techniques, most metastatic sites are possible to sample by FNA. However, as significance and clinical implications of the longitudinal tracking of tumor clonal composition in a patient are still largely unknown, re-biopsy of metastasis should (for now) be only recommended when there is a change in response to treatment or a new metastatic site is diagnosed. Nevertheless, we envision this practice recommendation to change as the mechanisms of tumor evolution are better understood. Newer clinical trials are being redesigned to accommodate this knowledge about evolution and longitudinal analysis of tumors. This will ultimately lead to better understanding of treatment resistance development and will help to uncover therapeutic choices that will prolong the survival and enhance the quality of life of patients with metastatic cancer. Therefore, we are confident that cytopathology is a discipline with a central role in state-of-the-art practice of diagnostic and treatment of metastatic disease.

References

1. American Cancer Society. Cancer facts & figures 2016. Atlanta: American Cancer Society; 2016.
2. Ferlay J, Steliarova-Foucher E, Lortet-Tieulent J, et al. Cancer incidence and mortality patterns in Europe: estimates for 40 countries in 2012. Eur J Cancer. 2013;49(6):1374–403. https://doi.org/10.1016/j.ejca.2012.12.027.
3. Klein CA. Parallel progression of primary tumours and metastases. Nat Rev Cancer. 2009;9(4):302–12. https://doi.org/10.1038/nrc2627.

4. Collins VP, Loeffler RK, Tivey H. Observations on growth rates of human tumors. Am J Roentgenol Radium Therapy, Nucl Med. 1956;76(5):988–1000. https://doi.org/10.1016/j.ijthermalsci.2004.09.006.

5. Steel GG, Lamerton LF. The growth rate of human tumours. Br J Cancer. 1966;20(1):74–86.

6. Friberg S, Mattson S. On the growth rates of human malignant tumors: implications for medical decision making. J Surg Oncol. 1997;65(4):284–97. https://doi.org/10.1002/(SICI)1096-9098(199708)65:4<284::AID-JSO11>3.0.CO;2-2[pii].

7. Huyge V, Garcia C, Alexiou J, et al. Heterogeneity of metabolic response to systemic therapy in metastatic breast cancer patients. Clin Oncol. 2010;22(10):818–27. https://doi.org/10.1016/j.clon.2010.05.021.

8. Baldus SE, Schaefer KL, Engers R, Hartleb D, Stoecklein NH, Gabbert HE. Prevalence and heterogeneity of KRAS, BRAF, and PIK3CA mutations in primary colorectal adenocarcinomas and their corresponding metastases. Clin Cancer Res. 2010;16(3):790–9. https://doi.org/10.1158/1078-0432.CCR-09-2446.

9. Folprecht G, Gruenberger T, Bechstein WO, et al. Tumour response and secondary resectability of colorectal liver metastases following neoadjuvant chemotherapy with cetuximab: the CELIM randomised phase 2 trial. Lancet Oncol. 2010;11(1):38–47. https://doi.org/10.1016/S1470-2045(09)70330-4.

10. Aparicio S, Caldas C. The implications of clonal genome evolution for cancer medicine. N Engl J Med. 2013;368(9):842–51. https://doi.org/10.1056/NEJMra1204892.

11. Sequist LV, Waltman BA, Dias-Santagata D, et al. Genotypic and histological evolution of lung cancers acquiring resistance to EGFR inhibitors. Sci Transl Med. 2011;3(75):75ra26. https://doi.org/10.1126/scitranslmed.3002003.

12. Navin N, Krasnitz A, Rodgers L, et al. Inferring tumor progression from genomic heterogeneity. Genome Res. 2010;20(1):68–80. https://doi.org/10.1101/gr.099622.109.

13. Navin N, Kendall J, Troge J, et al. Tumour evolution inferred by single-cell sequencing. Nature. 2011;472(7341):90–4. https://doi.org/10.1038/nature09807.

14. Maley CC, Galipeau PC, Finley JC, et al. Genetic clonal diversity predicts progression to esophageal adenocarcinoma. Nat Genet. 2006;38(4):468–73. https://doi.org/10.1038/ng1768.

15. Almendro V, Cheng YK, Randles A, et al. Inference of tumor evolution during chemotherapy by computational modeling and in situ analysis of genetic and phenotypic cellular diversity. Cell Rep. 2014;6(3):514–27. https://doi.org/10.1016/j.celrep.2013.12.041.

16. Ciriello G, Miller ML, Aksoy BA, Senbabaoglu Y, Schultz N, Sander C. Emerging landscape of oncogenic signatures across human cancers. Nat Genet. 2013;45(10):1127–33. https://doi.org/10.1038/ng.2762.

17. Schmitt FC, Longatto-Filho A, Valent A, Vielh P. Molecular techniques in cytopathology practice. J Clin Pathol. 2008;61(3):258–67. https://doi.org/10.1136/jcp.2006.044347.

18. Schmitt F, Barroca H. Role of ancillary studies in fine-needle aspiration from selected tumors. Cancer Cytopathol. 2012;120(3):145–60. https://doi.org/10.1002/cncy.20197.

19. Di Lorito A, Schmitt FC. (Cyto)pathology and sequencing: next (or last) generation? Diagn Cytopathol. 2012;40(5):459–61. https://doi.org/10.1002/dc.21691.

20. Schmitt FC, Soares R, Cirnes L, Seruca R. PCR amplification of DNA obtained from archived hematoxylin-eosin-and giemsa-stained breast cancer aspirates. Diagn Cytopathol. 1998;19(5):395–7. https://doi.org/10.1002/(SICI)1097-0339(199811)19:5<395::AID-DC19>3.0.CO;2-4.

21. Nagel H, Schulten HJ, Gunawan B, Brinck U, Füzesi L. The potential value of comparative genomic hybridization analysis in effusion-and fine needle aspiration cytology. Mod Pathol. 2002;15(8):818–25. https://doi.org/10.1097/01.MP.0000024521.67720.0F.

22. Gailey MP, Stence AA, Jensen CS, Ma D. Multiplatform comparison of molecular oncology tests performed on cytology specimens and formalin-fixed, paraffin-embedded tissue. Cancer Cytopathol. 2015;123(1):30–9. https://doi.org/10.1002/cncy.21476.

23. Kanagal-Shamanna R, Portier BP, Singh RR, et al. Next-generation sequencing-based multigene mutation profiling of solid tumors using fine needle aspiration samples: promises and

challenges for routine clinical diagnostics. Mod Pathol. 2014;27(2):314–27. https://doi.org/10.1038/modpathol.2013.122.

24. Karnes HE, Duncavage EJ, Bernadt CT. Targeted next-generation sequencing using fine-needle aspirates from adenocarcinomas of the lung. Cancer Cytopathol. 2014;122(2):104–13. https://doi.org/10.1002/cncy.21361.

25. Shah RH, Scott SN, Brannon AR, Levine DA, Lin O, Berger MF. Comprehensive mutation profiling by next-generation sequencing of effusion fluids from patients with high-grade serous ovarian carcinoma. Cancer Cytopathol. 2015;123(5):289–97. https://doi.org/10.1002/cncy.21522.

26. Zheng G, Lin M-T, Lokhandwala PM, et al. Clinical mutational profiling of bone metastases of lung and colon carcinoma and malignant melanoma using next-generation sequencing. Cancer Cytopathol. 2016;124(10):744–53. https://doi.org/10.1002/cncy.21743.

27. Piqueret-Stephan L, Marcaillou C, Reyes C, et al. Massively parallel DNA sequencing from routinely processed cytological smears. Cancer Cytopathol. 2016;124(4):241–53. https://doi.org/10.1002/cncy.21639.

28. Beca F, Schmitt F. MicroRNA signatures in cytopathology: are they ready for prime time? Cancer Cytopathol. 2016;124(9):613–5. https://doi.org/10.1002/cncy.21728.

29. Nishino M. Molecular cytopathology for thyroid nodules: a review of methodology and test performance. Cancer Cytopathol. 2015;124(1):14–27. https://doi.org/10.1002/cncy.21612.

30. Tayari M, Winkle M, Kortman G, et al. Long noncoding RNA expression profiling in normal B-cell subsets and Hodgkin lymphoma reveals hodgkin and reed-sternberg cell–specific long noncoding RNAs. Am J Pathol. 2016;186(9):2462–72. https://doi.org/10.1016/j.ajpath.2016.05.011.

31. Su X, Malouf GG, Chen Y, et al. Comprehensive analysis of long non-coding RNAs in human breast cancer clinical subtypes. Oncotarget. 2014;5(20):9864–76. https://doi.org/10.18632/oncotarget.2454.

32. Pauli C, Puca L, Mosquera JM, et al. An emerging role for cytopathology in precision oncology. Cancer Cytopathol. 2015;124(3):167–73. https://doi.org/10.1002/cncy.21647.

33. DeRose YS, Wang G, Lin Y-C, et al. Tumor grafts derived from women with breast cancer authentically reflect tumor pathology, growth, metastasis and disease outcomes. Nat Med. 2011;17(11):1514–20. https://doi.org/10.1038/nm.2454.

34. Zhao X, Liu Z, Yu L, et al. Global gene expression profiling confirms the molecular fidelity of primary tumor-based orthotopic xenograft mouse models of medulloblastoma. Neuro-Oncology. 2012;14(5):574–83. https://doi.org/10.1093/neuonc/nos061.

35. Reyal F, Guyader C, Decraene C, et al. Molecular profiling of patient-derived breast cancer xenografts. Breast Cancer Res. 2012;14(1):R11. https://doi.org/10.1186/bcr3095.

36. Beca F, Schmitt F. Growing indication for FNA to study and analyze tumor heterogeneity at metastatic sites. Cancer Cytopathol. 2014;122(7):504–11.

37. Cancer Genome Atlas Network. Comprehensive molecular portraits of human breast tumours. Nature. 2012;490(7418):61–70. https://doi.org/10.1038/nature11412.

38. Amir E, Miller N, Geddie W, et al. Prospective study evaluating the impact of tissue confirmation of metastatic disease in patients with breast cancer. J Clin Oncol. 2012;30(6):587–92. https://doi.org/10.1200/JCO.2010.33.5232.

39. Wilking U, Karlsson E, Skoog L, et al. HER2 status in a population-derived breast cancer cohort: discordances during tumor progression. Breast Cancer Res Treat. 2011;125(2):553–61. https://doi.org/10.1007/s10549-010-1029-2.

40. Simmons C, Miller N, Geddie W, et al. Does confirmatory tumor biopsy alter the management of breast cancer patients with distant metastases? Ann Oncol. 2009;20(9):1499–504. https://doi.org/10.1093/annonc/mdp028.

41. Martins D, Beca F, Schmitt F. Metastatic breast cancer: mechanisms and opportunities for cytology. Cytopathology. 2014;25(4):225–30. https://doi.org/10.1111/cyt.12158.

42. Beca F, Polyak K. Intratumor heterogeneity in breast cancer. In: Stearns V, editor. Novel biomarkers in the continuum of breast cancer. Cham: Springer; 2016. p. 169–89. https://doi.org/10.1007/978-3-319-22909-6_7.

43. Zhou M, Yu P, Hou K, et al. Effect of RAS status on anti-EGFR monoclonal antibodies+5-FU infusion-based chemotherapy in first-line treatment of metastatic colorectal cancer: a meta-analysis. Meta Gene. 2016;9:110–9. https://doi.org/10.1016/j.mgene.2016.05.001.

44. Tabernero J, Van Cutsem E, Diaz-Rubio E, et al. Phase II trial of cetuximab in combination with fluorouracil, leucovorin, and oxaliplatin in the first-line treatment of metastatic colorectal cancer. J Clin Oncol. 2007;25(33):5225–32. https://doi.org/10.1200/JCO.2007.13.2183.

45. André T, Blons H, Mabro M, et al. Panitumumab combined with irinotecan for patients with KRAS wild-type metastatic colorectal cancer refractory to standard chemotherapy: a GERCOR efficacy, tolerance, and translational molecular study. Ann Oncol. 2013;24(2):412–9. https://doi.org/10.1093/annonc/mds465.

46. Lièvre A, Bachet J-B, Boige V, et al. KRAS mutations as an independent prognostic factor in patients with advanced colorectal cancer treated with cetuximab. J Clin Oncol. 2008;26(3):374–9. https://doi.org/10.1200/JCO.2007.12.5906.

47. Lièvre A, Bachet JB, Le Corre D, et al. KRAS mutation status is predictive of response to cetuximab therapy in colorectal cancer. Cancer Res. 2006;66(8):3992–5. https://doi.org/10.1158/0008-5472.CAN-06-0191.

48. Oliveira C, Velho S, Moutinho C, et al. KRAS and BRAF oncogenic mutations in MSS colorectal carcinoma progression. Oncogene. 2007;26(1):158–63. https://doi.org/10.1038/sj.onc.1209758.

49. Stoffel EM, Erichsen R, Frøslev T, et al. Clinical and molecular characteristics of post-colonoscopy colorectal cancer: a population-based study. Gastroenterology. 2016;151(5):870–878.e3.

50. Pang NKB, Nga ME, Chin SY, et al. KRAS and BRAF mutation analysis can be reliably performed on aspirated cytological specimens of metastatic colorectal carcinoma. Cytopathology. 2011;22(6):358–64. https://doi.org/10.1111/j.1365-2303.2010.00812.x.

51. Cai G, Wong R, Chhieng D, et al. Identification of EGFR mutation, KRAS mutation, and ALK gene rearrangement in cytological specimens of primary and metastatic lung adenocarcinoma. Cancer Cytopathol. 2013;121(9):500–7. https://doi.org/10.1002/cncy.21288.

52. Pelliccioni S, Lupi C, Sensi E. Anaplastic lymphoma kinase gene rearrangements in cytological samples of non-small cell lung cancer comparison with histological assessment. Cancer Cytopathol. 2014;122:445–53. https://doi.org/10.1002/cncy.21418.

53. Smouse JH, Cibas ES, Jänne PA, Joshi VA, Zou KH, Lindeman NI. EGFR mutations are detected comparably in cytologic and surgical pathology specimens of nonsmall cell lung cancer. Cancer Cytopathol. 2009;117(1):67–72. https://doi.org/10.1002/cncy.20011.

54. Khode R, Larsen DA, Culbreath BC, et al. Comparative study of epidermal growth factor receptor mutation analysis on cytology smears and surgical pathology specimens from primary and metastatic lung carcinomas. Cancer Cytopathol. 2013;121(7):361–9. https://doi.org/10.1002/cncy.21273.

55. Billah S, Stewart J, Staerkel G, Chen S, Gong Y, Guo M. EGFR and KRAS mutations in lung carcinoma: molecular testing by using cytology specimens. Cancer Cytopathol. 2011;119(2):111–7. https://doi.org/10.1002/cncy.20151.

56. Ulivi P, Romagnoli M, Chiadini E, et al. Assessment of EGFR and K-ras mutations in fixed and fresh specimens from transesophageal ultrasound-guided fine needle aspiration in non-small cell lung cancer patients. Int J Oncol. 2012;41(1):147–52. https://doi.org/10.3892/ijo.2012.1432.

57. Treece AL, Montgomery ND, Patel NM, et al. FNA smears as a potential source of DNA for targeted next-generation sequencing of lung adenocarcinomas. Cancer Cytopathol. 2016;124(6):406–14. https://doi.org/10.1002/cncy.21699.

58. Centeno BA, Enkemann SA, Coppola D, Huntsman S, Bloom G, Yeatman TJ. Classification of human tumors using gene expression profiles obtained after microarray analysis of fine-needle aspiration biopsy samples. Cancer. 2005;105(2):101–9. https://doi.org/10.1002/cncr.20737.

59. Wei S, Lieberman D, Morrissette JJD, Baloch ZW, Roth DB, McGrath C. Using "residual" FNA rinse and body fluid specimens for next-generation sequencing: an institutional experience. Cancer Cytopathol. 2016;124(5):324–9. https://doi.org/10.1002/cncy.21666.

60. Jayson GC, Kohn EC, Kitchener HC, Ledermann JA. Ovarian cancer. Lancet. 2014;384(9951):1376–88. https://doi.org/10.1016/S0140-6736(13)62146-7.
61. Marchetti C, Palaia I, De Felice F, et al. Tyrosine-kinases inhibitors in recurrent platinum-resistant ovarian cancer patients. Cancer Treat Rev. 2016;42:41–6. https://doi.org/10.1016/j.ctrv.2015.10.011.
62. Jang S, Atkins MB. Which drug, and when, for patients with BRAF-mutant melanoma? Lancet Oncol. 2013;14(2):e60–9. https://doi.org/10.1016/S1470-2045(12)70539-9.
63. Davies H, Bignell GR, Cox C, et al. Mutations of the BRAF gene in human cancer. Nature. 2002;417(6892):949–54. https://doi.org/10.1038/nature00766.
64. Grob JJ, Amonkar MM, Karaszewska B, et al. Comparison of dabrafenib and trametinib combination therapy with vemurafenib monotherapy on health-related quality of life in patients with unresectable or metastatic cutaneous BRAF Val600-mutation-positive melanoma (COMBI-v): results of a phase 3, open-l. Lancet Oncol. 2015;16(13):1389–98. https://doi.org/10.1016/S1470-2045(15)00087-X.
65. Mandala M, Merelli B, Massi D. Nras in melanoma: targeting the undruggable target. Crit Rev Oncol Hematol. 2014;92(2):107–22. https://doi.org/10.1016/j.critrevonc.2014.05.005.
66. Murali R, Thompson JF, Uren RF, Scolyer RA. Fine-needle biopsy of metastatic melanoma: clinical use and new applications. Lancet Oncol. 2010;11(4):391–400. https://doi.org/10.1016/S1470-2045(09)70332-8.
67. Hookim K, Roh MH, Willman J, et al. Application of immunocytochemistry and BRAF mutational analysis to direct smears of metastatic melanoma. Cancer Cytopathol. 2012;120(1):52–61. https://doi.org/10.1002/cncy.20180.
68. Bernacki KD, Betz BL, Weigelin HC, et al. Molecular diagnostics of melanoma fine-needle aspirates: a cytology-histology correlation study. Am J Clin Pathol. 2012;138(5):670–7. https://doi.org/10.1309/AJCPEQJW3PLOOZTC.

Clinical Integration of Molecular Results on Cytology (Post-analytical Phase)

Perry Maxwell, Fernando C. Schmitt, and Manuel Salto-Tellez

14.1 Why Clinical Integration Is Necessary

We conceptualised in 2004 the framework for molecular diagnostics in cytopathology, primarily in the areas of solid tumours and haemato-oncology which, during the course of the years, have become part of our molecular diagnostic understanding. The area of "Diagnostic Molecular Cytopathology" [1] central to many developments in personalised/precision medicine was governed then by two main provisos, namely, (1) that almost any molecular test that could be applied to formalin-fixed, paraffin-embedded (FFPE) material could also be applied to any cytology sample and (2) that the adoption of a genotypic dimension to the phenotypic diagnostic routine would change the way that many practising pathologists operated. Such changes have become both a challenge and opportunity. With this opportunity came also the responsibility to provide due diligence in the pre-analytical aspects of such tests and that each test be specifically optimised and validated for cytology samples. Subsequently we have seen the development of cancer immunology, amounting to a revolution in oncology that has also deeply transformed the way in which we practise pathology for both tissue and cytology samples, benefiting from more precise sampling procedures such as endobronchial ultrasound (EBUS)-generated sampling. In

P. Maxwell (✉) · M. Salto-Tellez
Northern Ireland Molecular Pathology Laboratory, Queen's University Belfast,
Belfast, UK
e-mail: P.Maxwell@qub.ac.uk

F. C. Schmitt
Department of Pathology, Medical Faculty of Porto University,
Porto, Portugal

I3S, Instituto de Investigação e Inovação em Saúde, Universidade do Porto,
Porto, Portugal

IPATIMUP, Institute of Molecular Pathology and Immunology of Porto University,
Porto, Portugal

© Springer International Publishing AG, part of Springer Nature 2018
F. C. Schmitt (ed.), *Molecular Applications in Cytology*,
https://doi.org/10.1007/978-3-319-74942-6_14

addition, there are occasions in which molecular testing is the ideal way of bringing extra diagnostic relevance to challenging areas in cytopathology with a high level of diagnostic uncertainty, such as pancreatic FNAs or thyroid aspirates. Today, we are immersed in a broad technology transformation, with technologies such as next-generation sequencing (NGS) or gene expression (GE) arrays leading a "second revolution".

With this in mind, it would appear that the cytopathologist or cellular pathologist should have the knowledge to carry out a certain degree of morpho-molecular integration in their reports.

14.2 Levels of Clinical Integration

It may be perceived that a cellular pathologist is the obvious choice to be the integrator of the morphological with the molecular. As a competent tissue morphologist, does this qualification, however, lead naturally to being an integrator of the molecular? There are two types of integration to be achieved: *diagnostic* (aiming to establish a diagnosis in the context of an accepted taxonomic classification) and *therapeutic*. A haemato-oncology histopathological report exemplifies the former where the result of clonality testing or the presence of a translocation can confirm/refute a diagnosis of malignancy and provide a clear diagnostic certainty. Moreover, neuropathology and sarcoma/soft tissue pathology share such a paradigm, the latter with some application to cytopathology—see Chap. 12.

The skill set required for *therapeutic integration*, however, whilst adding molecular information on therapeutics, does not influence the cytopathology diagnosis but adds levels of molecular complexity to inform a therapeutic decision. Specifically this requires very broad knowledge and very specific training in interpretative molecular diagnostics and clinical genomics, whereas diagnostic integration occurs in a simpler paradigm. Some key aspects of modern molecular testing include the following: there is the need to understand the technologies that generate the result; judge if a specific test is satisfactory from a technical point of view and have the option to suggests modes to troubleshoot a suboptimal test run; understand the biological variables that some of these tests may bring to the forefront in some cases; have the appropriate knowledge to manage increasingly complex data (i.e. bioinformatics); and, indeed, be aware of the clinical relevance of any biological variable that these tests may produce. Clinical integrity may be compromised should any of these aspects be misjudged and the morpho-molecular "integrator" needs to be as versed in molecular diagnostics as in morphology.

We would argue that lacking appropriate subspecialty training, cellular and tissue pathologists (exceptions aside) cannot drive therapeutic integration. As cellular pathologists, for too long we have been trained exclusively in the morphological. Recent attempts to redefine training are too timid especially if we take into account the degree of "genomic complexity that is coming to us: crafting NGS reports with the necessary skills to translate specific mutations in hundreds of genes into therapeutic recommendations with different levels of certainty. Who will drive the expertise in "interpretative genomics"? Some will argue that the integration of knowledge necessary to translate complex genomics information into credible therapeutic options should happen at the multidisciplinary team or tumour board, and not beforehand, by a broad group of competent individuals, and not by practitioners who are, essentially, morphologists. In any case, in an area of medicine such as "clinical genomics" that is currently being defined empirically, empowering cytopathologists with genomic knowledge appears to be a key element for future training programmes.

14.3 Clinical Integration: Is the Material Technically Adequate?

Clinical integration in the post-analytical phase reviews robust quality metrics, themselves indicative of the quality of the analysis incorporated within the pre-analytical and analytical phases. All molecular tests therefore must undergo a rigorous validation process in order to account for pre-analytical factors, which influence the analytical. We have extended this conceptual framework to immunocytochemistry (ICC, [2]).

At time of writing, national endeavours to introduce robust NGS to the routine laboratory are failing in a significant number of clinical samples for two reasons: lack of sufficient nucleic acids to run a satisfactory test (quantity) and suboptimal preservation of the sample (quality). The latter is translated into morphological aspects of suboptimal cytological integrity (preprocessing ischaemia time, suboptimal fixation, etc.). The former simply relates to the number of cells available for testing.

14.3.1 Total Cellularity

Total cellularity—an assessment of cellularity, irrespective of cell type as all contribute to the total DNA (or RNA) yield. Sensitive single gene QPCR tests can manage with yields of as low as 2 ng, whereas routine NGS chemistries for targeted sequencing can manage with 10 ng, and for some NGS platforms, a minimum of 20 ng may be required. Of course, this also depends on the means of yield assessment; NanoDrop technology will detect not only single intact DNA but also double-strand fragments, whereas technologies such as QUBIT are more single strand DNA specific, the latter methodology being used for NGS platforms.

The practical translation of this is clear; extractions of samples with numbers of cells in the low hundreds assessed by sensitive technologies such as QUBIT are likely to provide a large number of fails in NGS testing. The determination of minimum cellularity for successful NGS library preparation will, therefore, depend on the many factors outlined above.

How many cells are necessary to be truly representative of a cancer in a cytology specimen? Unfortunately the answer is not simple and would depend on many factors: the type of test, the percentage of tumour cells in the overall sample cellularity, the sensitivity of the test and the expected "hit rate" (i.e. the percentage of positive malignant). The issue of total cellularity, therefore, surfaces again, where knowledge of the total cells within a sample is relevant to what we call "therapeutic immunocytochemistry". There is a clear need for a precise assessment of the total cells. Indeed tests such as for PDL1 clearly specify the minimum requirement of 100 malignant cells to generate a confident report (Dako PDL1 training data).

14.3.2 Percentage of Malignant Cells

Percentage of malignant cells—the lower limit of detection as stated in our molecular diagnostic tests is a definition of the lowest malignant cell content in a background of wild-type content. In order to understand the context of a "no mutation detected" result, we cite this lower limit of detection as part of the clinical report. The lower limit of detection is dependent upon the type of platform used, the detection chemistry in the case of ICC or the number of cycles used in any PCR amplification step ahead of NGS library preparation. Examples include that of microsatellite instability analysis requiring as much as 30% malignant cell content [3] down to 2% for some NGS sequencing methods [4].

In cytology samples this is made more difficult as, traditionally, cytopathologists are able to recognise a population that is "unequivocally malignant", a population "unequivocally benign" and an "atypical" cellular component. Indeed, when an accurate percentage of "positive malignant cells" is the goal, and, therefore, an accurate perception of all the malignant cells in the cytology sample is necessary, our experience has shown that reviewing IHC results of markers such as TTF1 in lung cytopathology ahead of percentage malignant cell estimates may be crucial for an accurate calculation. Such reviews, therefore, form a key component in crafting the final molecular report and stating with confidence when a test is truly detecting no mutation and when the result may represent a borderline value. Better sampling would improve the confidence by which it is achieved should the opportunity and clinical utility arise.

14.3.3 Certainties in the Original Cytopathological Diagnosis

Certainties in the original cytopathological diagnosis—this can be subdivided into two assumptions: (a) the diagnosis is correct; and (b) the material submitted (perhaps further sections from a cell block) is representative of the sample that generated the original diagnosis. This is where a hybrid type of cytopathologist is required, where the cytopathologist with the relevant experience and knowledge can truly integrate the technological, morphological and associated pre-analytical and analytical metrics to form the robust clinical report molecular pathology required today. In the absence of these individuals, reliance must continue on the essential cooperation between cytopathologists and molecular diagnosticians.

14.4   Where Training Is the Solution

We therefore propose that the integrator of the molecular report should be a trained integrator. This may be a morphological cellular pathologist, trained in the technologies used and the sometimes complex genomic interpretation of the results and fully conversant with pre-analytical and analytical factors contributing to the result. We have proposed the "Belfast model" for pathology trainees where consolidation of knowledge regarding molecular biology throughout the training period with its application to current diagnostic molecular pathology practice is key to the development of a cellular pathologist, competent to integrate morphological with the molecular [5]. Such a basic knowledge-led curriculum is aimed at trainees in their first 2 years of training which in the UK and will prepare them for the first part of the Royal College of Pathologists (RCPath) examination. This allows the candidate to demonstrate theoretical knowledge underpinning molecular diagnostics. Interactive educational sessions are led by the academic lead and other members of the molecular pathology team. Specialist elements involve laboratory accreditation, test validation, digital pathology, new and emerging technologies and tests, research ethics and governance.

By extending training periods, trainees undertake an aspect of original research and take responsibility for their own learning, within the framework of managing their time between assessing and annotating samples, assessing diagnostic cases and working on the research project.

A period of sub-specialisation is offered upon the trainee's successful completion of the second part of the RCPath examination. This is a period of focus on independent reporting and professional development, which may take the form of molecular diagnostic test sign-out, participation in the development and/or validation of new tests, the management of the laboratory and training junior trainees in their first stage of molecular diagnostic training as outlined above. This gives the trainee the unique opportunity amongst their peers where training is within a framework of current practice and future practice in molecular pathology. Alternatively, the trainee may undertake a "super-specialty", gaining experience and competence in both the classic morphological aspects and the relevant molecular tests for an organ or system. An academic pathway may also be cultivated by the trainee through the uptake of extending their original research and within their current training, exploring whether or not a higher academic qualification may be desirable.

A key element in the delivery of such a training programme is the need for close working relationships between the clinical environment and the academic world. We would argue that such healthcare-academic coalitions are ideally placed to provide the technical expertise and clinical trial experience sometimes essential at the forefront of molecular diagnostic development; this liaison is also key for access to samples and clinical information, which is the backbone of academic translational medicine. The need, therefore, is for both to work together and in so doing, provide a hybrid approach which can deliver a model such as outlined here for training the future pathologist.

Through this model, the training is incorporated within the current curriculum as far as possible and seeks to provide a trained cellular pathologist capable of integrating the morphological with the molecular, understanding the limitations of both disciplines and translating this knowledge into a comprehensive morpho-molecular report.

14.5   Where There Is a Minimal Report Content

Minimum reporting guidelines, often translated into reporting templates or "LIMS canned texts", are usually adopted by accredited laboratories, often following the feedback of organisations such as UKNEQAS Molgen (minimum clinical report content). Taking all into account, therefore, one can derive some basic rules to clinical molecular pathology reporting as a guide to the cellular pathologist integrator.

A clinical report which integrates morphology with molecular diagnostics would consist of the following constituent properties: those required for patient identification such as a minimum number of patient identifiers, those for clerical functionality such as page numbering, those for clinical context of both the request and report, those for technical context in which the result may be understood and those for incidental findings which may occur due to multigene testing.

There should be a minimum of two unique patient identifiers plus a unique laboratory identifier clearly at the top or bottom of each report pages, each of which is numbered sequentially. The results should be stated in a brief manner. The remainder of the body of the report should then place in context these results. There should be an integration of the molecular results with clinical context in which the request is made. In the example of the report in Fig. 14.1, the report examples the results from a lung adenocarcinoma. We state that the malignant cells showed immunoreactivity for *TTF1* and napsin A and as such an adenocarcinoma and should be tested for *EGFR* mutations. We reflex test for *ALK* translocations and *PDL1* protein expression. Some laboratories add tests for *ROS1* translocations. A description of the procedure used highlights the malignant cell content as a percentage of neoplastic cells which formed the test material for DNA extraction, what tests were applied and what regions were tested. Finally, limits of the test are identified in the lower limit of detection and test sensitivity. A clinical comment puts in context the findings and the impact of the result on potential therapy. A signature and date of the reporting team are included. Many formats are available, but following these basic rules such as the above and using HGVS nomenclature of specified variants leads to a more coherent report which can be understood by different centres.

In this example, we see how the cellular pathologist can directly input their morphological experience in not only placing in context the request for testing but also in the assessment of malignant cell content as described in Sect. 14.3.2.

Moving onto the report for the NGS result, the same rules apply with the addition of total cell input as described in Sects. 14.3.1 and 14.3.2. There is a temptation to describe the test in full, but it should be remembered that clinical colleagues require the result and a statement by which they can gain confidence in the integrity of the

<table>
<tr><td>Patient Name:</td><td>Hospital Number:</td></tr>
<tr><td>Date of Birth:</td><td>Gender:</td></tr>
</table>

CLINICAL HISTORY:

Pleural effusion showing malignant cells positive for *TTF1* and Napsin A (C/R Report# and block identifier and if appropriate: cell block).

TEST RESULTS:

The specimen was representative of tumour, containing approximately 35% neoplastic nuclei.

EGFR Exon 19 deletion detected

ALK overexpression not detected

PDL1 protein detected of equal to or greater than 50% of malignant epithelial cells

CLINICAL COMMENT:

An ***EGFR* exon 19 deletion was DETECTED**.

This patient may benefit from *EGFR* TKi treatment. In particular, there is clinical evidence that tumours carrying exon 19 deletions are particularly sensitive to *EGFR* TKi treatment in the first line setting.

No evidence of an *ALK* protein overexpression was observed. Current clinical evidence does not support the use of *ALK* inhibitor treatment in *ALK*-negative tumours

PD-L1 protein expression of equal to or greater than 50% detected. This result indicates that this patient may benefit from anti-PDL1 therapy in either a first or second line setting.

TEST DETAILS:

DNA was extracted using the cobas® DNA extraction kit (Roche). Mutation testing was conducted using cobas® 4800 Real-Time PCR (Roche)

EGFR: The cobas® *EGFR* mutation test v2 detects >95% of commonly occurring mutations in *EGFR* exons 18, 19, 20 and 21 with a limit of detection of 5%. This test may not distinguish between specific sequence variants within some exons or codons [reference cDNA sequence: NM_005228.4].

***ALK* IHC and FISH**: *ALK* fusion protein overexpression tested using antibody (D5F3 clone) from Ventana. FISH for *ALK* gene rearrangement testing conducted in positive or equivocal IHC cases using Abbot Vysis *ALK* Dual Colour Breakapart FISH probe *ALK* rearrangement cut off >15% positive tumour cells for FISH * *there may be other indicators of response to ALK inhibitors such as translocations involving the ROS1 gene.*

***PDL1* IHC:** *PDL1* protein tested using antibody (SP263 clone) from Ventana.

Signed: Date:

Fig. 14.1 Illustration of the minimum content for a molecular cytopathology report, which integrates clinical context of both the request and result. Note that we have included clinical comment impact statements on EGFR, ALK and PDL1 as these, at the time of writing, are standard of care target genes

result to begin treatment. Some laboratories provide web links to describe in full their tests, reserving the space available in the report for the clinical relevance and briefly describing the limitations of the test and how the metrics stated ensure that (a) a result describing the absence of a detectable mutation can be trusted and (b) the result describing an actionable mutation detected can be actioned. Such parameters are dealt with in detail elsewhere in pre-analytical and analytical reporting and measurement of uncertainty principles [6].

References

1. Salto-Tellez M, Koay ES. Molecular diagnostic cytopathology: definitions, scope and clinical utility. Cytopathology. 2004;15:252–5.
2. Maxwell P, Salto Tellez M. Validation of immunocytochemistry as a morphomolecular technique. Cancer Cytopathol. 2016;124:540–5.
3. Berg KD, Glaser CL, Thompson RE, Hamilton SR, Griffin CA, Eshleman JR. Detection of microsatellite instability by fluorescence multiplex polymerase chain reaction. J Mol Diagn. 2000;2:20–8.
4. Jennings LJ, Arcila ME, Corless C, Kamel-Reid S, Lubin IM, Pfeifer J, Temple-Smolken RL, Voelkerding KV, Nikiforova MN. Guidelines for validation of next-generation-sequencing-based oncology panels. J Mol Diagn. 2017;19:341–65.
5. Flynn C, James J, Maxwell P, McQuaid S, Ervine A, Catherwood M, Loughrey MB, McGibben D, Somerville J, McManus DT, Gray M, Herron B, Salto Tellez M. Integrating molecular diagnostics into histopathology training: the Belfast model. J Clin Pathol. 2014;67:632–6.
6. Mattocks CJ, Morris MA, Mathijs G, Swinnen E, Corveleyn A, Dequeker E, et al. A standardized framework for the validation and verification of clinical molecular genetic tests. Eur J Hum Genet. 2010;18:1276–88.

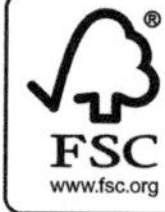